The Physiological Mechanisms of Motivation

The Physiological Mechanisms of Motivation

Edited by
Donald W. Pfaff

With 125 Figures

Springer-Verlag
New York   Heidelberg   Berlin

Donald W. Pfaff
Professor of Neurobiology
    and Behavior
The Rockefeller University
1230 York Avenue
New York, New York 10021
U.S.A.

Library of Congress Cataloging in Publication Data
Main entry under title:
The physiological mechanisms of motivation.
   Includes bibliographies and index.
   1. Motivation (Psychology)—Physiological aspects.
I. Pfaff, D. W. (Donald W.)   [DNLM: 1.
Motivation—Physiology.   BF 683 P578]
BF503.P49   599.01'88   81-18467   AACR2

© 1982 by Springer-Verlag New York Inc.
All rights reserved. No part of this book may be translated or reproduced in any
form without written permission from Springer-Verlag, 175 Fifth Avenue, New
York, New York 10010, U.S.A.
The use of general descriptive names, trade names, trademarks, etc., in this
publication, even if the former are not especially identified, is not to be taken as a
sign that such names, as understood by the Trade Marks and Merchandise Marks
Act, may accordingly be used freely by anyone.

Printed in the United States of America

9 8 7 6 5 4 3 2 1

ISBN 0-387-**90650-9** Springer-Verlag New York Heidelberg Berlin
ISBN 3-540-**90650-9** Springer-Verlag Berlin Heidelberg New York

Preface

To scientists engaged in research on the cellular mechanisms in the mammalian brain, concepts of "motivation" seem to be a logical necessity, even if they are not fashionable. Immersed in the detailed, time-consuming research required to deal with mammalian nerve cells, we usually pay scant attention to the more global brain–behavior questions that have arisen from decades of biological and psychological studies. We felt it was time to confront these issues—namely, how far has neurobiological investigation come in uncovering mechanisms by which motivational signals influence behavior?

At Rockefeller University, we have recently held a course on this subject. We restricted our treatment to those motivational systems most tractable to physiological approaches, and invited scientists skilled in both behavioral issues and physiological techniques to participate. This volume results from that course. The deans and administration at Rockefeller University provided much help in planning the course, and the staff of Springer-Verlag assisted in planning the book. Gabriele Zummer helped organize both the course and the processing of book chapters. They all deserve our thanks.

December 1981

Donald W. Pfaff
Professor of Neurobiology
and Behavior
Rockefeller University

Contents

List of Contributors

ALAN N. EPSTEIN   Joseph Leidy Laboratory of Biology, University of Pennsylvania, Philadelphia, Pennsylvania 19104, U.S.A.

SUSAN E. FAHRBACH   The Rockefeller University, 1230 York Avenue, New York, New York 10021, U.S.A.

HARVEY GRILL   The Rockefeller University, 1230 York Avenue, New York, New York 10021, U.S.A.

JOEL I. GRINKER   The Rockefeller University, 1230 York Avenue, New York, New York 10021, U.S.A.

RONNIE HALPERIN   Department of Psychiatry, Bronx V.A. Hospital and Medical Center, 130 West Kingsbridge Road, Bronx, New York 10468, U.S.A.

DAVID J. MAYER   Department of Physiology, Medical College of Virginia, MCV Station Box 551, Virginia Commonwealth University, Richmond, Virginia 23298, U.S.A.

NEAL E. MILLER   The Rockefeller University, 1230 York Avenue, New York, New York 10021, U.S.A.

RALPH NORGREN   The Rockefeller University, 1230 York Avenue, New York, New York 10021, U.S.A.

DONALD W. PFAFF   Neurobiology and Behavior, The Rockefeller University, 1230 York Avenue, New York, New York 10021, U.S.A.

CARL PFAFFMAN   The Rockefeller University, 1230 York Avenue, New York, New York 10021, U.S.A.

DONALD D. PRICE   Department of Anesthesiology, Medical College of Virginia, MCV Station Box 695, Virginia Commonwealth University, Richmond, Virginia 23298, U.S.A.

EVELYN SATINOFF   Department of Psychology and Program in Neural and Behavioral Biology, University of Illinois, Champaign, Illinois 61820, U.S.A.

GERARD P. SMITH   Department of Psychiatry, Cornell University Medical College and The E.W. Bourne Behavioral Research Lab, New York Hospital-Cornell Medical Center, Westchester Division, White Plains, New York 10605, U.S.A.

RICHARD L. SOLOMON   Department of Psychology, University of Pennsylvania, 3815 Walnut Street, Philadelphia, Pennsylvania 19104, U.S.A.

ELIOT STELLAR   Institute of Neurological Sciences, School of Medicine, University of Pennsylvania, Philadelphia, Pennsylvania 19104, U.S.A.

Part One

Concepts

Chapter 1

Motivational Concepts: Definitions and Distinctions

DONALD W. PFAFF

Suppose an organism, studied in a particular context, is presented with a well-defined stimulus and the well-defined response expected does not occur. A short time later (too soon for changes in maturation) the same organism in the same context at the same time of day is presented with the same stimulus, and the response does occur. What explains the response on the second trial? A change in the organism, called motivation, may be inferred. As an intervening variable, the concept of motivation identifies a logically required cause of behavioral change.

Treatments of motivation concepts have ranged from spare, logical treatments similar to that above, to rich elaborations, especially when dealing with human psychological states, emphasizing relations to arousal and emotion. Problems have arisen in use of the concept. For example, a relatively simple one bears on the question of response definition. The behavioral response whose occurrence leads to the inference of a motivational change must be defined at a molar level so that the idea of "motivation" is not used to explain small variations, for example, in the amplitude of a monosynaptic reflex.

A more serious problem in the history of behavioral research was that presumed motivations were assigned arbitrarily and multiply as free variables, to supply false explanations in the absence of systematic experimentation. This in turn justified a scholarly reaction, for example, in the words of B. F. Skinner (1953):

> In traditional terms an organism drinks because it needs water, goes for a walk because it needs exercise, breathes more rapidly and deeply because it wants air, and eats ravenously because of the promptings of hunger. Needs,

wants, and hungers, are good examples of the inner causes. . . . Sometimes the inner operation is inferred from the operation responsible for the strength of the behavior—as when we say that someone who has had nothing to drink for several days "must be thirsty" and probably will drink. On the other hand, it is sometimes inferred from the behavior itself—as when we observe some-one drinking large quantities of water and assert without hesitation that he possesses a great thirst. In the first case, we infer the inner event from a prior independent variable and predict the dependent variable which is to follow. In the second case, we infer the inner event from the event which follows, and attribute it to a preceding history of deprivation. So long as the inner event is inferred, it is in no sense an explanation of the behavior and adds nothing to the functional account. (pp. 143-144)

However, the mere fact of inference is not enough to justify discarding a scientific concept. Well-known laws (prominently, Newton's second law, $F = MA$) contain variables whose value and units depend absolutely on the other variables (measurable) in the equation. Whether the concept of motivation can be allowed depends on its heuristic value: Does it fruitfully and efficiently explain stimulus–response relations? Experiments that produce variations in the response of interest under controlled conditions allow us to evaluate the stimulus–response relations that potentially can be explained by a motivational concept. Neal Miller (1967) has emphasized the use of a variety of techniques for altering a potentially "movitated response." These amount to the use of convergent operations in the sense that if variations in the response are to be explained by a single intervening variable, then there should be perfect correlations between the effects on the response of a variety of different manipulations (Miller, 1959). For example, consider the animal whose variations in eating might be explained by the motivational concept of "hunger." In the first place, the response— amount of food consumed—must be defined clearly and heuristically: Should we deal with total food intake over a long time, or a measure approaching instantaneous rate? Is account being taken of the animal's normal pattern of food intake (eating in relation to drinking)? What schedule of food presentation following approach responses should be used to alter the effects of satiety?

With the response well defined, in the case of food intake, Miller (1967) lists a variety of manipulations by which to produce changes in response that might be explained efficiently by the single concept "hunger." These include manipulations of the stimulus, changes of the organism, and alterations in the difficulty of an experimentally defined approach response. Regarding changes in the stimulus, if the organism's hunger is higher, we predict certain regular changes in the effect of stimulus palatability on the amount of food consumed. For example, if the animal with supposedly low motivation requires a highly pal-atable diet (e.g., sweet food), an animal with higher motivation would not only be expected to take in greater amounts of that food but would also be expected to be impeded less in its food intake by the addition of quinine, which makes the food bitter. The dimension of palatability yields families of experiments whose results should be understandable in terms of variations in hunger. Next, some operations manipulate the organism itself. Systematic changes in hunger should be able to be produced as a function of time of food deprivation. On the same theoretical "hunger" dimension, satiation can be produced by freely feeding, or experimentally by stomach loading, or can be mimicked by stomach distension. Finally, regarding the response, experimental variations in the circumstances of operant responses arbitrarily chosen to be required for food presentation can be studied. For instance, if an animal's hunger is increased, its rate of bar pressing or running speed (if these are chosen as approach responses) may be expected to be increased. Similarly, if the animal's motivation is increased, the effort it will spend in difficult responses in order to approach food may be expected to be greater. Finally, with increased hunger the frequency with which the animal will tolerate pain, as from the electric shock during crossing a grid, will be increased. Each of these aspects of arbitrary response requirements can be used parametrically to generate sets of experiments for potential explanation by the motivational concept of hunger.

If the methods of converging operations (Miller, 1959, 1967) provide one type of solution to the problems for motivational concepts posed by Skinner and others, a second, new, and exciting approach derives from modern work on the biology of behavior. Whereas decades ago intervening motivational variables might have been inferred and only that, physiological techniques now allow us directly to observe presumed motivational variables and to alter them directly. The main purpose of this book is to see how far modern neurobiological and other physiological work of this sort has brought us in specifying what motivation is. The paragraphs that follow provide introductions to chapters that present some of the better studied motivational systems. I have tried to organize this brief historical introduction to motivational concepts in such a manner as to distinguish clearly among them.

Motivation: A Brief Review of Concepts

Initial Impetus for Developing Concepts

Historically, the oldest approaches to motivational theories attributed the behavior of human beings to rational mental processes. Reasoning about the characteristics of such mental processes included much teleology (Bolles, 1975). In Bolles' view the mechanist's approach to behavioral explanations (as opposed to the teleological approach) included determinism: the assumption that the world of physical events would provide lawful explanations for all phenomena, including behavior. Thus, hypothetical constructs, presumably corresponding to real physiological variables, were assumed to intervene, in order to explain variability of behavior under apparently constant environmental conditions. In order to be empirically sound, they have been required to be tied experimentally to two or more external, measurable events.

Why bother about motivational concepts? Bolles (1975) considers that the impetus for motivational theorizing was to achieve economic explanations of entire classes of behavioral categories. Simple restatements of large bodies of otherwise apparently disparate behavioral data are not adequate.

From studies of animal behavior, also, the concept of instinct was introduced to explain adaptability of behavior patterns of lower animals under changing environmental circumstances without attributing a degree of intelligence to those animals that did not seem reasonable (Bolles, 1975, p. 86). Unfortunately, the very open-endedness and flexibility of the instinct concept allowed it to be used as a false explanation. There were so few limiting factors in its definition and limiting facts from empirical observations that it could be applied indiscriminately. In some cases (William James, 1890) instinct was used in the sense of an organism's acting in order to obtain certain goals. In that case, the definition had a teleological component. In other cases, especially with McDougall (1914), instincts were used to explain motivation in all cases, with a new instinct being postulated to "explain" each new response. Thus, the explanatory power of the concept was nil.

More useful has been the concept of instinct as applied by ethologists (e.g., Lorenz, 1950). On the one hand, instinct amounts to the name given to the relationships between particular releasing stimuli and particular fixed action patterns. In this case, it is a summary of stimulus-response relationships. On the other hand, the hydraulic theory of motivation (Lorenz, 1950), resulting from the ethologist's concept of instinct, amounts to a model for systematic physiological investigation.

Getting Along Without Motivational Concepts

For many modern neurobiological researchers (Thompson, 1975), motivation does not refer clearly to a real process, but rather to a set of problems for physiological analysis. What neural or humoral changes explain variations in responsiveness to environmental stimuli available in constant form? Thus, for Thompson (p. 295 ff. in Thompson, 1975) the physiologist searches for "organism variables" operating in circumstances containing well-defined stimuli and reflex responses. With this approach, hypothesized internal states that cannot be verified physiologically and manipulated selectively are merely false explanations.

Other authors have admitted the meaningfulness of motivational concepts in purely behavioral terms but have felt that their definitions are so blurred that theoretical terms cannot be recognized clearly and distinctly (Bindra, 1959). Bindra clearly avoids the older theoretical traps of trying to explain the initiation of behavioral responses by referring to "instincts" indiscriminately. Where there are no ways of using converging empirical observations to focus on an instinct and where there are not direct physiological observations of its "quantity," Bindra recognizes that using the idea of instinct is merely an example of circular logic: "Why did the behavior occur? Because of the instinct. How do we know there is an instinct? Because the behavior occurred." The residual questions that motivational research tries to answer, for Bindra, have to do with why an organism is active at all and, given activity, why some responses emerge rather than others. Beyond these broad considerations Bindra is unwilling to go.

Indeed, it is interesting that authors with great experience in the analysis of animal behavior can describe comprehensively the biology of a wide range of behavior patterns with no reference to the term "motivation" (e.g., Marler and Hamilton, 1966). Instead of using such concepts as "drive," these authors simply describe behavioral sequences for their own sake, and catalog what is known about the biological control mechanisms for each of them. They can describe in intricate detail, for instance, that in feeding and drinking behaviors, alternate approach response sequences can often be used by the same organism to achieve a given end. Multiple control mechanisms for what we think of as "motivated behavioral responses" provide means for achieving particular commodities safely; one can be used when another is blocked. Importantly, this very diversity may be used to explain lacks of exact correlations among different behavioral measures of motivation. Again, Marler and Hamilton (1966) can treat specific hungers but instead of referring to "drive," they discuss the exact nature of external stimuli, receptors, thresholds, and response sequences. This framework is adequate to make comparisons among major zoological groups. Hormones, also, can be referred to in terms of their roles vis-à-vis other behavioral influences and in terms of their mechanisms, rather than as "motivational signals." Here the impressively long sequences of sexual and parental behaviors can be described, as can their correlations with long-term environmental cycles. In other treatments of animal behavior, also, the means of regulation of particular types of behavioral responses are discussed without explicit reference to motivation, but instead with reference to "feedback signals" and homeostasis (Davis, 1966). Similarly, variations in insect behavior (Roeder, 1963) are attributed to variations in "endogenous activity" which could correspond to motivational mechanisms but are not described that way. Instead, the regulation of overall activity and specific behavioral types tends to be attributed to exogenous factors, oscillators, and so forth.

Nor does the avoidance of motivational concepts derive from a specific period or theoretical climate. In 1935, thoroughly within an American traditional psychology point of view, Maier and Schneirla concerned themselves with the modifiability of behavior, but almost entirely emphasized learning and (in complicated organisms) "higher mental processes." Motivation was thought of simply as one of the factors determining performance and learning (Maier & Schneirla, 1935, pp. 407–420). With independent variables such as food deprivation used for producing changes, for example, in error rate during a maze-running task, motivation was simply a "performance variable." Thus, the concept of motivation was entirely linked to that of reward.

One type of substitute for motivation as such was presented by Dawkins (in Bateson & Hinde, 1976) in the form of goal hierarchies. Attempting to use well-defined "algorithms for detecting patterns in behavior," Dawkins found that the most complete and precise descriptions would reduce goal-directed behaviors to cybernetic computer-like programs. Here he is realizing in greater detail ideas presented generally by Miller, Galanter, and Pribram (1960) in their test-operate–test-evaluate program. When goal-directed behaviors are conceived of as resulting from programs of action rules and stopping rules, their teleological mystery is removed.

The other way of avoiding motivational concepts is to discuss the internal causes of behavior, focusing exclusively on physiological mechanisms with no theory allowed (e.g., Scott, 1958). Thus, Scott discussed internal causes by cataloging specific cues for satiety-controlling feeding behavior, and hormonal cues related to sexual responses and maternal behavior (Scott, 1958, pp. 75–104). One of the earlier attempts to do this specifically, for example, dealt simple with correlations between stomach contractions and feelings of hunger, suggesting that afferent input from the stomach would be an important motivational cue for hunger, although the authors did not describe it that way (Cannon & Washburn, 1912).

Approaches Through Ethology

Nevertheless, some modern ethologists have recognized the potential unifying power of motivational theories and integrated them with traditional terms in the field of animal behavior (Eibl-Eibesfeldt, 1970). Here, examples of motivational influences are seen in the lowering of thresholds for fixed action patterns in response to certain releasing stimuli. While cyclicities such as circadian rhythms might lead to regular alterations in general motor restlessness, Eibl-Eibesfeldt's emphasis on motivation refers to variations in appetitive behavior strength in specific "releasing situations." Mechanisms regulating such variations would be taken as physiological mechanisms of motivation. Good examples come, for example, from studies of sticklebacks and from the development of reproductive and maternal behavior in the ringdove. Although the most the author would hazard in the discussion of actual physiological mechanisms of motivation (p. 59) was "an accumulation of a central nervous excitatory potential as the basis for instinctive behavior," presumably the charge for neurobiological research is to add much needed physiological detail.

In other treatments, motivated behavior is treated as a form of stereotyped behavior in parallel with the discussion of instinct (Dethier & Stellar, 1961, pp. 63–80). From taxes, Dethier and Stellar build systematically to more complicated processes, featured primarily by more complicated contingencies. Thus, these authors construct a kind of continuum from taxes through reflexes through instinctive and motivated behavior patterns, reflecting increasing complication of stereotyped decision trees. Dethier and Stellar note that in the past instinctive behaviors were defined as unlearned, adaptive, and characteristic of a species, but that since the first two of these criteria were difficult to prove, old arguments about classification gave way to simple, direct experimental investigation of the behavior patterns themselves.

The analysis of motivational concepts received more impetus from American psychologists, who included the idea of drive states and satiety as drive reduction. For Dethier and Stellar these concepts led naturally to studies of hypothalamic mechanisms for natural, stereotyped behavior patterns.

In some treatments within the context of experimental and physiological psychology (Kling and Riggs, 1971, pp. 793–794) motivational theories are allowed, but are taken more to relate to nondirected, generalized drive states that energize behavior without guiding it. Concepts of "activation and arousal" are prominent as general energizers that have no steering properties. Then, drive reduction under specific response contingencies is taken to guide behavior in particular ways. For example, motivational effects are shown in this way during experiments measuring running speed toward water as a function of the number of hours of water deprivation. Here, thus, motivation as an intervening variable is used to explain the energization of responses, and decreases in motivation reinforce immediately preceding specific responses.

Approaches Through Physiology

Given the history of psychological studies of motivation, the manner of approaching and using motivational concepts through physiology is obvious. Thus, the main impetus has lain with experimental physiological work aimed at identifying the nature and neural effects of motivational signals. In the case of behavioral systems that are "regulatory," motivational signals have the role of feedbacks helping to keep biologically important variables at set points. Here, for example, many studies have dealt with identifying satiety signals following food intake, and much neurophysiological work has described the neural detection and effects of changes in temperature. Other well-studied motivational systems are not regulatory in this sense, but are biologically crucial, such as those having to do with reproduction and parental care. There, motivational variables whose chemistry is well known, steroid hormones, drive stimulus–response chains in well-described behavioral sequences.

We must note that striking progress in some cases toward the identification of the chemical or physical nature of a motivational signal, the discovery of its neural effects, and the elucidation of the neural circuitry for the behavior thus motivated has not dissolved the need for motivational concepts but simply explains their physiological basis. The neuroanatomical, electrophysiological, neurochemical, and neuroendocrine techniques used for these analyses are laborious. Further, not all motivational systems are equally accessible for neurophysiological or neuroendocrine study. Thus, the use of potentially unifying motivational terms offers the possibility that when one motivational system is explained physiologically, others will be too.

Drive

If "motivation" refers to the energizing of behavior, generally, and to response choices that account for the directionality of behavior, the term "drive" refers to a specific theory of how this occurs.

Historically, before 1930, organisms were regarded as inactive unless specifically aroused (Hebb, 1955). The sources of arousal could be regarded as motivating influences and could also be used to explain the strengthening of certain stimulus–response connections. During the period between 1930 and 1950, however, the view in which motivation could be reduced to (biological drive + learning) declined, and the idea of "spontaneous activity" in the central nervous system (and therefore, endogenous activity of the organism) was accepted. But this did not account for the selection of some behavioral responses over others.

Drives could not only be held to energize behavior in general, but also, since they were considered to be derived from specific biological needs (departure from a zero state of motivation), could be used to explain the occurrence of some behavioral acts in the absence of others. If, as Cannon supposed, organisms have a homeostatic tendency to reduce specific biological needs, concepts surrounding drive theory lead us quickly to physiological experimentation. As a result of important biological deprivations, causing a deviation from a state of homeostasis (i.e., a state of zero bodily need), animals will not only become more active but will engage in particular types of activity that have the effect of approaching the goal that will reduce that bodily need. For example (Warden et al., 1931), rats will cross electric grids with greater frequency to obtain particular goals, as a function of the amount of time of deprivation of those goals. The frequency with which an animal overcomes a barrier to approach a particular environmental object was taken, therefore, as a measure of drive resulting from a biological deprivation. In this vein, an important development was the obstruction method apparatus (Jenkins, Warner, & Warden, 1926). The rat was required to get from a starting box to a goal box by transversing a compartment whose floor was a grill that could be electrified. Among the parameters that could be varied were the duration of the electric shock, the exact time of the shock, its intensity, the overall amount of time the rat was required to spend in that compartment, and so on. Using this apparatus, Warner claimed a quantification of "sex drive" in rats (Warner, 1927), and also studied the effect of time of food deprivation on "hunger drive" (Warner, 1928). In the latter study, for example, the frequency with which rats crossed the electrified grid increased sharply over short periods of deprivation, then leveled off, and finally fell slightly as a function of very long periods of food deprivation. With a different apparatus and response measure, Heron and Skinner (1937) also attempted to quantify "hunger" as a function of food deprivation. Their procedure was to use a conditioned response with periodic reinforcement (keeping the level of food consumption down and thus avoiding modification of the drive as a result of its measurement), as a function of time of food deprivation. Rates of bar pressing increased monotonically from period of deprivation of 0–5 days. While viewing operant response rate during low fixed-ratio reinforcement schedules as ideal for accurate measurement of drive. Heron and Skinner (1937) agreed with the view, later stated precisely by Miller, that converging operations for the measurement of hunger drive would be necessary, for instance, if different drives were to be compared in strength.

In the most detailed theoretical use of the concept of drive, Hull (1943) defined the idea such that it would contribute to the energy of behavior—its initiation and maintenance. Then, depending on the definitions of specific drive states, the concept could also be taken in plural form to explain the directionality of behavior with respect to the environment. According to Hull (1943), drive is theoretically linked to and operationally manipulated by variations in animals' biological needs. By Hull's theory, drive reduction is reinforcing. Thus, a behavioral response would have to be explained in at least two steps. A body need would arise as a result of a deprivation or change in bodily circumstance, producing an increased drive state. With the existence of this drive state explaining the occurrence of some responses and not others, those behavioral responses followed by drive reduction will increase in frequency under future conditions where the same drive is imposed.

Following these historical developments, Hebb (1955) treated relations between motivation and the central nervous system with concepts of the mid-fifties. By this time there were many neurophysiological data available on the arousal system in the reticular formation, which influenced not only the EEG but also the overall state of alertness of the animal. Hebb proposed that this arousal is synonymous with the level of general drive. Derived from this, he talked about optimal levels of arousal (i.e., nonspecific cortical bombardment) for the performance of any given response. (See "Emotion" section later in this chapter.) At this time, neuroanatomical data were convincingly supportive of the view that the directionality of behavior could be accounted for by specific drives—for example, hunger, pain, and sex—mediated by different nerve cell groups (Stellar, 1954).

In the more general context of experimental psychology (Kling and Riggs, 1971) primary drives were defined as unlearned drive sources: Although processes variously called boredom, curiosity, or exploration were considered, the examples easiest to accept usually included hunger, thirst, aversive stimuli, sex, thermal regulation, and perhaps maternal drive. In those circumstances, with antecedent conditions that could be manipulated unambiguously, experimental psychologists were confident of being able to "set up the drive," that is, operationally to induce a state of bodily need (pp. 800–801). In contrast, "secondary sources" of drive were defined as learned or acquired drives. The best examples came from sets of drives derived from strong aversive stimuli. Previously neutral stimuli paired with aversive stimuli quickly acquired aversive properties such that animals would work to avoid them. As counseled by the theoretical approach of Neal Miller to these questions, consummatory (escape) responses and operant (avoidance) responses were involved in converging operations to arrive at an empirically well-anchored definition. Similarly, with approach responses such as food intake, measures of drive included consummatory activity (e.g., total amount of goal object consumed, rate of goal-object consumption, muscular vigor of the goal response), all of which could be shown to vary systematically as a function of the time of deprivation. Then of course the other sets of measures would derive from the arbitrarily large set of operational responses that could be used experimentally to see how hard the animal would work to obtain the goal object. From a more ethological viewpoint (Dethier & Stellar, 1961), interpretations of their data by American psychologists achieved an analysis of motivational concepts that essentially took ideas like instinct and transformed them into the idea of a drive toward a goal, with successful consummatory responses resulting in satiety.

The idea of drive continues to find use by current researchers skilled in modern physiological techniques (Thompson, 1975). For Thompson, motivations derive from unsatisfied needs that result in drives. We have the best physiological information on needs and drives that come from easily understood biological determinants such as hunger, thirst, sex, and thermal motivation. In line with the experiments and theories referred to above, the strength of drive is inferred by depriving the organism to create a state of need, and measuring behavioral changes with a variety of measures of consummatory and operant responses. Thompson also treats the distinction between basic tissue needs (primary needs) and other, derived sources of need (Thompson, 1975, p. 296ff.). From this, he derives the concept of reinforcement.

Drive concepts are not alien to ethological theory (Bateson & Hinde, 1976). The idea of fixed action patterns was associated with the building up of specific tensions that sought release (e.g., Lorenz, 1950; Tinbergen, 1951). The building up of this tension would correspond to increased drive, and the selection of behavioral responses that reduce the drive state would express the idea of a fixed action pattern. The dependence of the release of a fixed action pattern on the occurrence of a particular sign stimulus simply corresponds to relatively inflexible stimulus–response connections in a traditional psychological framework. The most famous experiments linking ethological interpretations of drive to brain physiology were done by von Holst and St. Paul (1963). They used electrical stimulation of the brain in domestic fowl to localize what they called particular driving functions in the central nervous system. Clearly, they took their cue from the results of Hess (1954), who used this approach with great success for analysis of the neurophysiological control of autonomic function. They found that electrical stimulation of particular locations led to shifts in drive state, inferred from increased frequencies of particular behavioral responses. Interactions among behavior patterns (including averaging, alternation, and masking) could be interpreted as interactions among different drive states.

Bindra (1959) points out, in line with cautions from Thompson (1975), that the primary shortcoming of all drive concepts lies in potential logical circularity. Such circularity is broken where there are independent measures to experimentally establish drive state existence, and, still better, where drives processes can be studied physiologically.

Reinforcement, Reward

In experimental psychology (Kling and Riggs, 1971, p. 796), decreases in motivation are taken to be sufficient for the phenomenon of reinforcement. In fact, in some experiments the fact of reinforcement is

14   D. W. Pfaff

taken as partial evidence of a foregoing motivational state. Inversely
(p. 798), punishment, defined as a decrease in the frequency of preceding responses, is taken to be due to an increase in motivational state.
In the most highly developed theory (Hull, 1943), drive reduction is
the essential element of a reinforcing event. Thus, for Hull, those responses which are followed immediately by drive reduction tend to
increase their frequency under similar conditions in the future.

Operationally, a stimulus is reinforcing if, presented immediately
after a behavioral response, the subsequent frequency of that response
is increased (Skinner, 1938, p. 62). From this definition, and from
Hull's theoretical considerations, it is clear that organisms in particular
motivational states would be particularly susceptible to certain forms of
drive reduction, or reinforcement. According to Bindra (1959), the
strongest relations of reinforcing concepts to motivation came through
the drive reduction hypothesis. Given that a state of need exists in an
animal, any event which reduces that need (or drive) will be positively
reinforcing. Conversely, an increase in the response strength of those
responses which precede such reinforcers is taken as an indirect index
of the initial drive state of that animal.

In a physiological tradition (Thompson, 1975), reinforcement must
be derived from tissue needs. Reductions either in basic tissue needs
(primary needs) or other, derived sources of need will be reinforcing
(Thompson, 1975, pp. 296–297). While mechanistically oriented biolo-
gists strive to analyze the neural effects of differing need states in direct
physiological experiments, this effort is not opposed to psychologically
oriented drive reduction theory. Instead, we are merely examining the
exact neurobiological means by which need reduction results in reward
or reinforcement (operationally defined as an increase in frequency
foregoing behavioral responses).

One discussion of reinforcement or reward (Milner, 1970) is heavily
physiological and links these concepts to the phenomenon of self-
stimulation. For Milner, discussions of motivation begin with physiological analyses of biological regulatory mechanisms, and he distinguishes
between "regulatory" and "nonregulatory" motivational systems.
Another, orthogonal distinction among motivational systems is largely
anatomical and based on the model of Olds (Olds, 1962; Olds & Olds,
1965). According to that model, motivational systems based on activity
in the medial hypothalamus and upper brain stem were largely based on
somatosensory input and were adrenergic and aversive. Those systems
derived from activity in the lateral portion of the hypothalamus and
upper brain stem were more dependent on olfaction and cholinergic
activity, and were related to approach responses. Although this particular neuroanatomic model is oversimplified, mechanistic approaches of
this sort in general are not antagonistic to zoological theories of reinforcement presented by Glickman and Schiff (1967) or, from an etho-

logical tradition, by Tinbergen (1951). Their concern was to show how motivational systems could act by eliciting certain natural patterns of species-specific consummatory responses. In ethological terms, their approach would emphasize how motivational effects (operating through internal stimuli and hormones) alter the ability of innate releasing stimuli to activate fixed action patterns.

Nowhere are the phenomena of motivation and reinforcement discussed more extensively in a physiological vein than in treatments of intracranial self-stimulation (Milner, 1970). Olds and Milner (1954) demonstrated, in male rats, the reinforcement of instrumental responses by electrical stimulation of the septum. Stimulus points in the cingulate cortex and midbrain tegmental region were also effective, whereas control points in the medial lemniscus, medial geniculate body, corpus callosum, and caudate nucleus gave negative results. Further experiments (Olds & Olds, 1962) gave a more extensive neuroanatomical mapping and focused on interactions between approach points and escape points in the tegmentum and hypothalamus of rats. Clearly, some electrodes yielded much higher results with reward tests whereas others yielded higher results with escape tests. It seemed clear, therefore, that there might be separate appetitive and aversive motivational systems. Olds and Olds seemed to favor interactions through a one-way inhibition: that tegmental escape electrodes would inhibit the effects of hypothalamic approach ones.

In circumstances where intracranial electrical stimulation would markedly increase the frequency of foregoing instrumental responses, Olds clearly favored the interpretation of a purely positive reinforcing effect: that electrical stimulation at such points would reduce drive and thus be rewarding and even pleasurable. In Deutsch's theory of self-stimulation (Deutsch, 1960; Deutsch & Deutsch, 1966), the initial decrement in motivational energy due to the response comprises a reward which will facilitate the occurrence of the next response, but in addition the electrical stimulus causes increased motivational levels required for activating the next response. This theory is supposed to account for the necessity of a "priming" stimulation and for the rapid extinction shown in self-stimulation. For example, the experiments of Howarth and Deutsch (1962) were based on the hypothesis that, because of the requirement for a "priming function" of the immediately preceding electrical stimulus, the termination of electrical intracranial self-stimulation should be a decreasing function of time. Their results showed, indeed, that the number of trials required for extinction was a simple decreasing function of the time that the lever for self-stimulation was unavailable. The authors took these results to confirm Deutsch's theory that part of the "drive" for intracranial self-stimulation is a direct effect of the electrical pulses, which therefore cause motivational excitation as well as reward (Deutsch, 1960).

Incentive

Theories of Hull (1943) included the idea that reinforcer magnitude may be a function not only of deprivation state but also of the direction by stimuli of specific goal responses. Characteristics of the goal object, therefore, could cause variations in the intensity or vigor of goal responses. This is defined as the incentive value of those stimulus characteristics. The strength of the goal response covaries with changes in deprivation and changes in the stimulus characteristics (incentive) of the goal object or reinforcer.

As summarized by Bolles (Bolles, 1975, pp. 291–300), the initial theory of incentive motivation (Hull, 1931) was that the consummatory response, or goal response, is elicited by the joint action of deprivation and specific stimuli (such as those emanating from food). Whereas drive depends on internal events, incentive is a property of external events, primarily stimuli associated with the goal objects. Bolles suspects that the physiological explanation of drive, related to measurable variables such as levels of known chemical in the blood, will be easier than the untangling of incentive properties of stimuli in view of the complicated coding in some sensory physiological systems. The most extensive use of the concept of incentive for the explanation of motivated states came from the theory of Mowrer (1960).

How do drive and incentive interact? Hull (1952) proposed that the two of them multiply to determine total motivation, whereas Spence (1956) thought that they add.

Some theorists have given a major role to incentive motivation in their overall view of this field. In the view of Bindra (1959), the only important theoretical basis for distinguishing among motivational activities would be in terms of the environmental objects with respect to which these activities are organized: food, mates, and so forth. Thus, for Bindra, motivational phenomena must be understood by considering the goals toward which motivational responses are directed. A big problem with his approach is the assignment of "purpose" to behavioral responses where purpose has subjective connotations and is even further away from direct physiological realization than most other behavioral concepts. Nevertheless, Bindra classifies goals as a subset of the category of objects and events called incentives. Incentives are defined as objects and events that affect an organism's behavior radically and reliably. So, "a goal is an incentive that is chosen by the investigator as a reference point for describing observed behavior" (Bindra, 1959, p. 54). Two decades later these definitions seem unnecessarily to be based in teleology, to be overly broad and overlapping.

In an approach that is both more modest and more physiological, Milner (1970, p. 406) simply says that incentive motivation explains those responses elicited in the apparent absence of biological drive, while Thompson (1975, p. 298) recognizes that the exact nature of sensory stimuli (their incentive value) determines behavioral responses along with the amount of biological need.

Arousal

In the 1950s, the concept of arousal was often discussed in the context of motivational questions. An enthusiastic theorist along these lines was Bindra (1959). Roughly speaking, a state of high arousal is recognized in an organism that is awake, excited, tense, showing a high degree of "energy mobilization" or "activation." In all cases, the idea of arousal refers to the energy or excitation level of an organism, and roughly may be treated as a dimension of behavior. As such, we may refer to humoral and neural processes which underlie variations in an animal's response along this dimension.

Among the measures of arousal (Bindra, 1959, p. 213ff.) are muscle tension in various parts of the body, electroencephalographic arousal, galvanic skin response, heart rate, vasomotor changes, respiration rate, oxygen consumption rate, and simple behavioral observations (e.g., awake versus asleep). These measures are not always well correlated with each other, and even within a measure there may be complexities. For instance, muscles may be tense and active in one part of the body and not another.

Among factors which can bring about changes in arousal level are environmental changes, reduction in sensory variation, task performance, noxious stimulation, and drugs. Bindra considers that effects of anxiety, stress, frustration, and monotony on arousal level can be explained through their effects on degree of stimulus variation, environmental change, need for task performance, or noxious input.

Can variations in arousal explain variations in the occurrence of responses? Bindra (1959, pp. 246–249) offers two generalizations. First, there is an optimum range of level of arousal within which a given measure of performance will reach its highest value, and the greater the deviation from the optimum arousal range, the greater the decrease in the performance measure. Second, with increased practice at performing an activity or task, there will be an increase in the range of the optimum level of arousal as well as the range within which the activity occurs at all.

From the point of view of traditional experimental psychology (Kling and Riggs, 1971, pp. 826–832), there were questions about the relations between arousal level and "general drive." Such authors emphasized the variety of experimental measures of an organism's "general activation": heart rate, EEG, and so forth.

Intuitively, from all of these treatments, there seems to be some relation between an animal's arousal and measures of motivation. But from neither a physiological nor an experimental psychological viewpoint has there been shown a necessary identification of the concepts of arousal and motivation.

Emotion

Comparing the roles of motivational and emotional processes makes sense in the realms of both neuroanatomical and zoological (evolutionary) thought. Motivational signals, especially humoral signals, have major impact upon hypothalamic neurons. These hypothalamic neurons control behavioral, endocrine, and autonomic states that recognize the bodily needs signaled by the motivational influences and drive skeletal and autonomic behavioral acts to acquire from the environment substances which will reduce those needs. Emotional states are adaptive in being associated with muscular readiness and autonomic readiness (often in support of anticipated muscular action) to initiate those behavioral responses required to obtain the environmental commodities called for by motivational (regulatory or hormonal) influences. These emotional states also lead to signs that we call emotional expressions and as such betray the state of emotion of the organism and can be used as expressive signals in animal communication. Many emotional states depend on neural activity in limbic system structures in phylogenetically ancient portions of the forebrain. With the conceptualization of motivational and emotional states given above, the meaninfulness of the close neuroanatomical connections between limbic system and hypothalamus becomes clear. Not only do limbic structures project heavily to medial hypothalamic cell groups; medial hypothalamic neurons also project back to the limbic system. The parallel with these obvious reciprocal neuroanatomical connections is the adaptive coupling of emotional and motivational states.

In our book explicit references to the relations of motivational influences with emotional experience will be found in the chapter by Eliot Stellar (Chapter 13).

One of the older physiological theories of emotion was the James–Lange theory: Here, the role of visceral factors in emotion was emphasized, with the claim that they mediate both the behavioral and the experiential effects. "We feel afraid because we run." That is, according to James, our feeling of the bodily changes *is* the emotion. Proponents of the Cannon–Bard theory of emotion criticized by the James–Lange theory, particularly because emotional behavioral responses can be observed after the viscera have been surgically removed. Thus, sensations from them could not be essential for causing emotional states. Instead, the Cannon–Bard theory emphasized that mechanisms underlying emotion must derive primarily from central neural states.

From a more current, neurophysiological point of view, Thompson (1975, p. 368ff.) avoids discussing aspects of emotional experience which by definition are purely subjective. Instead, he concentrates on features of objective emotional behaviors, especially easily identified in their most extreme forms: anger, fear, joy, and so on. Approachable with experimental physiological techniques are the roles of the autonomic nervous system in the generation and expression of emotional responses (Thompson, 1975, p. 374ff.). Here the concept of emotionality can be measured through variables controlled by the autonomic nervous system, such as galvanic skin response, heart rate, blood pressure, pupil size, depth of respiration, rate of respiration, rate of eye blinking, intestinal motility, muscle tension in various parts of the body, amount of peripheral blood flow, and changes in salivary fluid composition. When correlated with emotional states some of these measures may be causes of emotional changes and others merely reflections of emotional state.

A more single-minded approach to the neurophysiology of motivation came when Hebb (1955) emphasized the role of the ascending reticular activating system in desynchronizing the cortical electroencephalogram correlated with increases in the overall state of alertness. Then, for any particular behavior required, increases in alertness or arousal from an optimal range would lead to emotional states characterized by disturbance and anxiety and interfere with response performance, whereas decreasing arousal from the optimal range would lead to harmfully low levels of interest or emotional activation.

Schlosberg (1954) mapped a psychological theory of emotionality which attempted to indicate in three-dimensional space the dimensions of this concept. Included were provisions for plotting positive and negative affect, both orthogonal to an intensity dimension. In Schlosberg's thought, remarkably little attention is given to the physiological nature or the biological adaptiveness of emotional states.

Bindra (1959) warns that many of the situations associated with emotional changes also cause motivational phenomena. Because of this, he decried a lack of clear differentiating criteria which would allow the distinction between emotion and motivation. Simply because both sets of response patterns are controlled by "interactions between internal and environmental conditions," he mistakenly discarded the possibility of maintaining distinctions between them.

In recent ethology, perhaps the most extensively treated and certainly most popularly discussed emotion state is that of aggression. Lorenz (1963, pp. 40–59) identifies three evolutionary adaptive functions of aggression: balanced distribution of conspecifics across space, selection of the strongest animals by fighting, and defense of the young. He also identifies aggression as an emotional pressure which sometimes explains behavior patterns that appear to have nothing to do with aggression itself. Lorenz hastens to show that aggression, far from being purely detrimental to a species, when functioning in the right way can be essential for its preservation. That is, he thinks that "orderly, stimulus-bound aggression will function according to useful evolutionary principles, while spontaneous aggression can be quite dangerous." According to Lorenz, if pressure for the release of an aggressive emotional state builds without expression in normal, zoologically regulated form, it might eventually be released without proper environmental stimuli, to the detriment of the species.

Motivation Is a Unitary Behavioral Concept with Multiple Neurophysiological Mechanisms

From the beginning of this chapter we see that the concept of motivation is logically required for the efficient explanation of large categories of behavioral changes. At the behavioral level, "motivation" can be used in a fashion uniform across particular need states: It is always an intervening variable used fruitfully to demonstrate lawfulness of certain behavioral responses. But does that mean that neurobiological mechanisms are also constant across particular motivational states?

The purpose of this book is to examine those motivational conditions which have been best studied with neuroanatomical, neurophysiological, and neurochemical techniques. How far has modern neurobiology brought us in the reductionistic explanation of motivational changes?

Comparisons across chapters in the book show a clear multiplicity of physiological mechanisms of motivation. While at the behavioral level the concept of motivation is a "warm blanket" (unitary and comforting), the physiological analysis of the impacts of motivational signals on the central nervous system remind one of a "patchwork quilt." The multiplicity of biological mechanisms is consistent with the view that they evolved separately in an ad hoc manner to meet specific regulatory and other adaptive needs.

Among the regulatory behavior patterns, behavioral responses return biologically important variables to set points for the maintenance of homeostasis. Some of these have the character of a "positive motivation": The motivated behaviors are approach responses or actual consumption. A well-studied example is the case of hunger. Carl Pfaffmann (Chapter 4) covers neurophysiological analyses of sensory input related to food intake. Only rarely does the firing rate of a particular gustatory-responsive nerve cell predict the behavioral valence of the tasty substance used. Thus, we must look centrally for much of the explanation of the behavioral changes connoting hunger. Ralph Norgren's neuroanatomical and electrophysiological studies are striking for their emphasis on mechanisms in the lower brain stem and limbic forebrain, in a field of discourse where the hypothalamus has been the most frequently studied structure. For hunger, an obvious opportunity for biological analysis comes in the study of satiety signals that turn off feeding. The exquisite review by Gerard Smith (Chapter 5) shows at least three sources of satiety signals. Grinker (Chapter 6) considers the implications of modern results with chemical and cellular techniques for the understanding of human obesity.

Even comparing hunger with another form of ingestive behavior, drinking, shows a lack of uniformity among neurobiological mechanisms. In turn, within the field dealing with physiological regulations on water intake and salt balance, we deal with mechanisms triggered by changes in blood volume as well as blood sodium concentration. Alan Epstein's chapter (Chapter 7) reviews elegant analyses of the humoral and neural mechanisms controlling water intake.

In some cases it is not obvious that motivational signals can be divided into freestanding "positive" and "negative" (or approach versus avoidance, or "pleasant" versus "aversive") categories. The concept of linked opponent processes in motivation, analogous to those proposed for color vision, was created by Richard Solomon and is reviewed in Chapter 11. A similar type of idea played a role in Deutsch's approach to the motivational phenomenon of intracranial self-stimulation, reviewed here (in Chapter 12) by Halperin and Pfaff in the setting of hypothalamic and autonomic physiology.

An undeniably "negative" form of motivation, which is "regulatory" in the sense that motivated responses remove the animal from aversive conditions, is the response to pain. David Mayer and Donald Price review the neurophysiology, neuroanatomy, and neuropharmacology of pain response systems in Chapter 15, providing the opportunity to compare physiological experiments in animals with experiential conditions in humans. Along these lines, Eliot Stellar compares animal and human responses in situations dealing, for example, with thermal comfort (Chapter 13). The use of experiments on arousal and stress to deal with questions of aversive motivation is included in the chapter by Neal Miller (Chapter 14).

A different set of motivational mechanisms, including important cellular changes in the preoptic area, manages the animal's response to changes in body temperature. The logical analysis of hierarchies of thermoregulatory responses comes in Evelyn Satinoff's chapter (Chapter 8).

The biological bases of some motivational systems lie in bioligically crucial, well-documented steroid hormone effects not associated with the obvious regulation of a homeostatic variable. Perhaps the best analyzed physiological mechanisms for motivation concern the impact of steroid sex hormones on the central nervous system (Pfaff, 1980). Farbach and Pfaff (Chapter 9) review the steroid hormonal and neural mechanisms for maternal behavior in the rat. Data in the chapter by

Pfaff (Chapter 10) indicate that the neural and endocrine analyses of
the mechanisms for sexual responses have indeed uncovered mechanisms of sexual motivation.

References

Bateson, T. P. G., & Hinde, R. A. *Growing points in ethology.* Cambridge, England:
Cambridge University Press, 1976.
Beach, F. A. Neural and chemical regulation of behavior. In H. F. Harlow & C. N.
Wilsey (Eds.), *Biological and biochemical bases of behavior.* Madison, Wis.:
University of Wisconsin Press, 1958.
Bermant, G. Response latencies of female rats during sexual intercourse. *Science,*
1961, *133,* 1771-1773.
Bermant, G., & Westbrook, W. H. Peripheral factors in the regulation of sexual con-
tact by female rats. *Journal of Comparative and Physiological Psychology,* 1966,
61, 244-250.
Bindra, D. *Motivation, a systematic reinterpretation.* New York: Ronald Press, 1959.
Bolles, R. C. *Theory of motivation* (2nd ed.). New York: Harper & Row, 1975.
Bolles, R. C., Rap, H. M., & White, G. C. Failure of sexual activity to reinforce
female rats. *Journal of Comparative and Physiological Psychology,* 1968, *65,*
311-313.
Cannon, W. B., & Washburn, A. L. An explanation of hunger. *American Journal of
Physiology,* 1912, *29,* 441-454.
Cicala, G. A. *Animal drives.* Princeton, N.J.: Van Nostrand, 1965.
Davis, D. E. *Integral animal behavior.* New York: Macmillan, 1966.
Dawkins, R. Hierarchical organization: A candidate principle for ethology. In
T. P. G. Bateson & R. A. Hinde (Eds.), *Growing points in ethology.* Cambridge,
England: Cambridge University Press, 1976.
Dethier, V. G., & Stellar, E. *Animal behavior.* Englewood Cliffs, N.J.: Prentice-Hall,
1961.
Deutsch, J. A. *The structural basis of behavior.* Chicago: University of Chicago
Press, 1960.
Deutsch, J. A., & Deutsch, D. *Physiological psychology.* Homewood, Ill.: Dorsey
Press, 1966.
Eibl-Eibesfeldt, I. *Ethology: The biology of behavior.* New York: Holt, 1970.
French, P., Fitzpatrick, D., & Law, O. T. Operant investigation of mating preference
in female rats. *Journal of Comparative and Physiological Psychology,* 1972, *81,*
226-232.
Glickman, S. E., & Schiff, B. B. A biological theory of reinforcement. *Psychological
Review,* 1967, *74,* 81-109.
Hebb, D. O. *The organization of behavior.* New York: Wiley, 1949.
Hebb, D. O. Drives and the CNS. *Psychological Review,* 1955, *62,* 243-254.
Heron, W. T., & Skinner, B. F. Changes in hunger during starvation. *Psychological
Record,* 1937, *1,* 51-60.
Hess, W. R. *Das Zwischenhirn.* Frankfurt, Germany: Schwabe, 1954.
Howarth, C. I., & Deutsch, J. A. Drive decay: The cause of fast extinction of habits
learned for brain stimulation. *Science,* 1962, *137,* 35-36.

Hull, C. L. Goal attraction and directing ideas conceived as habit phenomena. *Psychological Review*, 1931, *38*, 487–506.

Hull, C. L. *Principles of behavior.* New York: Appleton, 1943.

Hull, C. L. *A behavior system.* New Haven: Yale University Press, 1952.

James, W. *Principles of psychology.* New York: Holt, 1890.

Jenkins, T. N., Warner, L. H., & Warden, C. J. Standard apparatus for the study of animal motivation. *Journal of Comparative Psychology*, 1926, *6*, 361–382.

Kling, J. W., & Riggs, L. A. (Eds.). *Woodworth and Schlosberg's experimental psychology* (3rd ed.). New York: Holt, Rinehart & Winston, 1971.

Lorenz, K. The comparative method in studying innate behavior patterns. *Symposia of the Society for Experimental Biology*, 1950, *4*, 221–268.

Lorenz, K. *On aggression.* New York: Bantam Books, 1963.

Maier, N. R. F., & Schneirla, T. C. *Principles of animal psychology.* New York: McGraw-Hill, 1935.

Marler, P., & Hamilton, W. J. *Mechanisms of animal behavior.* New York: Wiley, 1966.

McDougall, W. *An introduction to social psychology.* Boston: Luce, 1914.

Miller, G., Galanter, E., & Pribram, K. *Plans and the structure of behavior.* New York: Holt, 1960.

Miller, N. E. Liberalization of basic S-R concepts: Extensions to conflict behavior, motivation and social learning. In S. Koch (Ed.), *Psychology: A study of a science* (Study 1, Vol. 2). New York: McGraw-Hill, 1959.

Miller, N. E. Behavioral and physiological techniques: Rationale and experimental designs for combining their use. In C. F. Code & W. Heidel (Eds.), *Handbook of physiology*, Section 6: *Alimentary canal* (Vol. 1, *Food and water intake*). Baltimore: Williams & Wilkins, 1967.

Milner, P. M. *Physiological psychology.* New York: Holt, Rinehart & Winston, 1970.

Mowrer, O. H. *Learning theory and behavior.* New York: Wiley, 1960.

Olds, J. Hypothalamic substrates of reward. *Physiological Review*, 1962, *42*, 554–604.

Olds, J., & Milner, P. Positive reinforcement produced by electrical stimulation of septal area and other regions of rat brain. *Journal of Comparative and Physiological Psychology*, 1954, *47*, 419–427.

Olds, J., & Olds, M. E. Drives, rewards and the brain. In *New directions in psychology* (Vol. 2). New York: Holt, Rinehart & Winston, 1965.

Olds, M. E., & Olds, J. Approach–escape interactions in rat brain. *American Journal of Physiology*, 1962, *203*, 74–89.

Pfaff, D. W. *Estrogens and brain function.* New York: Springer-Verlag, 1980.

Richter, C. P. Animal behavior and internal drives. *Quarterly Review of Biology*, 1927, *2*, 307–343.

Roeder, K. D. *Nerve cells and insect behavior.* Cambridge, Mass.: Harvard University Press, 1963.

Schlosberg, H. Three dimensions of emotion. *Psychological Review*, 1954, *61*, 81–88.

Scott, J. P. *Animal behavior.* Garden City. N.Y.: Doubleday, 1958.

Sheffield, F. D., Wulff, J. J., & Backer, R. Reward value of copulation without sex drive reduction. *Journal of Comparative and Physiological Psychology*, 1951, *44*, 3–8.

Skinner, B. F. *The behavior of organisms: An experimental analysis.* New York: Appleton-Century, 1938.

Skinner, B. F. *Science and human behavior.* New York: Macmillan, 1953.

Spence, K. W. *Behavior theory and conditioning.* New Haven: Yale University Press, 1956.

Stellar, E. The physiology of motivation. *Psychological Review,* 1954, *61,* 5-22.

Thompson, R. F. *Introduction to physiological psychology.* New York: Harper & Row, 1975.

Tinbergen, N. *The study of instinct.* Oxford, England: Clarendon Press, 1951.

von Holst, E., & St. Paul, U. On the functional organization of drives. *Animal Behavior,* 1963, *11,* 1-39.

Warden, C. J., et al. *Animal motivation: Experimental studies on the albino rat.* New York: Columbia University Press, 1931.

Warner, L. H. A study of sex behavior in the white rat by means of the obstruction method. *Comparative Psychology Monographs,* 1927, *4* (No. 22).

Warner, L. H. A study of hunger behavior in the white rat by means of the obstruction method. *Journal of Comparative Psychology,* 1928, *8,* 273-299.

Chapter 2

Instinct and Motivation as Explanations for Complex Behavior

ALAN N. EPSTEIN

Few behaviors are truly reflexive, and those that are are not the behaviors with which most animals make their livings. If you have any residual doubt about that assertion, recall the characteristics of reflexes as studied by Sherrington early in this century (reprinted in 1947). They are innate, they lack spontaneity, are stimulus bound, and stereotyped. That is, a particular set of them occurs in all animals of the same kind as the outcome of their genome and its realization in normal development (innateness). Reflex effects (exitatory or inhibitory) are always elicitable from an intact nervous system by some combination of the duration and repetition of their stimulus provided that the stimulus is the right kind ("adequate" in Sherrington's terminology) and strong enough (stimulus binding).[1] And the afferent input is necessary; without it the behavior does not occur (no spontaneity). The stimulus determines the frequency and form of the behavior, and the form is the same from episode to episode of its elicitation and across animals of the same kind (stereotypy). The taxes and kineses of the older animal behaviorists (see Fraenkel & Gunn, 1961) are the same kinds of behavior in all respects.

---

[1] When appropriately combined, inhibitory reflexes can render those that are excitatory nonelicitable by even high intensities and long durations of their adequate stimuli. Both, nevertheless, remain stimulus bound. That is, the frequency and intensity of the inhibition are a direct consequence of the frequency and intensity of its adequate stimulus, and once that stimulus is removed, the excitatory effect is revealed to have been active and under the control of its adequate stimulus throughout the inhibition. See Sherrington's studies of reciprocal and flexor inhibition for examples.

Admittedly, reflexes are not trivial for behavior. They keep the domestic machinery of the animal operating automatically and flawlessly,
and they are necessary elements of overt behavior. Movements of all
kinds would be disordered or impossible without them. Ingestion could
not occur or would be catastrophic without reflex swallowing and
gagging. Reflexes provide defense against predators and prevent injury;
and afferent feedbacks from them are potent and classical reinforcers
(Pavlov, 1927). But its tight stimulus control, stereotypy, and lack of
spontaneity make the reflex inadequate as an explanation of complex
behavior. What, for example, are the adequate stimuli for the three
most common behaviors of the rat: sleeping, grooming, and locomotion? Are they bound in frequency and form to a particular kind of
afferent input? And do they have no spontaneity? On the contrary,
they all exhibit impressive freedom from external stimulus control. I
am not saying that they are entirely free of such control. That would be
absurd. But I am saying that when you recall what we know about the
cerebral machinery of sleep and waking (Jouvet, 1967), about the mechanisms of circadian running (Moore, 1978), and about the central
programming of grooming (Fentress, 1973) in mammals, you will admit
that the reflex is not the model-concept for these behaviors. These behaviors are emitted by mechanisms within the central nervous system
that include stimuli as modifiers, but they are not elicited by stimuli
from an essentially passive nervous system. And if you consider behaviors like ingestion and reproduction, with which many of us here are
concerned, the defects of the reflex model are even more obvious. The
important fact for this discussion is that food and fluid, or a sexual
partner, are almost always *inadequate* for elicitation of intake or sex.
An appropriate stimulus object is of course necessary for the behavior,
but it is not by itself sufficient to elicit it. The animal's internal state
makes food or fluid adequate for ingestion or a conspecific adequate
for copulation, and because the state waxes and wanes the stimuli are
adequate only periodically and then only briefly. In the case of reproductive behavior the internal state is overwhelmingly important. It not
only makes the behavior possible but it converts it from one form to
another. Consider the female mammal's (Adler, 1981) or insect's (Loher
& Huber, 1966) response to a sexually aggressive male, which she will
attack when she is not in the appropriate hormonal state but will accept
if she is. Or in the case of another behavior, recall that the adult ringdove with a crop that is not distended may kill rather than feed a squab
if solicited by it (Lehrman, 1955). Moreover, it is characteristic of these
behaviors that when the potentially adequate stimulus objects are absent (and reflexes are therefore impossible) new behaviors, sometimes
quite novel and idiosyncratic, can be strung together as a prelude to
encounters with them (Teitelbaum, 1966).
   In order to understand how animals generate behaviors with these

characteristics we need concepts that are more complex and neurological mechanisms that are more endogenous than those for the reflex.
Motivation and instinct are such concepts. They are needed for this
purpose, and in this chapter I want to give you my views on how they
can be made more useful.

Some Key Terms Defined

First I need to avoid some conceptual snares by telling you what I mean
by the key words I have already used. Begin with "animals." I use it in
its biological sense to mean all of them that we know about, not just
the handful of domestic pets or pests and the few primates that so
many of us work with. I mean all the animals, both great and small, in
their 20 or 25 phyletic divisions (depending on how many extinct phyla
you count) within which they have been isolated from each other
genetically for at least 400 million years (the chordates are the most
recent, having arisen in the Ordovician). Although genetic and cellular
mechanisms have been conserved across phyla, animals within a phylum
are each a particular kind having ancient and conspicuous differences
from those in all the others. Many of these differences are fundamental
for behavior. Differences in body format (radial or bilateral symmetry,
e.g.) and body size (the largest insect is approximately the size of the
smallest mammal), number (ranging from none to several hundreds),
arrangement and form of appendages, nature of skeletal support (none,
internal, or external), modes of locomotion, receptor equipment, strategies of feeding, reproduction, and defense, and mechanisms of thermoregulation are examples. All are based on a separate genetic descent that
has left each phylum, after its eons of isolation, very different from all
the others, and I for one am uncomfortable with generalizations across
them unless the behavior being compared is very ancient, ubiquitous,
and very similar in its essential characteristics. Habituation and sensitization appear to be behaviors for which this can be done (Kandel, 1979).
   Within phyla, species have succeeded not because they have been the
same but because they have evolved structural and behavioral solutions
to the peculiar demands of a particular habitat. Think of locomotion
and how different it is as a behavioral problem in an animal with no
limbs living in the earth (an earthworm, e.g.), or in one with eight limbs
living in the sea (octopus) or in the air (spider), and even among these
we should be careful not to lump the spiders and the octopi, which are
very likely to have different neurological schemes for the control of
their limbs. Or consider the special case of flying, which has evolved
in all the vertebrate orders and is also a talent of many insects. Is the
mechanism by which mosquitoes fly (beating their wings at 400–500
Hz) the same, in essence, as it is in birds? And even among evolutionary

neighbors where the theme may be the same we should be cautious that the variations on it may not be trivial. Birds (and extinct reptiles) fly with their arms, and most of them do so in daylight using visual guidance; bats fly with their hands at night using sonar; reptiles and amphibians are gliders; and fish propel themselves with their whole bodies. Is this just a series of minor variations on a single theme? Can we understand flying in all vertebrates by studying it in only one kind?

The best analyzed example I know of this problem of fundamental differences in superficially similar phenomena is the ontogeny of sexual behavior. Courtship and copulation are in many insects activated by hormones (see Truman & Riddiford, 1974) and are therefore not different in principle from what is happening in animals like ourselves (Pfaff, 1980), but the development of their sex behavior is another matter. An insect's sexual role, at least in moths, bees, ants (Whiting, 1932), and flies (Benzer, 1973), is determined entirely by the genetics of its brain. Insect mosaics that are gynandromorphs (composed of parts that are genetically male and others that are female) with male heads and female bodies court females and attempt male copulation with their ovipositors! Contrast this with rodents in which neonatal hormones can defy genotype and can produce a behaviorally competent (but sterile) adult whose behavior is the opposite of its genotype. Not so in insects. The genotype of the brain determines sex behavior regardless of the kind of body (including its glands and gonads) with which it has to work. In animals like us the ontogeny of gender also depends on genotype, of course, but in addition it depends on hormones at a critical stage in development, whereas in animals like moths and flies it does not. So for me "animals" means creatures of enormous diversity both in the kinds of behaviors that they exhibit and in their underlying mechanisms. When we deal with animals from different phyla (or even from different orders) we should expect diversity and, like Noah, should respect it. Different mechanisms may have evolved within them for complex behaviors and these may be disguised by the superficial similarities imposed on complex behavior by convergent evolution. I think it's time to make some distinctions, to do some splitting and less lumping, or we may do with the behavior of moths and rats what we are warned not to do with the flavor of apples and oranges.

No doubt the stunning success of the biochemists and geneticists in revealing the universal themes of metabolism and heredity is responsible, in large part, for the tendency to lump animals in the study of behavior. If the behaviors being compared are similar, it is assumed that they will share common underlying mechanisms even if the animals being compared have only an ancient and obscure genetic relationship.

But eagerness to find the basic machinery of behavior appears to have led to an insensitivity to the warning that, in addition to being conservative of cellular function (the genetic and metabolic biochemistry of cells), evolution has been opportunistic and inventive and that its capacity for novelty is most apparent for complex functions such as behavior. Consider the sequence: cellular respiration → ventilation → vocalization → language. It is an evolutionary sequence in which the more recent functions (to the right) depended for their emergence on the establishment of each of the earlier or antecedent functions listed to its left. All cells, both plant and animal, must exchange gases with their ambient fluid across their membranes. All cells do it, and there is impressive conservatism across kinds of cells and kinds of organisms in the gases exchanged and in the cellular mechanisms by which the exchanges take place. But now consider the relation between cellular respiration and vocalization. They are linked in evolution through ventilation. The simplest animals (protozoa, sponges, coelenterates) respire directly across their cell membranes. More complex animals (crustacea, mollusks, fish) have respiratory appendages such as gills that often require ventilation by positive-pressure pumping or fanning in order to move the ambient water over the respiratory membranes. Ventilation is not a cellular process localized to the gills. It is ordered movement of several body parts controlled by the central nervous system. With this innovation behavior is added and the basic cellular process of respiration is now served by a novel and more complex function whose mechanisms cannot be understood, or even predicted, from those of respiration itself. The next transition, that from ventilation to vocalization, required an additional innovation. It awaited the emergence of animals that respire in air. They do so either with trachea (some worm-like animals, insects) or with lungs that require a behavioral pump which, in reptiles, birds, and mammals, depends for its action on a negative-pressure thorax (a novelty in its own right that is not a simple elaboration of the mechanism by which gills are ventilated). Behavior continues to be essential for respiration and now in combination with a new process—air moving through tubes—provides an opportunity for sound production, an opportunity that was exploited by birds and mammals in particular. Reviewing this sequence, I think you will agree that cellular respiration and ventilation are the evolutionary antecedents of vocalization, but would you accept them as the basic processes by which vocalization can be understood? Would you recommend that someone wishing to understand birdsong study gill ventilation in crabs or fish? And when we include the ultimate innovation in this evolutionary sequence my point is made emphatically. Vocalization is antecedent to language. Language could not have evolved if there had not been animals that respired by moving air through tubes, thereby providing an apparatus for sound production. Everyone, I think, would recognize the futility of using pulmonary ventilation as a "simple model" for understanding the basic mechanisms of language. Language is a biological novelty dependent on mechanisms that are simply not inherent in breathing, and was confined in its emergence to a small group of animals. There is no model system for its analysis. It must be studied in animals that have it.

I want the same set of ideas applied to less esoteric behaviors, to motivated behaviors in particular. I think that they have also been formed in evolution by a combination of conservatism and innovation so that, for example, the eating (the consumption of food that is already sensed) done by all animals is not the same as the motivated feeding (the arousal of the central state of hunger and the search for and selection of food) done by only some. The problem for my argument is that, unlike respiration and language, which hardly need to be distinguished, eating and motivated feeding look so much alike. In fact, motivated feeding culminates in eating and there are reasons to believe that the basic mechanisms of eating have been conserved among a large number of very different kinds of animals. For example, eating is inhibited by afferents from the gut in animals as diverse as insects (Dethier & Bodenstein, 1958), mollusks (Susswein & Kupfermann, 1975), and mammals, both in infant rats (Lorenz, Ellis, & Epstein, 1982), and in adult primates (McHugh & Moran, 1979). But I don't believe that motivated feeding is an evolutionary relic that can be studied in any animal that eats. To me it looks very different from its antecedents, and in what follows I will emphasize its complex and novel aspects, hoping that you will agree that a rat that is feeding is doing things that a slug or a bug simply does not do when it eats.

So much for animals. How, then, am I using the word "behavior"? Without too much formality I can give you my sense of the meaning of behavior as follows: Behavior is the organized effector actions (largely by muscle and glands) with which animals (and some plants) relate to themselves, conspecifics, external resources, and other sensible aspects of the environment. By "effector actions" I mean visceral and glandular effects as well as somatic. In short, behavior is what animals do to make their livings. Individual instances of behavior arise, in all animals, from three quite different processes. I think of them as the components whose interactions result in what animals do. Each is a class. One or several of the items within each, but not all of the items named below, will participate in the control of the particular behavior at issue. They are (1) an *endogenous component*—the animal's genome and its realization in development (the kind of animal that is behaving), and the animal's neural, humoral, and energetic state at the time the behavior is performed (what is happening inside the animal with respect to its state of arousal, its mood, its energy stores and temperature, its hormones); (2) an *acquired component*—the retained effects of the animal's individual past history. Here I take the broadest possible view. These may be the result of rearing conditions, use and disuse, sensory adaptation, acclimatization, habituation or sensitization, conditioning, learning, or aging, or may even be the effects of past pathology (addiction and taste-aversion learning are good current examples). It is only necessary that they have been part of the behaving animal's past history and that they be carried forward in some form into the current behavior setting; and (3) a *reactive component*—the stimulus events and their afferent consequences that are operating to trigger, guide, and terminate the behavior. Here I am referring to all of the processes by which stimuli affect behavior. Less needs to be said of this component because it is the subject of the extensive literature on the stimulus control of behavior.

It is inconceivable to me that behavior can occur without the cooperative interaction of these three components, except for reflexes in which an acquired component may be absent, particularly if there has been no immediately prior stimulation. Behavior cannot occur without an actor, a particular kind of animal whose phenotype sets limits on what it can, and cannot, do. The behaving animal will have an internal state and a unique individual history, and it will be utilizing afferent input at some stage in its behavioral performance. Even the most thoroughly endogenous of behaviors, such as circadian locomotion in mammals or flight in locusts, are controlled by sensed information in their natural expressions. Circadian running is entrained by light, and locusts' flight is triggered by and guided by mechanoreceptors.

I emphasize this concept of components of behavior because I do not want to be misunderstood in what is written below to be attributing some behaviors to pure innateness and others to pure learning. I do not want to waste time on the old nature/nurture issue. Innateness will always play a role in behavior (after all, what an animal can do is a consequence of the kind of animal it is), and learning will, if it can. It is far more interesting to me, first, to expand the discussion to include all of the most interesting determinants of behavior (the items that I have included within the description of each component are my suggestions in this regard); second, to view them as falling naturally into three classes of qualitatively different processes; and third, to assess for each behavior how the components interact in its expression.

"Complex behaviors" are those in which all three components play a major role. These behaviors are the principal concern of this discussion. They are those in which internal states are operating and are therefore drive induced, and in which stimuli trigger, guide, and terminate the behavior but are not sufficient by themselves to arouse it. And these behaviors are organized in most instances into appetitive and consummatory phases (in aversive behaviors the appetitive phase appears only after repetition of the noxious stimulus). I use "appetitive" and "consummatory" (and "aversion") as they were defined by Craig (1918) in his discussion of appetites and aversions in the behavior of doves. He wrote

An appetite [which he calls elsewhere "a certain readiness to act"] . . . is a state of agitation which continues so long as a certain stimulus, which may be called the appeted stimulus, is absent. When the appeted stimulus is at length received it stimulates a consummatory reaction [which he calls elsewhere "the end action of the series"], after which the appetitive behavior ceases and is succeeded by a state of relative rest. . . . An aversion is a state of agitation which continues so long as a certain stimulus, referred to as the disturbing stimulus, is present; but which ceases, being replaced by a state of relative rest, when that stimulus has ceased to act on the sense-organs.

Surprisingly, "stimulus" is a word that needs some defense. Many, some of whom should know better, use it in the layman's sense to mean anything that causes behavior. I use it in its technical sense: afferent inputs aroused by receptor action that are effective in controlling behavior. The outcome may be to arouse or suppress behavior. The important thing is that a stimulus be a receptor-activated input that makes a difference for what an animal is doing.

Instinct and Motivation Compared

With this introduction I can return to my main theme, namely, that we need concepts that take account of the complexities of behaviors that are not reflexive. Motivation and instinct do so, but they need to be distinguished in order to make them more useful as explanations of complex behavior. The distinction is difficult because instinct and motivation are so similar. So much so that others (Lashley, 1938; Tinbergen, 1974) have discussed them as if they were the same. I believe that there are important differences between them, differences both in the kinds of animals in which they occur and in the characteristics of the behaviors that are described by each concept. I am convinced that motivated behavior is biologically less common and psychologically more complex than instinctive behavior. And I believe that the differences deserve emphasis, because they are diagnostic of differences in underlying neurological mechanisms and therefore ought to be respected when we choose species for study of the brain mechanisms of motivated behavior.

Most of what follows is hypothetical. I am convinced that it is a valuable description of the nature of complex behavior, but my conviction is based on intuition more often than on evidence and when it is I use the word "belief" hoping that it will be read literally. Those who do not share my convictions, and I expect that there will be many, should take my ideas as suggestions for debate and ultimately for research.

The Similarities

First, consider the similarities. Historically the concepts of motivation and instinct arose as explanations for the spontaneity of behavior and for its inconstancy in frequency and form in response to constant stimulus conditions. Both of these phenomena require a concept of changeable internal states that generate the readiness for behavior.

Behavior is strikingly spontaneous. Much of what animals do is done without immediately preceding stimulation. This is true from protozoa to primates. Jennings' descriptions of the behavior of colonies of paramecia beating their way constantly through their medium are what I have in mind (Jennings, 1962), each animal making its own way through the water unsynchronized with its neighbors. I am also thinking of the detailed descriptions that we now have of the spontaneous behaviors of the great apes in the wild (Schaller, 1964). Richter put the issue before us with exactly the right breadth of mind and elegance of expression in his introduction to a review of his studies of the periodic behaviors of the undisturbed rat (1927) in which he wrote:

> One of the most fundamental of all the phenomena which characterize animal life and distinguish it from plant life is the spontaneous mobility of the animal organism. A few plants, to be sure, especially certain forms of marine vegetation, do move about, but these few are exceptions in the plant kingdom. The activity of animals, on the other hand, although it varies widely in form and extent from species to species, is an ordinary phenomenon which one anticipates under normal circumstances. We may ask, then, what it is that sets off the diverse performances which animals display. Ordinarily we think of most of their activity as being due to some form of external stimulation. We know, however, that all animals, from the lowest uni-cellular organism to man, are active even when all external stimuli have been eliminated. And since this spontaneous mobility, just as any other kind of mobility, must have a definitive cause, it must be due to some natural factor within the organism.

The phenomenon of spontaneity requires that behavior be conceived of as the outcome of states within animals that generate or suppress action, that it be thought of as essentially endogenous.

Second, the ideas of instinct and motivation were invented to account for the inconstancy of behavior in response to constant stimulation. I have already given examples and have emphasized that these are the behaviors of greatest interest for those of us who wish to understand how animals make their livings. This characteristic of altered responsiveness to unaltered stimulus conditions also requires a concept of behavior as the outcome of endogenous states, but in this case the states must be thought of as determining both the readiness of the animal to respond and the form of the behavior. Because of the spontaneity of behavior and because so much of it is essentially unpredictable from the stimulus characteristics alone, instinctive and motivated behaviors have not been thought of as mere reactions to concurrent stimulation. They have instead been attributed to the operation of changeable internal states that have been variously referred to as tendencies, moods, urges, central motive states, or most often as drives.

There are other prominent similarities between instinctive and motivated behaviors. Each includes a phase of wandering or of search and approach that precedes a phase of ultimate and terminating behavior (Craig's appetitive and consummatory phases). Instinctive and motivated behaviors often serve the same functions for the animal, that is, locomotion, communication, thermoregulation, reproduction, nutrition, predation, and defense. They have similar physiological mechanisms that employ hormones, pheromones, and endogenous pattern generators and oscillators. They are governed by deficit signals and servomechanisms and the performance of the behavior leads in many instances to the achievement of homeostasis or self-regulation (Richter, 1942-1943). In both instinct and motivation the behavior itself may be compounded of innate and acquired responses—the maternal behavior of the digger wasps is *not* entirely innate (from Baerends, 1941, as cited by Tinbergen, 1974), and the maternal behavior of the rat is clearly *not* entirely acquired (Rosenblatt & Lehrman, 1963). And in animals with sufficiently complex nervous systems, the mechanisms underlying both instinctive and motivated behaviors reside within the brain. With the similarities enumerated it is not surprising that instinct and motivation have so often been used as names for the same thing.

The Differences

But now consider the differences. Instinctive behavior is, in my view, by far the more common of the two. Remember, I am including all animals in this discussion, not just those that psychologists refer to rather grandly as "organisms." Remember also that the birds and mammals, which tend to preoccupy our thinking, are only the top layers of one of the smaller phyla (the Chordata) in both size and diversity of species, a group that is elite in complexity but modest in number. The entire phylum Chordata is only half the size of the Mollusca in number of species, and is an order of magnitude smaller than the Arthropoda. Fish are the most common vertebrates (twice as many species as birds and mammals combined), and the rodents are the most common mammals. The point here is threefold. First, there are different kinds of animals, and the overwhelming majority of them are different from us and our most common subjects in ancestry and design. Second, all have behavior including, in almost every instance known to me, what I am calling complex behavior, and it seems most unlikely that they would all be governed by the same underlying mechanism. And, third, animals of the other phyla, even those in our own that do not have hair or feathers, are not only different from us but are also simpler than us, and simpler animals are likelier to depend on simpler mechanisms for the execution of complex behaviors than do we and our favorite subjects.

The Characteristics of Instinct

It is my contention that instinct, which has the following distinguishing characteristics, is simpler than motivation, and that most animals employ it to make their livings. It is largely a heritable phenotype; that is, it is the outcome of genome realized in development, and is therefore essentially innate. Consequently it is species specific both in efferent program and in releasing and guiding stimuli (see Fraenkel & Gunn, 1961, for many examples). It occurs typically in small-brained, short-lived animals that live in isolation and exhibit the behavior infrequently (sometimes only once) in crucial situations in which it must be performed flawlessly. Examples abound. Many invertebrates mate only once (and this includes the behaviors of mate selection, copulation, and oviposition), and among those that require a blood-meal for maturation of their eggs many suck blood only once, silk moth larvae spin only one cocoon and eclose from it only once, the octopus copulates only once, and birds hatch only once. In other instances the instinctive behavior is repeated but is nevertheless perfect at its debut. Orb weaving by spiders, flying by insects, prey capture by squid, nipple attachment and licking behavior by rats, and several aspects of visual and auditory perception in cats and ducks are examples. But in the distinction that I am proposing here, instinct need not be entirely innate and I do not want to revert in this discussion to the old and largely useless distinction between instinct and motivation that was based on differences in their dependence on learning. Acquired components can contribute to the performance of instinctive behavior. Habituation and sensitization are common, as are sensory adaptation and the effects of rearing conditions, and the behavior can be shaped by associative learning, but the acquired elements tend to be admixed with otherwise innate behaviors (Tinbergen has referred to these as instances of "localized" learning). This is exemplified by the place learning of the digger wasp that has just dug a new nursery chamber and, before flying off to seek prey, memorizes the local geography of its location (Tinbergen & Kruyt, 1938, as cited by Tinbergen, 1974), and by the fact that immediately upon hatching, squid attack only small crustacea and do so competently but then diversify their prey choices as they acquire experience with other small marine animals (Wells, 1962). Learning of this kind does not diversify the behavior of individuals of the same species; on the contrary, in cooperation with genetic endowment and developmental history it reduces diversity and assures the species uniformity of instinctive behavior.

Finally, I believe that instinctive behavior is displayed by animals that are blind to its ends. This must be true whenever the behavior is performed only once, and is illustrated by the behavioral traps in which many animals can be caught whenever an unmodifiable determinant of their behavior is exploited so that it becomes self-destructive or absurd. Several examples come to mind. The light seeking of many flying insects is a familiar one. The demonstration (Gelperin & Dethier, 1967) that blowflies will starve to death by selecting very sweet but metabolically useless fucose instead of less sweet but nutritious sorbitol is another.[2] Others are the fact that the larvae of some herbivorous insects hatch from eggs laid in the ground and are negatively geotaxic, thereby assuring that they will ascend the stems of plants and encounter the leaves on which they feed. If they are mounted on a continuous horizontal track (such as the edge of an ordinary tumbler) they walk on it to exhaustion, being unable to climb downward; and the fact that the pupas of some moths will perform their lengthy and complex program of eclosion despite being removed from the pupal case before the behavior begins (Truman, 1978). In another example, newly hatched squid that, as I have already mentioned, capture shrimplike prey on first encounter with them will damage themselves by repeated collisions with the sides of a glass vessel while persisting in attempts to attack shrimp that have been confined within the vessel (Wells, 1962). And, as a last example, recall the pathetic spectacle, illustrated in Figure 2-1 taken from Tinbergen (1974), of an oystercatcher attempting to brood a giant artificial egg while ignoring eggs of normal size. Here the use of a supersign stimulus demonstrates that rather than being directed toward successful hatching, the brooding behavior is rigidly controlled by the stimulus characteristics of the egg. It is difficult to grant the characteristic of goal-directedness to behaviors in which an animal traps itself, and I believe that in most instances of instinctive behavior the animal literally does not know what it is doing. But this is an inference and many of you will take it for little more than an assertion. Fortunately, as I suggest below, it is testable. If a goal or some representation of it is implicit in the mechanism of the behavior, then it should be revealed by the characteristic of expectancy.

The cocoon spinning of the silkmoth larva (Van der Kloot & Williams, 1953) is an ideal illustration of what I mean by instinctive behavior, even to the inclusion of a possible role for an acquired component. At each of its larval molts prior to cocoon construction the caterpillar spins a flat molting pad and therefore has spun silk several times before

---

[2]The analogous experiment has not yet, to my knowledge, been done in the rat. When their food intake is decreased (Carper & Polliard, 1953) or is absent (Teitelbaum & Epstein, 1962) rats drink more of both nonnutritive sweet (saccharin) and nutritive carbohydrate (glucose) solutions. They drink roughly twice as much of the glucose, suggesting that they are responsive to both its taste and its nutritional consequences. But a supersweet solution with no nutritional value paired with a merely sweet liquid food have not been offered to a rat that must switch its preference for the supersweet to the food in order to avoid starvation.

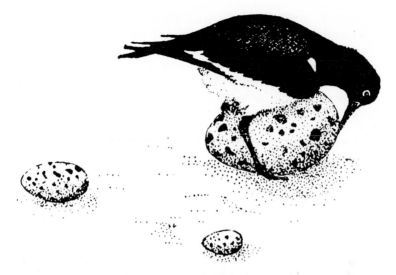

Figure 2-1. A female oystercatcher attempting to retrieve the largest available "egg" (a dummy provided by the experimenter) while ignoring her real egg, which lies in the foreground. (From Tinbergen, 1974.)

performing the ultimate behavior. Having reached an appropriate stage of development in complete isolation from all of its conspecifics and being prepared by appropriate changes in hormonal state (a decline in juvenile hormone and an increase in ecdysone), the mature larva evacuates its gut and wanders away from the leaves it has been eating, settling after some hours in a suitable site for spinning. It then spins a cocoon for the first and only time. It does so for half a day or more by executing an elaborate sequence of specialized movements that draw silk from its glands and form it into a three-dimensional double-layered, and therefore effectively insulated, cocoon within which the larva pupates and overwinters, and from which it ultimately emerges as an adult. Like the webs of spiders, the cocoons are records of the species-specificity of the behavior. The kind of larva that is about to spin predicts the details of the behavior it will display, and these details of behavior produce a cocoon whose size and shape are as diagnostic of the species of moth that produced it as is the animal itself. The emergence of the adult depends, in the species studied by Van der Kloot, on the mutual alignment of the loosely woven upper poles (called valves) of the inner and outer envelopes of the cocoon. The correct alignment of the valves is assured by a negative geotaxis that keeps the animal head up throughout the spinning episode. If the animal and the outer envelope it has just spun are turned 180 degrees just before it proceeds to the spinning of the inner envelope, the larva rights itself within the outer envelope, leaving the valve at what is now its lower pole. The animal then proceeds to spin its inner envelope with its valve normally upright, and thereby entombs itself within its own cocoon. Or, if the larva is removed from the outer envelope that it has just spun, it will continue to construct its cocoon but will enclose itself in only an inner envelope, within which it will very likely freeze to death during the ensuing winter. This, then, is instinctive behavior and it is in my view the dominant, even exclusive, form of complex behavior among animals of all phyla except ours. See Wigglesworth (1964) and Wells (1968) for reviews of the ubiquity and variety of instinctive behavior, and Evans (1973) for an affectionate description of the elaborate behaviors of one family of insects.

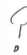

The Characteristics of Motivated Behavior

Motivated behavior, on the other hand, is, I believe, more complicated and more rare. In addition to being drive activated and to sharing with instinct the characteristics previously described (divisible into appetitive and consummatory phases, employing a variety of endogenous mechanisms including central programs and oscillators, contributing to homeostasis, serving a variety of functional ends), it has additional characteristics that are not those of instinctive behavior. It occurs in big-brained long-lived animals that typically live in social groups. It is exhibited repeatedly after an ontogeny during which its performance is improved. Like instinct it is subject to habituation and sensitization, but unlike instinct it is dominated by instrumental learning, particularly in its appetitive phase. Animals displaying it do so while anticipating its ends and it is therefore truly goal directed. And, finally, animals displaying it behave with affect. It therefore has characteristics that it does not share with instinctive behavior and that make it psychologically more complex.

Two of these characteristics are outcomes of learning. The first is *individuation of* the appetitive phase, that is, individual differences of approach, search, and selection are acquired in prior episodes of the behavior and are employed as operants thereafter (see Teitelbaum, 1966, for an earlier discussion), thus leading to diversification of the behavior among individuals of the same species and liberating them from the stereotype of species-specific performance. There is a genuine distinction here between neurological mechanisms for behavior that must employ a fixed efferent program (reflexes and instinct) and those which by associative learning acquire options for their expression; between those whose final common paths are predetermined and unchangeable, and those whose paths become specified by the animal's individual past history and remain changeable with changing circumstances of reinforcement. To understand my meaning, contrast the

feeding behavior of the blowfly (Dethier, 1978) with that of the rat.
The fly ordinarily eats by lowering its proboscis into liquids and by
sucking them into its foregut. It has very few options. It cannot lower
its head to the food droplet before it has extended its proboscis, and
it cannot bring the food to its mouth with its wings or other limbs. It
cannot, in fact, learn an operant (locomotion to a particular place has *set*
been tried) in order to obtain access to food. Once aroused, the neurological state of hunger in the fly's brain must be expressed through
the efferent program that begins with proboscis lowering and ends with *learned*
sucking. The rat, in contrast, can use its limbs to bring food to its
mouth, can negotiate mazes to obtain food, and can employ operants
by which it can be made to "go shopping" for food in a variety of im-
probable ways. Its feeding behavior, in its appetitive phase, is not
species-specific. Rather, it can be individuated. Add to the example
of feeding in the blowfly the egg retrieval of the greyleg goose (Lorenz
& Tinbergen, 1957). The "fixed action pattern" is precisely what I am
emphasizing here. The bird will not employ her other limbs to retrieve
the egg, will not leave the nest and push the egg home, cannot liberate
herself from the necessity to use her beak to roll the egg back to the
nest. It has no options other than downward scooping movements of
its bill. It can adjust with lateral movements to momentary changes in
the position of the egg, but it cannot use a qualitatively different efferent program. I am not referring here to simple variability of behavior
within a species-specific sequence; to the fact that the behavior will
adapt to changing stimulus circumstances (if a blowfly encounters
solid food, the lobes at the end of the proboscis are everted, exposing
teeth that scrape it in preparation for salivation that converts it into a
liquid[3]), or to the fact that from time to time an animal will fail to
complete the sequence of a fixed action pattern, or will back-and-fill
within it before finally coming to its end, or may even fail to initiate
it when presented with the appropriate releasing or adequate stimulus.
What I mean is that if the character of the behavior, in both its appetitive and consummatory phases, is the same across repetitions of it in *Instinct*
the same animals and must remain the same among animals of the same
kind regardless of environmental demands for altered appetitive behavior, then instinct is at work. But if qualitative differences in the efferent, *motivated*
program of appetitive behavior can be acquired by animals of the same
kind and are employed by them when they are engaged in behavior
that leads to the same terminal or consummatory stimuli, then the
behavior has become individuated and, as such, exhibits an essential
characteristic of motivated behavior. If motivation is inferred as underlying the expression of a particular instance of complex behavior,

[3]I am indebted to Vincent Dethier for this example, but he, I expect, does not
share my interpretation of it.

then it should, in my view, exhibit the capacity for individuation. Fortunately, one can test for this characteristic by arranging for the performance of the behavior in a setting that makes the use of the species-specific efferent program impossible. For instance, in the well-studied instance of mate selection by the silkmoth (see Kramer, 1978) in which the male flies to the source of a pheromone, encounters the female that is emitting it, and copulates with her, it would be important for its status as motivated behavior to know if the male could do something as apparently simple as walk to a pheromone-emitting female when his wings were immobilized.

A
Setting

The second learned characteristic of motivated behavior is *expectancy* or *anticipation of goals*. As the result of prior experience with goals, that is, with objects or situations that permit the performance of consummatory behavior that is appropriate to the animal's internal state, subsequent appetitive behavior is altered by the nature (value and location) of the previously encountered goal. When expectancy is operating, appetitive behavior changes in frequency, intensity, or form (as is the case for operant behaviors) in accord with the value of the goals to which it has already led the animal. Such changes in appetitive behavior are commonplace among mammals and birds. A very good example is Crespi's old experiments (1942) showing that the speed with which hungry rats run to the end of an alleyway is predictable from the amount of food that they have received there in prior trials. This can be seen in Figure 2-2, in which three groups of hungry rats were run in an alleyway for 256, 16, or only 1 morsel of food until the 20th trial, after which they were all given 16 morsels. Before the change, speed of running was a direct function of amount of reward, and afterward it changed abruptly and appropriately in the two groups that were switched (the 256 to 16 group, and the 1 to 16 group). Those animals for which the incentive for running was increased exhibited what Crespi called an "elation" effect; those which ran for less exhibited a "depression." He concluded that the appetitive behavior of his rats was not determined by the quantity of the incentive alone, but was also determined by prior experiences with them, and he was bold enough to suggest that "The elation and depression effects are an adequate experimental basis for defining a variable within the rat which may be termed on the basis of human analogy an 'expectation'."

Another example comes from the work of the Laceys (1980), which shows that a primary bradycardia, mediated by the vagus and independent of changes in respiration, accompanies the readiness of human subjects to respond to meaningful auditory or visual stimuli. As you can see in Figure 2-3, the cardiac deceleration (above) begins several seconds before the subject expects to make a response and deepens until the moment the response is made. This anticipatory bradycardia is highly reliable across subjects. It demonstrates that in manifesting

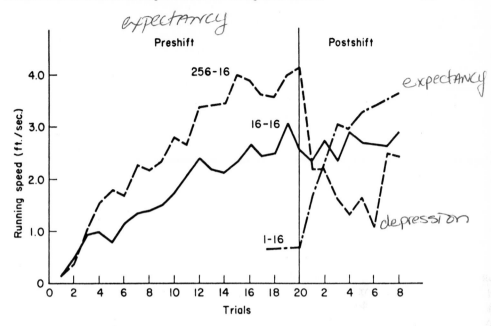

Figure 2-2. Speed of running by groups of rats in a runway as a function of amount of reinforcement. For the first 19 trials different groups were given 1, 16, or 256 pellets of food (acquisition data of the 1-pellet group are not shown). From trial 20 onward 16 pellets were given to all animals. (From Crespi, 1942, as adapted by Bolles, 1967.)

signs of expectancy the mammalian nervous system utilizes autonomic as well as somatic effector systems.

Endocrine changes have also been shown to occur prior to expected events. Rats that are trained to a feeding (or drinking) schedule secrete increased amounts of corticosterone just prior to the presentation of food (Krieger, 1974), and they do so even if the cup is empty and ingestion cannot occur (Levine & Coover, 1976). The increased adrenal secretion is accompanied by locomotion which is shifted by the expected ingestive behavior from the normal crepuscular peak to several hours before the scheduled feeding period. This was shown by Richter (1927) more than 50 years ago. And a last example comes from work that is closer to my own interests (Kriekhaus & Wolf, 1968). Rats that have had prior experience operating levers that deliver plain or salty water will, when made salt deficient for the first time, approach the "salty" bar from a distance in preference to the "water" bar, and will work at it more vigorously even when both bars deliver no fluid. That is, having learned where salt is and how to get it, the rat expects to find it there and will work for it when in need of salt for the first time. This incidentally provides an elegant example of the combination of inborn and learned elements in motivated behavior because the arousal of the

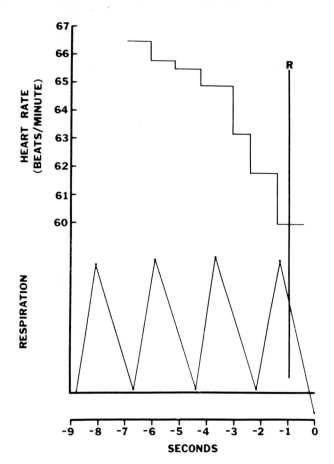

Figure 2-3. Computer-averaged curves for one typical subject showing cardiac deceleration in advance of self-initiated responses that resulted in a brief visual display. "R" shows the time of the subject's response. Respiratory curve shows the times of onset and duration of inspiration (upward deflection) and expiration (downward deflection). Note the lack of concomitant respiratory changes. (From Lacey & Lacey, 1980.)

appetite for salt, the prior condition for the heightened expectancy, is innate (Epstein & Stellar, 1955; Nachman, 1962).

These changes in appetitive behaviors depend on previous encounters with consummatory stimuli. The nature of those stimuli must therefore be remembered, and their memory must somehow be represented in the neurological mechanisms of the appetitive behavior itself. This representation, which in a neurological sense is the expectation, must then participate in the expression of the appetitive behavior and must do so before the animal reaches the stimuli that will terminate the behavioral sequence, that is, before it reaches its goal. Evidence for such anticipatory neurological events is as old as Walter's "contingent negative variation" or CNV (Walter, Cooper, Aldridge, McCallum, & Winter, 1964) and is as recent as Grastyan, John, and Bartlett's studies (1978) of the cerebral processing of conditioned stimuli during operant learning. The contingent negative variation is recorded from frontal scalp electrodes in humans observing successive visual or auditory stimuli. If the repetition of the pair of stimuli is monotonous, the EEG response to the second fades into background, but if it is made consequential (if, for instance, the subject is instructed to press a button exactly 10 sec after the appearance of the first signal in order to produce an interesting picture), a slow rise in the negative potential of the cortex begins just after the first signal and continues until the action is taken, when it terminates abruptly. The phenomenon appears after several repeated pairings of the stimuli and varies thereafter with the subject's mood and attitude. Grey Walter referred to it both as the CNV and as the E (or expectancy) wave because "it reflects the extent to which the subject expects the association between signals to be significant and intends to respond to them." In the more recent work (Grastyan et al., 1978) the evoked potentials from the geniculates of cats show changes in averaged wave form during operant training in a runway performance for food reward. These changes develop with training, are related to the significance of the stimuli (whether or not running will be rewarded), and occur just *before* the animal commits itself to the operant response.

Classical conditioning produces such changes readily and its major biological advantage may, in fact, be preparation for future consequential events. As training with the conditioned stimulus proceeds, the performance of the conditioned response comes to precede the onset of the unconditioned stimulus, the response is made in anticipation of reinforcement and may be employed to avoid it if it is noxious. The neurological events that underlie these anticipatory behaviors are being studied in the dentate gyrus of the rabbit hippocampus by Thompson and his colleagues (Thompson, Berger, & Berry, 1980). They precede the performance of the conditioned response (withdrawal of the nictitating membrane in anticipation of air-puff to the cornea) and the conditioned behavior follows them faithfully. According to Thompson:

> . . . under conditions . . . where behavioral learning will occur, unit activity in the hippocampus increases rapidly, initially in the UCS period, forms a temporal "model" of the behavioral response, and precedes it in time. . . . The growth of the hippocompal unit response is completely predictive of subsequent behavioral learning.

And he suggests that changes of this kind may be part of the neurological code for the goal-directedness of behavior.

Expectancy is, in my view, the characteristic that gives motivated behavior its quality of goal-directedness. And, as a phenomenon, it provides a test for the presence or absence of goal direction, a quality that should not be taken for granted or simply inferred for all complex behaviors. If the behavior is truly goal directed, repeated exposure of the animal to consummatory stimuli should result in progressive changes in its appetitive behavior. Recent studies of the eating behavior of *Aplysia*, a marine mollusk, are instructive in this regard (Susswein, Weiss, & Kupfermann, 1978). The animal eats seaweed and when deprived begins eating it promptly if it is stimulated by its taste or odor. Eating continues until it is suppressed by mechanical distension of the gut. Although short-term arousal, lasting about 30 minutes, of both biting and more generally of noneating behaviors such as siphon withdrawal is produced in food-deprived animals by contact with the food, repeated daily exposure to the food for five successive days did not accelerate the latency of the first biting response of the day. There is therefore no sign of expectancy in this behavior. In all of these respects, including *Aplysia*'s failure to acquire operants in order to obtain food that is not stimulating its chemoreceptors, its eating behavior is very much like that of the blowfly, and in both animals (perhaps in insects and mollusks generally) eating behavior appears to be governed by the simpler mechanisms of instinct.

The third distinctive characteristic of motivated behavior is *affect*. Motivated behavior is, I believe, often laden with affect, and affective expression should be expected of the internal state that is generating the behavior. Affect is expressed by very young animals and is often full fledged when first exhibited, as shown by Steiner's (1974) studies of the facial expressions of human infants. And it is typically species specific. For example, different sets of facial displays and body postures are stable characteristics of different species of vertebrates, including the primates (Chevalier-Skolnikoff, 1973).

Please appreciate that I am not lapsing here into 19th-century mentalism. Affect is an expression of an internal state that includes mood and feeling, but these can only be guessed at in all animals and even in man they can either be experienced privately or can be described secondhand. What I mean by affect is discernible patterns of somatic and autonomic–glandular (both exocrine and endocrine) responding that are expressed as integral aspects of appetitive–consummatory sequences of behavior. These patterns of affective responding regularly accompany the arousal of particular internal states and are recognizable expressions or signs of those states across animals of the same kind. Taken together, Ekman's demonstration (1973) of the effectiveness of human facial expressions as signs of emotion and of their universality of recognition in our cultural peers as well as among preliterate savages, and Averill's early experiment (1969) demonstrating differences in autonomic, respiratory, and thermal responding in humans watching mirth- or sadness-provoking films, illustrate what I mean.

I believe that whenever motivation is inferred as underlying a complex behavior, the exhibition of such patterns of responding should be expected. But to meet the criteria I am suggesting these cannot be only facial expressions, displays of limb or body movement, or changes in locomotion. They should be patterns of somatic, visceral, and glandular action; and within a particular kind of animal they ought to be richly complex and sufficiently diversified to express a variety of internal states. The somatic displays and sound emissions that are so common in communication among animals (the claw waving of Pacific crabs and the stridulation of crickets, e.g.) can be fractions of what I am describing as affect, as can the secretion of pheromones; but if they are not part of a distinctive pattern of responding that includes visceral and glandular effects, they should be thought of, it seems to me, as the nonaffective displays of instinctive acts.

Recent work of O. A. Smith and his colleagues (1981) is congenial to these ideas. They find that a distinctive pattern of cardiovascular responding, as measured by blood pressure, heart rate, and aortic and renal arterial flow, accompanies each of several behaviors in the baboon. These include alertness, sleep, leg exercise, and bar pressing for food and its conditioned emotional suppression. In the latter, a tone that had previously been paired with foot-shock evokes a distinctive pattern of cardiovascular responding and suppresses the baboon's bar pressing when it is sounded alone. It appears from this work that behaviors can indeed be characterized by distinctive overall patterns of responding even when only somatic and cardiovascular effects are considered.

Again, the criteria that I am suggesting for the diagnosis of motivation are subject to empirical test. Cricket stridulation or song is an instance of what I mean (Bentley & Hoy, 1974). The animals rub their wings together to produce it, drawing a scraper on the edge of one wing over a filelike specialization on the surface of the other. Cricket song is species-specific, sex-linked, and phenotypic behavior. Each species (there are more than 2,000) has its own songs, only the males sing them, and nothing more than a genetic program and normal development is necessary for their emission when the animal reaches adulthood. Most species have a small repertoire of songs: a calling song that the male sings when he has established a territory and which attracts sexually receptive females; a courtship song that precedes copulation; and a rivalry or aggressive song that is used when another male invades the territory. Vigorous fights result from these encounters and are even a spectator sport in some parts of the Far East, and the rivalry song is nearly always sung by the winner. How interesting it would be, from my point of view, to know, first, whether the patterns of visceral and glandular events inside a cricket are something more than those which would be expected from the mere physiological effort of stridulation;

and, second, whether the patterns are different when the cricket is simply calling from its territory, or is singing its "love song," or is facing off with another male in a territorial dispute and then singing its "victory song." The three kinds of song could, by analogy to birdsong, be accompanied by affect. If discernible and recognizable patterns of visceral–glandular responding were found to be integral aspects of their emission, then I would agree that crickets sing with "feeling." If not, then I would be confirmed in my belief that cricket song is another example of a biologically beautiful but cooly mechanical instinctive behavior.

I know of no better descriptions of the affective displays than those used by Darwin and Hess. In his book on the expression of the emotions (reprinted, 1965) Darwin's talented illustrator depicts cats and dogs in states of emotional expression and gives a clear indication of their variety and vividness, as the examples in Figure 2-4 show. Hess's cats displaying affect as the result of intracranial stimulation (Figure 2-5) illustrate their range from repose (above) to alert aggressiveness (his "affective defense reaction") and, in the latter (below), emphasize the autonomic effects (piloerection, pupillary dilatation, and on occasion, hypersalivation) that are integral parts of their expression (Hess, 1956). With evidence of this kind Hess was among the first to demonstrate how much of the mammalian brain is devoted to organizing such expressions.

To understand why I consider them so important for this discussion, contrast these graphic portraits with the behavior of a cockroach. If I allowed you to examine first a running dog and then a running roach but concealed from you in each case the conditions that triggered the locomotion and the behavior with which it terminated, I believe you would have no trouble discovering whether the dog was escaping a threat or approaching a safe shelter. But could you do the same for the roach? Could you tell from what it did while it ran whether it was threatened or eager? If I allowed you to observe the entire behavioral episode and you knew what had initiated the running and what the animal did at the end of the sequence, you might be tempted, as Darwin was and as some still are, to infer a mood or emotion underlying the roach's running behavior. But I believe that this would be pointless anthropomorphism unless when approaching shelter or escaping threat there were discernible differences in the visceral and glandular activity of the roach as well as in its overt behavior, as there are in the autonomic state and the overt behavior of the dog.[4] I believe,

[4] Insects (cockroaches, mostly) that have been shocked or been forced into hyperactivity exhaust the supply of neurosecretory material that is ordinarily found in the corpus cardiacum of their neuroendocrine system (Hodgson & Geldiay, 1959). But unlike the secretions of the vertebrate adrenal gland, the cardiacum material depresses both central nervous activity and locomotion (Özbas & Hodgson, 1958).

in other words, that motivated behavior is hedonic (see Stellar, Chapter 13, and Solomon, Chapter 11, for other discussions of this issue). It arises from mood, is performed with feeling, and results in pleasure

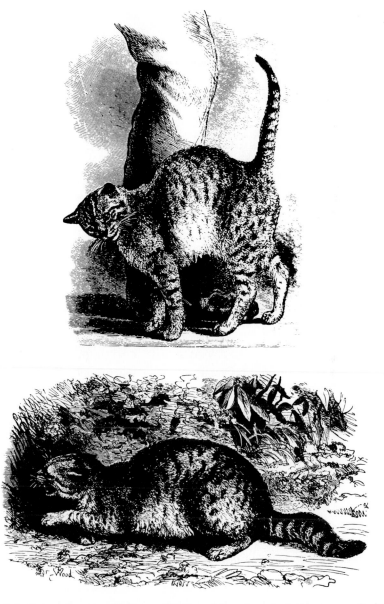

Figure 2-4. Darwin's cat soliciting affection (above) and stalking prey (below). Note the declaration in the animal's posture, facial expression (eyelids, mouth, vibrissae, and ears), and pelt (notice the difference in the hair of the tail) of the animal's affective state. (From Darwin, 1965.)

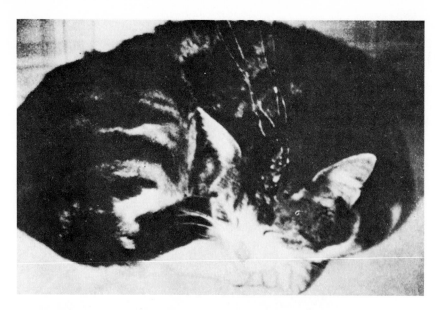

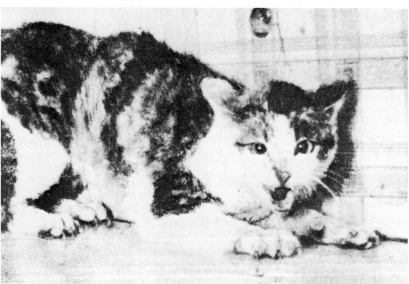

Figure 2-5. Hess's cats exhibiting affective states elicited by electrical stimulation of the brain. The animal sleeps (above) or is thrown into defensive rage (below), depending on which site is activated within the brain. (From Hess, 1956.)

or the escape from pain, and although the moods, feelings, and satisfactions themselves are private and beyond our reach as scientists, their overt expression in patterns of somatic, autonomic, and glandular responding is an important diagnostic characteristic of motivation.

A Summary of the Comparison: Its Virtues and Faults

It seems worthwhile at this point to summarize. I am advocating a distinction between instinct and motivation based on their observable characteristics, a kind of differential diagnosis of complex behaviors based on their distinctive signs. Table 2-1 summarizes the details. The characteristics or signs that instinct and motivation have in common are listed at the top, and their differences are given below. This scheme has several virtues that should make the concepts more useful. First, they should no longer be confused. The differential diagnosis that I am proposing offers a systematic and empirical way of distinguishing instinct from motivation. The question of the nature of complex behavior that has been so vexing in our literature can now be put to empirical test. If in manifesting a behavior the animal can employ operants, and if in the course of the behavior it displays signs of affect and expectancy, then the behavior cannot be instinctive. Imprinting in precocial birds and feeding in the blowfly provide very good examples of what I mean. Both have all the characteristics of instinctive behavior. But imprinting (Hoffman, 1969; Hoffman, Stratton, Newby, & Barrett, 1970) also has all three of the characteristics of motivation (the duckling will employ operants to reach the imprinted object; it does so affectively; and once having encountered the object, its subsequent appetitive behavior toward it is changed) and it is therefore a very nice instance of motivated behavior. Feeding in the fly, on the other

Table 2.1. A Comparison of Instinct and Motivation Based on Their Behavioral Characteristics

Common Characteristics
1. Both employ innate mechanisms for reaction (adequate and releasing stimuli) and action (final common paths, oscillators, and central programs).
2. Both employ acquired components.
3. Both are organized sequentially into appetitive followed by consummatory phases.
4. Both are drive induced.
5. Both contribute to homeostasis.

Differences	
Instinct	*Motivation*
Species-specific in releasing stimuli and efferent programs	Appetitive behavior can be individuated.
Appetitive behavior unmodified by expectancy	Anticipatory of goals
Nonaffective	Accompanied by expression of affect
Biologically common	Biologically uncommon

hand, has none of the characteristics of motivation (as I have already mentioned, a fly cannot individuate its appetitive behavior, and I am assuming that, when they are looked for, visceral and endocrine signs of affect will not be found in the fly) and it is therefore an instance of genuine instinct. Second, greater care can now be exercised in choosing instances of the two kinds of behavior for comparison and contrast, and if the examples chosen come from the different classes of behavior, then differences in their underlying mechanisms should be expected. Third, by calling attention to the greater complexity of motivated behavior, the distinction suggests additional options for its experimental analysis. We should now be alert to the neurological mechanisms that provide motivation with its instrumental, its goal-directed, and its affective aspects.

There are two caveats that must be given. First, the distinction I have drawn should *not* be read to mean that I believe that animals display *either* instinctive behavior *or* motivated behavior. There are two classes of animals, but not these two. There are, in my view, animals that display only instinct (most of those in the invertebrate phyla) and there are those, a smaller number but more complex and big brained, that display both. Birds provide some of the classic examples of instinctive behavior (the postural displays of shorebirds, egg rolling in the oystercatcher), but my concept does not deny them the capacity for motivation. On the contrary, I believe that the two kinds of behavior can coexist, and are, it seems, often admixed, in the same animal. Birds and mammals display what appear to be instincts, and these are most prominent early in their behavioral careers. For example, the food-begging and pecking behavior of newly hatched birds (Tinbergen & Kuenen, 1957; Hailman, 1967) and the nipple-attachment and sucking behavior of newborn rats (Blass, Hall, & Teicher, 1979; Lorenz, Ellis, & Epstein, 1982) seem to be quite instinctive at the outset. In neither case does the animal have an alternate efferent program for gaining food from the parent. In both cases an appropriate behavior appears phenotypically at hatching/birth and is molded to perfection by experience. The behavior is then stereotyped across individuals. As the animal matures the additional complexities of motivation are added, and when ontogeny is complete and it is fledged/weaned the instinct is replaced by motivated feeding behavior. This yielding in ontogeny of behaviors with instinctive characteristics to those that are fully motivational may be prototypical of birds and mammals. I believe that instincts may be rare in or entirely absent from the behavioral repertoires of adult homeotherms. The capacities of their nervous systems for instrumental learning, for affective expression, and for the acquisition of expectancies may make the distinction between instinct and motivation moot for animals of that kind, because in them motivation may be the principal form of complex behavior.

The question whether birds and mammals exhibit instincts will not be settled by what I say in this essay, but at least my proposal of a differential diagnosis of instinct and motivation makes it possible to put the question, whenever it arises, to empirical test. But this requires that the old and simple concept of instinct as unlearned behavior be abandoned, and that the characteristics of the two kinds of behavior that I have described here be accepted as experimentally useful.

By way of a second caveat, I have probably drawn the distinction too sharply. I believe that my dichotomy of instinct and motivation is useful for distinguishing between the behaviors of large classes of animals: between the behaviors of the vertebrates, on the one hand, which, having the most highly evolved nervous systems, seem to have specialized in motivation; and the behaviors of the mollusks and arthropods, on the other hand, which appear to have specialized in instinct. But remembering my own preaching about the prodigious diversity of animals and their behaviors, I may be oversimplifying in two different ways. First, there might be a need for more categories of complex behavior, more than just instinct and motivation. We should perhaps have one for organisms that behave but do so without nervous systems and are without associative learning (the protozoa, the sponges, and the behaving bacteria and plants), another for animals like the coelenterates, ctenophores, and echinoderms, whose nervous systems are built on an entirely different plan than those in animals that are bilaterally symmetrical and whose ancient geological histories have never, as far as we know, included life on land. And we may need still another category, at the other end of the evolutionary scale, for the precious few among all the animals that have language and technology.

I may also be drawing the distinction too sharply by not acknowledging nature's way of confounding, with her inventiveness, all armchair catalogs of behavior. Affect is certainly not an exclusive property of motivated behavior. The adequate stimuli for a variety of reflexes are in many instances inherently and innately affective. Pfaffmann and his colleagues (1977) have emphasized this aspect of the chemical senses, whose stimuli often have striking affective consequences resulting in acceptance or rejection. And, as I have mentioned above, the affects that many stimuli evoke are important for their effectiveness as unconditioned stimuli and reinforcers, and this is true for both acceptable and noxious stimuli. In animals like ourselves strong stimuli of many kinds evoke dual and opposing affects, as pointed out by Solomon (Solomon & Corbit, 1974), who has made these opponent affective processes the basis for an attractive theory of motivation. Expectancy is also not confined to instances of motivation. Behavior is anticipatory in ways that do not depend on learned changes in appetitive behavior, and these occur widely in the animal kingdom. Circadian locomotion is an example. It often results in the onset of activity (running, flying, crawling, or whatever means the animal uses) just before a photoperiodic change, and what an asset that must be to an animal (like the rat or cockroach) that lives in a burrow system where light–dark–light transitions are obscure or cannot be seen at all. Nicolaïdis has described several instances of anticipatory reflexes (1967). In the most extensively studied, secretion of ADH and an anti-diuresis occur in cats when they taste hypertonic solutions and well before there has been any change in the osmolarity of the blood. The directed out-flight of worker bees that have decoded the dance of their recently returned co-workers announcing the direction and distance from the hive of a food source appears to be another example.

And behavioral traps occur in big-brained animals. The oystercatcher attempting to retrieve a giant "egg" is an example. Whenever they are seen, a display of instinct should be suspected. Others occur as the result of bad habits or pathology. Young and Chaplin, for example, showed that rats that had been eating sucrose in preference to casein continued to do so, despite progressive protein starvation, when they were made protein deficient (1945).[5] And we know from the recent work of Teitelbaum and his colleagues (1981) that the behavior of brain-damaged or drugged rats is dominated by what they aptly call "independent motor subsystems" (for support, forward locomotion, head scanning, etc.) that can be aroused reflexively but which cannot be unified in the service of goal direction. They lead the animal into behavioral traps that are strikingly similar to those described above. In one, a rat that is not yet recovered from lateral hypothalamic lesions walks forward into a corner and cannot escape from it because the animal cannot add head scanning, which is necessary for turning, to forward locomotion.

I believe that these are not the same as the examples given earlier for invertebrates. They are, rather, motivated behaviors that are instinct-like because they have been subverted by conflicting habits (it should be remembered that when Young and Chaplin's animals were allowed to make their choice in a new environment in which their habitual choice could not control the behavior, they made the right choice and in-creased their intake of protein) or they are instinct-like because their neurological mechanisms have been degraded by damage or drugs. They seem to me to be either pathological atavisms in which the more com-plex mechanisms of motivated behavior are reduced to their instinct-like components, or idiosyncrasies of prior individual experience. They are not the native characteristics of all animals of the same kind.

[5] A similar example involving interference by sucrose preference with the choice of sodium chloride in adrenalectomized rats (Harriman, 1955) has not been con-firmed (Cullen & Scarborough, 1969).

Clearly, the characteristics of motivation are not exclusive to it. They can occur individually in simpler behaviors. I believe that it is the clustering of all three together, the constellation of instrumental behaviors, affect, and expectancy as aspects of the same behavior, that gives motivated behavior its special character. If that cluster occurred in the behavior of some phylogenetic neighbor, as well it might, I for one would have to admit that that kind of behavior was motivated.

Choosing Animals for the Study of Motivation

Now a last word about research strategy. Having emphasized the distinctions between the two forms of complex behavior, I think they should be respected when we choose species for the study of motivated behavior. Animals that cannot individuate their appetitive behavior, that show no evidence in it of expectancy, and that do not express affect are, in my view, not performing motivated behavior and are poor choices for its study. This excludes most animals, which may be unfortunate but should not be surprising. We should expect to find more complex neural and behavioral function in more complex animals. But it leaves us with a rich supply of mammals, birds, reptiles, and very likely with all of the remaining vertebrates except the simplest fishes. It does exclude most of the invertebrates either because they do not have brains or do not have the neural equipment for instrumental learning and affect. It also excludes the arthropods, some of whom may be brainy enough but who seem to have sacrificed the advantages of affective expression for those of a rigid exoskeleton.

The mollusks are a likely group, particularly because they include the brainiest of the invertebrates and have the advantage for affective expression of fleshy mobile bodies. But even here there are suggestions that they are limited to instinct and have not evolved the additional mechanisms necessary for motivation. First, like all other invertebrates they do not have an autonomic nervous system with which so much of affective expression is achieved. They do employ the same or very similar biogenic amines in their nervous system (Weiss et al., 1978) and their viscera are innervated by a separate neural apparatus, but this is hardly an autonomic nervous system, which is an anatomically widespread and highly reactive system that provides duplex and functionally antagonistic innervation to the viscera, smooth muscles, and glands, and is complemented by an adrenal gland that is under both neural control (mediated by the splanchnic preganglionics) and central hormonal control (mediated by the anterior pituitary). Second, although eating behavior (orientation to food odors, food grasping, biting, and swallowing) is being studied in the sea hare (Kupfermann, 1974) and its relatives (Reingold & Gelperin, 1980), I have already mentioned the facts that no one has yet succeeded in showing that these animals can learn an operant to obtain food, and there is no sign of expectancy in their appetitive behaviors. Recent work on their visceral responsiveness is only a little more encouraging (Dieringer, Koester, & Weiss, 1978). The behavioral arousal that is produced by eating is accompanied in aplysia by a tachycardia, especially in the starved animal, but it is not abolished by denervation of the heart, and the same is true when noxious stimuli elicit the arousal. Both eating and noxious stimuli therefore produce a tachycardia without neural mediation, apparently as the result of the metabolic cost of the behavioral activation. Food stimuli also result in a tachycardia even when eating is prevented (a basket of seaweed is hung in the aquarium), and this cardiac effect is reduced to one third by cardiac denervation without a reduction in biting behavior, demonstrating that neural activation of the viscera can occur in this animal independent of the metabolic consequences of vigorous behavior, and suggesting that it may have evolved at least a partial analog of affective reactivity. But even less can be said of the octopus, the biggest-brained of all the invertebrates, which may be little more than the most complex instrument for cool, instinctive behavior. Wells (1977) reported that no changes in heart rate or heartbeat amplitude could be detected in the male octopus during sexual arousal or even in the midst of copulation!

Because changing states within the brain are characteristics of both instinct and motivation, the investigation of the neurological bases of drive can be pursued in a great variety of animals with some hope of finding generalizations that will be useful across phyla. My own work on the induction of thirst by angiotensin is an example (Epstein, 1978, 1980). But the commonality of interest in drive and the other characteristics shared by instinct and motivation must not obscure the important differences that distinguish them. It is my belief that full understanding of the brain mechanisms of motivated behavior will not come from the study of animals that exhibit only instinctive behavior. It will come from the study of animals whose behavior is characterized by drive, by appetitive behavior marked by individuation and expectancy, and by expressions of affect.

Acknowledgments. The author's research and the writing of this essay were supported by Grant 03469 from the NINCDS.

My colleagues have been generous in their criticism of this review. Vincent Dethier, Charles Gallistel, Irving Kupfermann, Paul Rozin, Eliot Stellar, and Richard Solomon have been especially helpful in rescuing me from errors. Those that remain are entirely my own.

References

Adler, N. *Neuroendocrinology of reproduction: Physiology and behavior.* New York: Plenum Press, 1981.

Averill, J. R. Autonomic response patterns during sadness and mirth. *Psychophysiology*, 1969, *5*, 399-414.

Bentley, D., & Hoy, R. R. The neurobiology of cricket song. *Scientific American*, August 1974, pp. 84-96.

Blass, E. M., Hall, W. G., & Teicher, M. H. The ontogeny of suckling and ingestive behaviors. In J. M. Sprague & A. N. Epstein (Eds.), *Progress in psychobiology and physiological psychology* (Vol. 8). New York: Academic Press, 1979.

Carper, J. W., & Polliard, F. A comparison of the intake of glucose and saccharin solutions under conditions of caloric need. *American Journal of Psychology*, 1953, *66*, 479-482.

Chevalier-Skolnikoff, S. Facial expression of emotion in nonhuman primates. In P. Ekman (Ed.), *Darwin and facial expression.* New York: Academic Press, 1973, pp. 11-83.

Craig, W. Appetites and aversions as constituents of instincts. *Biological Bulletin*, 1918, *34*, 91-107.

Crespi, L. P. Quantitative variation of incentive and performance in the white rat. *American Journal of Psychology*, 1942, *55*, 467-517.

Cullen, J. W., & Scarborough, B. B. Effect of a preoperative sugar preference on bar pressing for salt by adrenectomized rat. *Journal of Comparative and Physiological Psychology*, 1969, *67*, 415-420.

Darwin, C. The expression of the emotions in man and animals. Chicago: University of Chicago Press, 1965. (First publication in 1872.)

Dethier, V. G. *The hungry fly.* Cambridge, Mass.: Harvard University Press, 1978.

Dethier, V. G., & Bodenstein, D. Hunger in the blowfly. *Zeitschrift für Tierpsychcologie*, 1958, *15*, 129-140.

Dieringer, N., Koester, J., & Weiss, K. R. Adaptive changes in heart rate of *Aplysia californica. Journal of Comparative Physiology*, 1978, *123*, 11-21.

Ekman, P. Cross-cultural studies of facial expression. In P. Ekman (Ed.), *Darwin and facial expressions.* New York: Academic Press, 1973, pp. 169-220.

Epstein, A. N. The neuroendocrinology of thirst and salt appetite. In W. F. Ganong & L. Martini (Eds.), *Frontiers in neuroendocrinology* (Vol. 5). New York: Raven Press, 1978, pp. 101-134.

Epstein, A. N. Angiotensin-induced water and salt intake. *Frontiers in Hormone Research*, 1980, *6*, 104-119.

Epstein, A. N., & Stellar, E. The control of salt preference in the adrenalectomized rat. *Journal of Comparative and Physiological Psychology*, 1955, *48*, 167-172.

Evans, H. E. *Wasp farm.* New York: Anchor Press, 1973.

Fentress, J. C. The development of grooming in mice with amputated forelimbs. *Science*, 1973, *179*, 704-705.

Fraenkel, G. S., & Gunn, D. L. *The orientation of animals.* New York: Dover Press, 1961.

Gelperin, A., & Dethier, V. G. Long-term regulation of sugar intake by the blowfly. *Physiological Zoology*, 1967, *40*, 218-228.

Grastyan, E., John, E. R., & Bartlett, F. Evoked response correlate of symbol and significate. *Science*, 1978, *20*, 168-171.

Hailman, J. P. The ontogeny of an instinct. *Behaviour*, Suppl. 15, 1967.

Harriman, A. E. The effect of a preoperative preference for sugar over salt upon compensatory salt selection by adrenalectomized rats. *Journal of Nutrition*, 1955, *57*, 271-276.

Hess, W. R. *Hypothalamus und thalamus.* Stuttgart: G. Thieme, 1956.

Hodgson, E. S., & Geldiay, S. Experimentally induced release of neurosecretory materials from roach corpora cardiaca. *Biological Bulletin*, 1959, *117*, 275-283.

Hoffman, H. S., Searle, J. L., Toffey, S., & Kozman, F. Behavioral control by an imprinted stimulus. *Journal of Experimental Analysis of Behavior*, 1966, *9*, 177-189.

Hoffman, H. S., Stratton, J. W., Newby, V., & Barrett, J. E. Development of behavioral control by an imprinting stimulus. *Journal of Comparative and Physiological Psychology*, 1970, *71*, 229-236.

Hotta, Y., & Benzer, S. Mapping of behavior in drosophila mosaics. *Nature*, 1972, *240*, 527-535.

Jennings, H. A. *Behavior of the lower organisms.* Bloomington: Indiana University Press, 1962. (First published in 1905.)

Jouvet, M. Neurophysiology of the states of sleep. *Physiological Reviews*, 1967, *47*, 117-177.

Kandel, E. *Behavioral biology of Aplysia: A contribution to the comparative study of opisthobranch molluscs.* San Francisco: W. H. Freeman, 1979.

Kramer, E. Insect pheromones. In G. L. Hazelbauer (Ed.), *Taxis and behavior, elementary sensory systems in biology.* London: Chapman and Hall, 1978, pp. 205-229.

Krieger, D. T. Food and water restriction shifts corticosterone, temperature, activity, and brain amine periodicity. *Endocrinology*, 1974, *95*, 1195-1201.

Kriekhaus, E. E., & Wolf, G. Acquisition of sodium by rats: Interaction of innate mechanisms and latent learning. *Journal of Comparative and Physiological Psychology*, 1968, *65*, 197-201.

Kupfermann, I. Feeding behavior in aplysia: A simple system for the study of motivation. *Behavioral Biology*, 1974, *10*, 1-26.

Lacey, J. I., & Lacey, B. C. The specific role of heart rate in sensorimotor integration. In R. F. Thompson, L. H. Hicks, & V. B. Shvyrkov (Eds.), *Neural mechanisms of goal-directed behavior and learning.* New York: Academic Press, 1980.

Lashley, K. S. Experimental analysis of instinctive behavior. *Psychological Review*, 1938, *45*, 445-471.

Lehrman, D. S. The physiological bases of parental behavior in the ringdove (*Streptopelia risoria*). *Behaviour*, 1955, *7*, 241-286.

Levine, S., & Coover, G. D. Environmental control of suppression of pituitary-adrenal system. *Physiology and Behavior*, 1976, *17*, 35-37.

Loher, W., & Huber, F. Nervous and endocrine control of sexual behavior in a grasshopper. *Symposium Society of Experimental Biology*, 1966, *20*, 381-400.

Lorenz, D., Ellis, S., & Epstein, A. N. Differential effects of upper gastrointestinal fill on milk ingestion and nipple attachment in the suckling rat. *Journal of Developmental Psychobiology*, 1982, in press.

Lorenz, K., & Tinbergen, N. Taxis and instinctive action in the egg-retrieving behavior of the greyleg goose. In C. H. Schiller (Ed.), *Instinctive behavior.* New York: International Universities Press, 1957, pp. 176-207.

McHugh, P. R., & Moran, T. H. Calories and gastric emptying: A regulatory capacity with implications for feeding. *American Journal of Physiology*, 1979, *236*, R254–R260.

Moore, R. Y. Central neural control of circadian rhythms. In W. F. Ganong & L. Martini (Eds.), *Frontiers in neuroendocrinology* (Vol. 5). New York: Raven Press, 1978, pp. 185–206.

Nachman, M. Taste preferences for sodium salts by adrenalectomized rats. *Journal of Comparative and Physiological Psychology*, 1962, *56*, 343–349.

Nicolaïdis, S. Early systemic responses to oro-gastric stimulation in the regulation of food and water balance. *Annals of the New York Academy of Sciences*, 1967, *157*, 1176–1203.

Özbas, S., & Hodgson, E. S. Action of insect neurosecretion upon central nervous system in vitro and upon behavior. *Proceedings of the National Academy of Sciences*, 1958, *44*, 825–830.

Pavlov, I. P. *Conditioned reflexes.* London: Oxford University Press, 1927.

Pfaff, D. *Estrogens and brain function.* New York: Springer-Verlag, 1980.

Pfaffmann, C., Norgren, R., & Grill, H. J. Sensory affect and motivation. *Annals of the New York Academy of Sciences*, 1977, *290*, Suppl. 18, 18–33.

Reingold, S. C., & Gelperin, A. Feeding motor programme in *Limax*. *Journal of Experimental Biology*, 1980, *85*, 1–20.

Richter, C. P. Animal behavior and internal drives. *Quarterly Review of Biology*, 1927, *2*, 307–342.

Richter, C. P. Total self-regulatory functions in animals and human beings. *Harvey Lectures*, 1942–1943, *37*, 63–103.

Rosenblatt, J. S., & Lehrman, D. F. Maternal behavior of the laboratory rat. In H. I. Reingold (Ed.), *Maternal behavior in mammals.* New York: Wiley, 1963, pp. 8–57.

Schaller, G. B. *The year of the gorilla.* Chicago: University of Chicago Press, 1964.

Sherrington, C. *The integrative action of the nervous system.* New Haven: Yale University Press, 1947.

Smith, O. A., DeVito, J. L., & Astley, C. The hypothalamus in emotional behavior and associated cardiovascular correlates. In A. R. Morrison & P. L. Strick (Eds.), *Changing concepts of the nervous system.* New York: Academic Press, 1981, in press.

Solomon, R. L., & Corbit, J. D. An opponent-process theory of motivation, I: Temporal dynamics of affect. *Psychological Review*, 1974, *81*, 119–145.

Stellar, E. Brain mechanisms in hunger and other hedonic experiences. *Proceedings of American Philosophy Society*, 1974, *118*(3), 276–282.

Susswein, A. J., Weiss, K. R., & Kupfermann, I. The effects of food arousal on the latency of biting in Aplysia. *Journal of Comparative Physiology*, 1978, *123*, 31–41.

Susswein, A. J., & Kupfermann, I. Localization of bulk stimuli underlying satiation in aplysia. *Journal of Comparative Physiology*, 1975, *101*, 309–328.

Teitelbaum, P. The use of operant methods in the assessment and control of motivational states. In W. K. Honig (Ed.), *Operant behavior: Areas of research and application.* New York: Appleton-Century-Crofts, 1966, pp. 565–608.

Teitelbaum, P. Disconnection and antagonistic interaction of movement subsystems in motivated behavior. In A. R. Morrison and P. L. Strick (Eds.), *Changing concepts of the nervous system.* New York: Academic Press, 1981, in press.

Teitelbaum, P., & Epstein, A. N. The lateral hypothalamic syndrome. *Psychological Review*, 1962, *69*, 74–90.

Thompson, R. F., Berger, T. W., & Berry, S. D. Brain mechanisms of learning. In R. F. Thompson, L. H. Hicks, & V. B. Shvyrkov (Eds.), *Neural mechanisms of goal-directed behavior and learning.* New York: Academic Press, 1980.

Tinbergen, N. *The study of instinct* (2nd ed.). New York: Oxford University Press, 1974.

Truman, J. W. Hormonal release of stereotyped motor programmes from the isolated nervous system of the cecropia silkmoth. *Journal of Experimental Biology,* 1978, *74,* 151-173.

Truman, J. W., & Riddiford, L. M. Hormonal mechanisms underlying insect behavior. *Advances in Insect Physiology,* 1974, *10,* 297-353.

Van der Kloot, W. G., & Williams, C. M. Cocoon construction in the cecropia silkworm. *Behavior,* 1953, *5,* 141-163.

Walter, G. W., Cooper, R., Aldridge, V. J., McCallum, W. C., & Winter, A. L. Contingent negative variation: An electric sign of sensorimotor association and expectancy in the human brain. *Nature,* 1964, *203,* 380-838.

Weiss, K. R., Cohen, J. L., & Kupfermann, I. Modulatory control of buccal musculature by a serotonergic neuron in *Aplysia. Journal of Neurophysiology,* 1978, *41,* 181-203.

Wells, M. J. Early learning by *Sepia. Symposium of the Zoological Society, London,* 1962, *8,* 149-169.

Wells, M. J. *Lower animals.* New York: World University Library, 1968.

Wells, M. J. *Octopus: Physiology and behaviour of an advanced invertebrate.* London: Chapman and Hall, 1977.

Whiting, P. W. Reproductive behavior of sex mosaics of a parasitic wasp, Habrobracon juglandis. *Journal of Comparative Psychology,* 1932, *14,* 345-363.

Wigglesworth, V. B. *The life of insects.* London: Weidenfeld and Nicholson, 1964.

Young, P. T., & Chaplin, J. P. Studies of food preferences, appetite and dietary habit, III: Palatability and appetite in relation to bodily need. *Comparative Psychology Monographs,* 1945, *18,* 1-45.

Part Two

Hunger and Thirst

Chapter 3

Taste: A Model of Incentive Motivation

CARL PFAFFMANN

This chapter is a subunit under the category of regulatory motivated behaviors, in particular, ingestive behavior, but it focuses on the incentive and reward value of gustatory sensory stimulation, including its hedonic properties. The main emphasis will be on those classes of stimuli, biologically and evolutionarily derived, which guide behavior in an appropriate manner leading to the procurement of important and necessary nutrients and ingredients from the environment, required for physiological well-being and the maintenance of life. On the other hand, there are series of other stimuli that are unattractive, indeed, aversive, some of which are toxic, that organisms do not seek but reject or avoid and work to reduce or eliminate. There is, thus, a bipolarity of stimuli as regards their behavioral value, from extremely positive, diminishing to zero, and then of increasing aversiveness.

Those stimuli which are positive (i.e., attractive in their own right) are sought after when first presented and do not require prior association with drive or need reduction or other more basic distress-relieving experiences to become positive. Their degree of positivity may be modulated, even modified, by such experiences but are not essential for their occurrence. Such stimuli function rather like ethologists' "releasers" of fixed action patterns of behavior, or like unconditioned stimuli for certain innate reflexive type behaviors leading to the ingestion of agents that are nutritious (and delicious). There is a coherence between biological utility, sensory effectiveness, and the hedonic quality aroused by these stimuli. Hedonic quality per se is subject to direct and independent assessment only in humans, but with proper observational and experimental ingenuity, it may also be validly attributed to animals. "Good tastes," however, are not automatic "go on every occasion" instigators because deprivation, both general and specific, influences these properties of taste stimulation.

The recognition that taste has particular significance for ingestive behavior in the generation of preference for one substance over another when choices of nutrients are available, indeed, "the pleasures of sensation" (Pfaffmann, 1960) have been recognized almost from the beginning of Western intellectual thought. In the first century B.C., Lucretius, in his long didactic poem "De Rerum Natura," wrote:

> so that you may easily see that the things which are able to affect the senses pleasantly, consist of smooth and round elements; while all those on the other hand which are found to be bitter and harsh, are held in connexion by particles that are more hooked and for this reason are wont to tear open passages into our senses. (Oates, 1940, pp. 98–99)

Aristotle observed that taste directs the choice of foods and beverages, and that the function of the pleasures aroused by taste was nutritive. Aristotle also remarked that "pleasantness and unpleasantness of the odor of food and drink belong to them contingently. These smells are pleasant when we are hungry, but when we are sated and not requiring to eat, they are not pleasant" (Aristotle, from Ross, 1906, p. 75). This was perhaps one of the earliest statements of what has more recently become a general theory of "alliesthesia" (Cabanac, 1971), which will be discussed in more detail later.

Wilhelm Wundt (1874) observed that hedonic tone or degrees of pleasantness–unpleasantness depend on stimulus intensity, and he propounded his well-known biphasic function, in which as stimulus intensity rises above threshold, pleasantness increases to a peak, then is followed by a turndown through indifference to increasing unpleasantness (see Figure 3-1). Early prototypic studies were Engel's studies of pleasantness ratings of taste solutions of increasing concentration.

Sugar shows much less falloff from the maximum, indeed, in some subjects no turndown at all; bitter, showing only a slight degree of pleasantness, is mostly unpleasant. His curves for salt and sour most clearly show the biphasic form and conform best to Wundt's schema (see Figure 3-2). These are average curves and Engel noted that individual data, albeit with the same general tendencies, may depart from these norms. For example, two subjects who found sugar increasingly unpleasant reported having excessively indulged in sweets and candies in childhood. Engel speculated on this as a possible cause for an acquired sweet aversion. Such individual differences permitted classifying individuals as either salt, sour, or bitter lovers; others as salt, sour, or bitter dislikers, their hedonic response functions departing in the appropriate manner from the average curves.

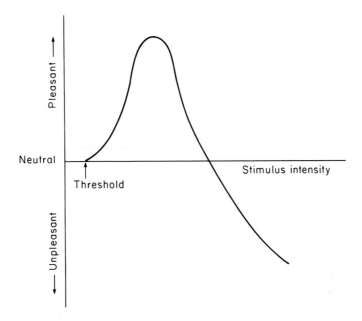

Figure 3-1. Wundt's biphasic scheme of hedonic value and sensory intensity. (From Pfaffmann, 1980.)

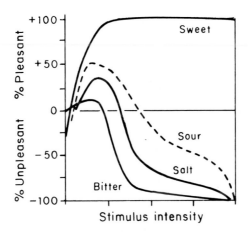

Figure 3-2. Degree of pleasantness of different taste solutions. Percentage of pleasant minus percentage of unpleasant judgments on the ordinate. Stimulus concentration is proportional to abscissa, the full length of baseline equaling 40% sucrose, 1.12% tartaric acid, 10% NaCl, and .004% quinine sulfate (by weight). (Replotted from Engel in Pfaffmann, 1980.)

Schneirla (1939, 1959, 1965), categorizing behavior objectively on an approach–withdrawal scale, measured A (approach) by the degree of an organism's movement closer to a stimulus source or W (withdrawal) by the objective increase in distance from an object, and elaborated a biphasic theory of response to stimulus intensity. In early ontogenesis, he said, low intensity of stimulation tends to evoke approach reactions of all organisms toward the source of stimulation; high intensities, withdrawal. When the earthworm, *Lumbricus terrestris L.*, for example, was stimulated at high intensity of illumination, prompt anterior shortening occurred in which movement (W) away from the source of stimulation predominated. At middle intensity, shortening was less prompt and with some increasing movement toward the source; at low intensity bodily extension and movement toward the source predominate. Deviations from this general rule seen in adult higher mammals Schneirla attributed to developmental changes during early ontogeny. The A (approach reaction) type of mechanism favors behaviors such as food getting, shelter getting, and mating; the W responses favor such adjustments as defense, huddling, flight, and other protective reactions. He (Schneirla, 1959, p. 3) then added:

> Doubtless the high road of evolution has been littered with the remains of species that diverge too far from these rules of effective adaptive relationship between the environmental conditions and response.

Berlyne (1967) attributed the pleasantness at medium but unpleasantness at high levels of intensity to arousal theory and believed that increased stimulus intensity increases arousal level directly. Moderate arousal is maximally preferred, high arousal aversive, so organisms normally strive to maintain an intermediate amount of arousal potential; hence, the biphasic character of response. Later Berlyne (1969) essentially adopted Schneirla's schema of two systems: The A system leads to increasing acceptance of a stimulus thar rises to a plateau, remaining there and of itself not turning down; the W system, with a somewhat higher threshold, also increasing with stimulus intensity but of opposite sign, counteracts the effects of A. The summation of these two systems algebraically yields a typical biphasic reaction curve.

In opposition to these trends toward objectivity, P.T. Young (1949, 1955, 1966) espoused a clearly hedonic factor in behavior. He contended that sensory stimulation per se is unidimensional, sensation magnitude increasing as stimulus intensity increases. Increasing sensory affect may have either an increasing positive (attractive) or a negative (aversive) value or the biphasic relation. The biphasic response, in particular, is taken as evidence of the distinction between stimulus sensory scales and hedonic values. That is, pleasantness of sensation at first rises in parallel with increase in sensation magnitude, but at a critical value pleasantness reaches a peak and begins to decrease, whereas sensation intensity continues to rise. Hedonically positive or pleasant stimuli are those toward which the organism moves or which it behaves to maintain. Those from which the organism retreats are hedonically negative and unpleasant. Young proposed that the hedonic process organizes and controls behavior and that it has an objective physiological substrate.

The intensity parameter alone is inadequate to account for differences between A and W (Pfaffmann, 1961). A major determinant of acceptance or rejection orthogonal to intensity is modality. Certain taste stimuli which arouse bitter sensations in weak concentrations are unpleasant, are avoided, and in increasing concentration lead only to increased rejection. Other stimuli causing sweetness are pleasant and under specified conditions are increasingly preferred as stimulus intensity increases. "The sweeter it is, the better it is." In a preference ingestion test, the biphasic response curve for sugar, where increases of concentration lead to increased intake up to a peak but then effect a turndown, the decline is only an apparent rejection.

Thus, in animals and man there appear to be certain innate determinants of the responses to taste; acids and quinine are mostly aversive, sugars preferred, salt most clearly biphasic. Although there is evidence for a true sensory aversiveness of strong salt, postingestive factors probably enhance its rejection. In the case of the physiological need for salt (NaCl), these aversive factors can be overridden, as in adrenalectomized rats or humans with adrenal pathology, so dramatically shown by Richter many years ago (1942). But it should be noted that there are species exceptions to these general rules. Hamsters, unlike rats, show little preference for salt normally (Carpenter, 1956) or when adrenalectomized (Salber & Zucker, 1974). Individual rhesus monkeys may show self-selection behavior on a salt-deficient diet if their internal homeostasis fails to maintain an adequate level of systemic salt (McMurray & Snowden, 1977). Whereas most organisms avoid quinine, Dua-Sharma and Smutz (1977) have reported that squirrel monkeys display a mild preference for weak bitter solutions before the aversion to stronger quinine solutions. Adult cats show little physiological evidence of taste sensitivity for sugar and no evidence of a sweet preference (Pfaffman, 1941; Carpenter, 1956).

The arousal of sensory affect (hedonic experience), acceptance and instigation of consummatory responses (or rejection), and the reinforcement of behavior are coherent (and related) properties of specific gustatory activation that probably involves the old brain and limbic structures (Pfaffmann, 1960) as elaborated in the remainder of this chapter.

Taste Hedonics and Behavior

Using a hedonic rating scale procedure with student volunteers who tasted solutions of sodium chloride and sugar of different concentrations, Pfaffmann (1961) confirmed Engel's average affective judgment curves for salt and sugar. Fractionating his groups into those subjects giving a large proportion of "dislike" judgments and those giving preponderantly "like" judgments, he found that 14 of 18 subjects showed an increased preference rating with increased concentration that leveled off at the highest value, that is, they liked sugar at all concentrations. Four, however, showed only dislike of sugar; the dislike increased as concentration increased. For NaCl, most subjects (13 of 18) reported an increasing dislike with concentration. Five, however, showed an increasing liking up to a peak preference and then a turndown for the strongest salt. Pangborn (1970), with a larger sample, found similar individual differences (see Figure 3-3). Moskowitz (1977) has made careful comparisons between the slope functions of category scales of taste sensory intensity and degree of pleasantness. He, like P.T. Young, emphasized that a breakpoint in hedonic scale shows that subjects are not merely rating sensory intensity by another name. Although judgment of both sweetness and pleasantness tends to increase monotonically, judgment of acids and salts where sensory intensity continues to increase monotonically show a pronounced hedonic breakpoint and thus a separation of the two values.

Besides individual differences in the relation between taste intensity and hedonic value (which might reflect past experiences with tastes, individual differences in current physiological status, or personal idiosyncracies), Moskowitz, Kumaraiah, Sharma, Jacobs, and Sharma

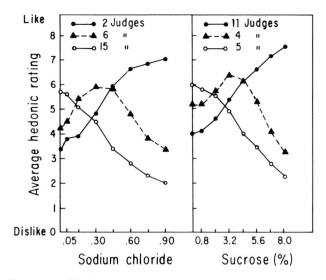

Figure 3-3. Relations of hedonic ratings to concentrations for sodium chloride and sucrose. The three different patterns show that different individuals respond differently as regards the taste pleasantness of these two commonly used substances. (Modified from Pangborn, 1970, with permission of the author.)

(1975) also demonstrated cross-cultural influences. A group of laborers from the Karnataka region in India, when tested with water solutions of glucose, sodium chloride, citric acid, and quinine, gave anomalously high pleasant ratings for citric acid and quinine. The Karnataka group scored glucose and sodium chloride much as do members of a Western population and as did a group of Indian medical students in the same locale tested by similar means. Karnataka laborers subsist on a sparse diet containing many sour foods including tamarinds, which are a slightly sweet but extremely sour fruit. The Karnataka diet generally tastes more strongly sour than Western diets.

Sensory pleasure or displeasure, said by Cabanac (1971, 1979) to be part of a basic physiological mechanism signaling the biological utility of a sensory stimulus, was shown to be influenced by the internal state of an organism. In one experiment in which subjects tasted and rated pleasantness of sugar solutions but did not swallow them, the rating of good pleasantness was unchanged throughout the series of trials. If, however, the subject swallowed each sucrose portion after tasting, judgments of pleasantness began to decrease and ultimately became increasingly unpleasant. The effect was not limited to taste alone. He also demonstrated a similar effect for thermal comfort. When body temperature was high, a cool stimulus applied to the skin felt pleasant; when body temperature was low, the cool stimulus felt unpleasant. Conversely, when body temperature was high, a warm stimulus felt unpleasant and the cool stimulus to the skin became pleasant. The capacity of a given stimulus to arouse pleasure or displeasure according to the internal state of the organism he termed alliesthesia, adding that pleasure was a sign of a stimulus useful to the subject, displeasure a sign of danger.

Cabanac (1979) further proposed a tridimensional theory of sensation: (1) a qualitative dimension (e.g., salt, sour, bitter, sweet, red, yellow) determined by the nature of the stimulus and the sense organs stimulated; (2) a quantitative dimension determined by the intensity of the stimulus; and (3) the affective or hedonic dimension. Taste and thermal stimuli display a more apparent hedonic dimension than do visual or auditory sensations, for example, but all sensory systems can vary in all three dimensions. Affective or hedonic dimensions are particularly striking in those senses playing a significant role in homeostasis.

The dramatic reversal of preference to an aversion (conditioned taste aversion), most thoroughly analyzed by Garcia, Hankins, and Rusiniak (1974) in animals, is so well known that it needs little elaboration here. The same effect is familiar to many humans after having dined or wined too lavishly or suffered a chance visceral gastric ailment after eating. Being sick to the stomach following a meal can change a previously desired food into a repellent one, not simply cognitively, but in affect;

it becomes obnoxious, tasting just horrible to the victims. Taste aversion conditioning has been studied experimentally in cancer patients undergoing chemotherapy, such therapy often being associated with subsequent malaise and other visceral distress. A group of children receiving chemotherapy were given a specially flavored ice cream as a test substance just before the treatment. They showed a conditioned aversion specifically to the flavored ice cream, but not to other flavors (Bernstein, 1978). Part of the anorexia often reported with cancer patients might be due to such conditioning (Morrison, 1978). Conversely, the enhancement of a preference by recovery from illness has also been demonstrated. A food preference can be enhanced by associating a particular flavor with physiologically beneficial nutrients (LeMagnen, 1967). Negative hedonic affect is associated with food aversions, unlearned or learned; positive affect with beneficial consequences.

Hedonic concepts have been especially criticized as explanations of positive responses toward stimuli for their inherent logical circularity when applied to subhuman species that cannot rate pleasantness–unpleasantness directly. Positive hedonic affect is said to lie behind the widespread preference for sugar solutions both inside and outside the laboratory. An organism is said to prefer A because it likes A, but we can only say it likes A because it takes A, an obvious circularity that critics contend adds nothing to the description of behavior. However, most recently Garcia (1981), on hedonics and learned taste aversions, observed:

> Rats can learn to use flavor to avoid shock, although they use the odor component more effectively than the taste component; in this case, the flavor becomes a sign for shock. When flavor is followed by illness, inhibition of drinking is much simpler because rats simply do not like the flavors; an affective change or hedonic shift occurs. . . . This distinction cannot be inferred from the quantity of fluid consumed, but it is quite obvious from the behavior of the rat: It gapes, retches, and rubs its chin on the floor.

And in 1917 Luciani in his *Textbook of Physiology* (p. 139) wrote:

> In daily life we make a distinction between the sapid substances, based on the affective impression they make upon us rather than on the quality of their tastes: thus we discriminate between agreeable, indifferent, insipid, and disagreeable tastes. Agreeable and disagreeable substances excite different expressional movements of the facial muscles; indifferent and insipid substances produce no facial movements, or at most arouse an expression of indifference or slight disgust. . . .
>
> By means of these expressional reactions it is possible even in babies of a few months old and in many animals to distinguish clearly between the sensations aroused by different tastes in the mouth. A sweet taste always gives them a pleasurable sensation, even when it is in excess. Other substances, on the contrary, give a disagreeable sensation in concentrated solutions, or are indifferent if they are dilute. In the first case the reaction is a movement of

sucking or licking; in the second there are efforts at repulsion and evidences of displeasure or disgust.

Jacob Steiner (1973) studied human neonates prior to any feeding experience when solutions of sugar, acid, or quinine were applied to the tongue surface. He observed and photographed specific gustofacial responses to a sweet solution (Figure 3-4A): a marked relaxation of the face, an expression resembling "satisfaction" often accompanied by a slight smile frequently followed by eager licking and sucking. A sour solution (Figure 3-4B) caused pursing of the lips, often accompanied or followed by nose wrinkling and eye blinking. A bitter fluid (Figure 3-4C) caused a typical arched mouth opening with the upper lip elevated; angles of the mouth were depressed, and the tongue protruded. These gestures were accompanied by a facial expression of disgust or

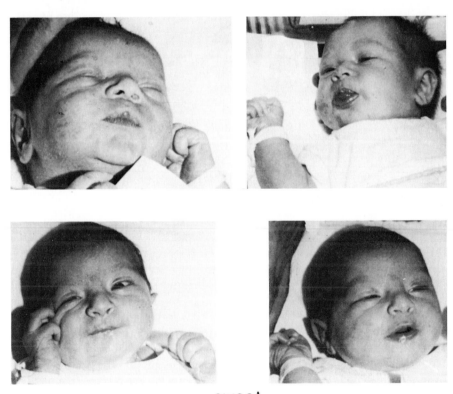

sweet

A

Figure 3-4. The gustofacial responses of normal infants to the administration of (A) sweet (25% sucrose), (B) sour (2.5% citric acid), and (C) bitter (.25% quinine sulfate) solutions. For (B) and (C), see next page. (From Steiner, 1973, with permission of the author.)

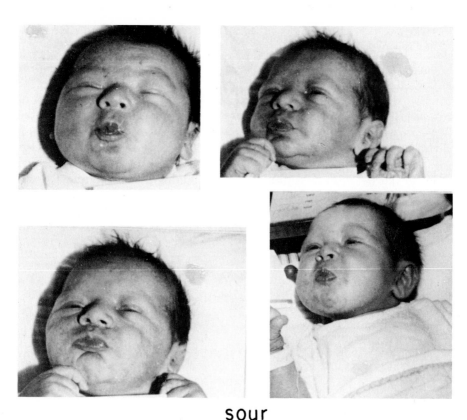

sour

B

Figure 3-4.

rejection, followed frequently by spitting or even vomiting. Such neonatal facial expressions to tastants in the very first hours of extrauterine
life prior to feeding indicates that these responses present at birth were
not acquired by life experience or learning.

Older infants between 1 and 3 days of age tested for their ingestion
of sugar solutions were found to consume more of the sweetened water
than plain water and did so in proportion to sweetness. Sucrose and
fructose proved more effective than lactose or glucose in increasing
intake (Desor, Maller, & Greene, 1977). To measure the strength of
sucking, Nowlis and Kessen (1976) used a specially designed nipple and
pressure transducer. The amplitude of anterior tongue pressure was a
direct function of sugar concentration, sucrose being more effective
than glucose in direct proportion to the relative sweetness, as measured
in psychophysical studies of adult humans.

Overall, most studies of unlearned taste hedonics with stimuli in

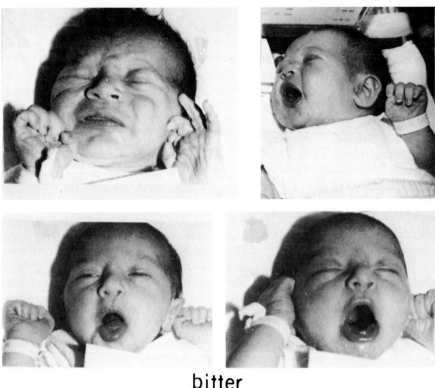

bitter

C

Figure 3-4.

aqueous solutions have found sweetness to be pleasant, and saltiness and sourness pleasant at low levels but unpleasant at higher values; but bitterness is mostly unpleasant, becoming increasingly so as concentrations rise. Generalization of such hedonic properties of these taste qualities to food flavors and beverages, especially to ethnic or gourmet delectables, must be made with caution. Bitterness in beer may indeed be an attractive flavor component, depending on one's favorite brew. The bite of chilies (hot peppers) and other condiments is highly prized but not by the young or uninitiated (Rozin, 1978). Implicit in the pleasant–unpleasant characterization is also the A–W relationship; pleasant tastes are accepted, unpleasant rejected (Moskowitz, 1974). The development and continued use of hedonic rating scales in food-survey research show these ratings to be significantly reliable indicators of what consumers actually prefer and select when actual food items or beverages are tested without regard to how or why such preferences have arisen (Meiselmann, 1977).

Correlating Taste Physiology and Behavior

Sensory electrophysiology of the chorda tympani taste nerve has been carried out on the human chorda tympani during otological surgery to free fixation of the stapes, but this was a rare and unusual opportunity that, after several studies, has not recurred since (Diamant & Zotterman, 1959; reviewed in Zotterman, 1971). Electrophysiological recordings from the nerves of taste in animals have been made in a wide variety of species from fish to monkey. In mammals, the chorda tympani nerve, which innervates the anterior tongue, has been the main source of information, with relatively few studies of the posterior tongue's glossopharyngeal nerve (IX). In frogs, the IXth nerve is the primary gustatory sensory nerve. Species differences in the chorda tympani reactivity of mammals are quite clear. For example, the cat has relatively little sugar sensitivity (Pfaffmann, 1941) and although rat's chorda shows responses to sugar (Hagstrom & Pfaffmann, 1959; Noma, Goto, & Sato, 1971), they are much weaker in the nerve as a whole than in the hamster, gerbil, dog, rabbit, and such primates as squirrel monkey and rhesus monkey (Pfaffmann, 1975; Jakinovich, 1976a, 1976b; Sato, Ogawa, & Yamashita, 1975).

In general, two methods of recording are used. One is multiunit neural activity, which can be given a quantitative measure by means of an electronic summator originally developed by Beidler (1953). This provides a running average (not true integration) over an adjustable time frame by adjusting the rise and fall time constants of the device, as shown in Figure 3-5. This gives only an overall view of neural activation but may be a biased sample, since the larger nerve fibers yield larger potentials than do smaller diameter fibers, thereby contributing more potential to the summator record. There is the possibility of a relation of fiber size to quality of stimulus, quinine receptors being said to innervate smaller diameter nerve fibers, but this relationship is not firmly established. The other method is the time honored single-unit recording requiring microdissection of nerve bundles until a single unit's typical response is seen on the cathode ray oscilloscope monitor. Frequency of response to stimulation in the form of a poststimulus histogram is a typical measure. Penetrating cell bodies of the geniculate ganglion by means of microelectrodes has also been used to record single taste afferent responses, a procedure much like that for recording unit or multiunit activity in CNS (Boudreau & Alev, 1973). In nearly all cases there is a monotonic increase of discharge in both number of fibers active and increased frequency of discharge therein. In the human studies there was a good correlation between perceived magnitude of the taste intensity and the magnitude of summated nerve activity (Zotterman, 1971).

A number of different behavioral measures have been employed with

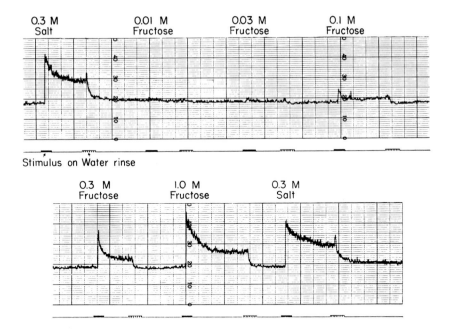

Figure 3-5. Summator records of responses in a squirrel monkey's chorda tympani nerve to an increasing concentration series of fructose. A reference salt stimulus, .3 M ammonium chloride, brackets the sugar series. (From Pfaffmann, 1966, with permission, Rockefeller University Press.)

animals. The classic is Richter's two-bottle preference test (Richter & Campbell, 1940; Richter, 1942). Typically, an individual living cage with a single animal is provided with two calibrated drinking tubes, one containing taste solution, the other plain water, for 24 hours. Preference (or aversion) thresholds are obtained by providing a successively increasing concentration series until a greater (or lesser) amount of solution than water is ingested. The magnitude of preference or aversion for suprathreshold concentrations is given by relative amounts of solution consumed over water intake. The behavioral response of albino rats to ascending concentrations of four basic taste stimuli is shown in the upper half of Figure 3-6. Acid and quinine solutions are rejected; the preference for salt and sugar, however, is a biphasic one: first, a preference that rises to a peak of maximal intake, than a turndown with decreasing intake, and ultimately rejection. The lower part of Figure 3-6 shows the summator response functions from the rat chorda tympani and IXth nerves combined. The sugar response is relatively less than that to acid, salt, and quinine, but the concentration ranges for neural activity and the aversion and preference–aversion functions coincide.

The salt and sugar preference–aversion functions superficially resemble a biphasic intensity function. High concentrations of both salt

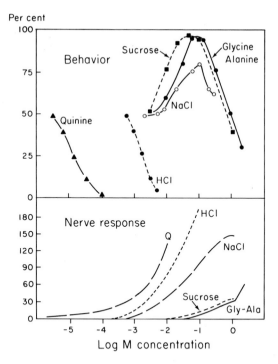

Figure 3-6. Correlation of behavioral preference or aversion with composite electrophysiological responses of chorda tympani and glossopharyngeal nerve to indicated solutions of tastants. The upper panel shows intake of indicated taste solution as a percentage of total fluid intake (solution + H_2O) in a two-bottle preference test. The lower panel shows neural responses to the same stimuli relative to the .1 M NaCl response. (From Pfaffmann, 1977.)

and sugar are hypertonic so that over a 24-hour period they would influence the animal's nutritional state and fluid balance and would interact with and influence behavioral preference. Behavioral methods based on operant conditioning on an intermittent schedule of reinforcement so that fluid intake can be limited to brief sips in the course of an hour test is one way of restricting volume of intake and thus minimizing the postingestive effects.

Behavior may be classified into two classes, consummatory and instrumental. Consummatory behavior, licking and swallowing, is the final act that brings the food or fluid object into the oral cavity and esophageal passageways. Instrumental behavior is such a response as reaching for a cup and bringing it to the mouth or pressing a bar or key that delivers the fluid at a delivery spout to be licked, or any of a number of other motor responses that obtain food or fluid. With proper apparatus arrangements, the relation between instrumental and consummatory responses in the behavior chain may be prolonged or temporally arranged according to a variety of different schedules. The consummatory response (i.e., ingestion of food or fluid) is said to provide the reinforcement for learning such instrumental responses. Reinforcement can be regular (i.e., every bar press pays off with fluid), or periodic (only every other, every 10th, or every 50th bar press pays off), or aperiodic on a random schedule, and so on. The distinction between consummatory and operant (i.e., instrumental) may be arbitrary as regards licking (Hulse, 1967). The act of licking may have an instrumental role, since it brings the fluid into the mouth so that the ultimate consummatory response, swallowing, can occur. At the same time, licking and tasting leading to swallowing may be considered an unconditioned stimulus–response reflex chain. Consummatory behavior is closely linked to reward or reinforcement; but in the act of licking and swallowing, gustatory stimulation usually occurs. For certain classes of stimuli, like sugar, the mere tasting (i.e., sensory stimulation) may be rewarding so that the sweet taste will reinforce bar presses and licking. Quinine will be aversive and will not reinforce ingestive behavior. The correspondence between pleasantness and reward or unpleasantness and nonreward is an agelong debate.

When sugar solution intake is restricted by an appropriate schedule, the functions for bar-press rate or lick rate do not show the biphasic turndown, but continue to rise toward and level off at a plateau of concentration values where ad-lib 24-hour intake measures turn down. The biphasic response function is only apparent and does not indicate a reduced preference or aversion to the sugar per se, but reflects other sensory or physiological factors.

Figure 3-7 shows the relation between bar pressing and lick rate in four different squirrel monkeys when sucrose concentration is varied on an operant intermittent reinforcement schedule (a fixed interval of 30) for a briefly presented sugar solution.[1] Lick rate varied with concentration for all four animals; bar pressing for only three animals. (It did not vary for Snoopy, the animal with the lowest lick rate.) None of the behavioral functions showed the turndown at the higher sugar concentration that showed when given the two-bottle preferential 24-hour intake test. Squirrel monkeys were avid for sugar, ingesting so much sugar solution that they became waterlogged and intake measures became erratic. The free-access period had to be reduced to 1 hour a day. The bar-press test periods were set at 20- or 30-minute durations each day.

Since different sugars—sucrose, fructose, glucose, lactose, and mal-

---

[1] Twenty-five licks occurred at each presentation (.01 ml per lick providing .25 ml per presentation) where continuous drinking occurred at the higher concentrations.

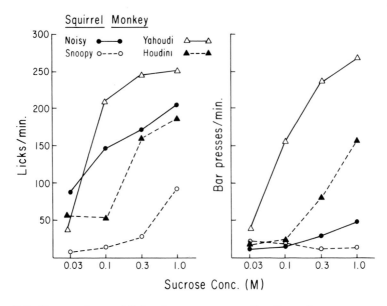

Figure 3-7. Bar-pressing and lick-rate measures as a function of sucrose concentration in four squirrel monkeys. (From Pfaffmann, 1965, data from Jay & Fisher; © 1965, Amer. Psychol. Assoc.; adapted with permission of the publisher.)

tose—differ in degree of sweetness to humans in that order, sweetness being greatest for sucrose, we tested the relative effectiveness of the sugars in the bar-pressing lick-rate task; it yielded an order of effectiveness: sucrose > fructose > maltose ⩾ lactose ⩾ glucose, as shown in Figure 3-8 (Ganchrow & Fisher, 1965; Pfaffmann, 1977). Lick rate in this case did not show as systematic a seriation of the different sugars. Such monotonic bar-pressing response functions for sugar solutions were first demonstrated in rats (Guttman, 1953).

The selection of the squirrel monkey was dictated by our interest in a species with good sugar electrophysiology and sugar preference. Single units in the squirrel monkey chorda tympani showed that there is a cluster of sugar-specific units that all responded in the order: sucrose > fructose > maltose ⩾ lactose ⩾ galactose ⩾ glucose. Thus the bar pressing and electrophysiology of taste input are in agreement certainly as regards relative order of sucrose > fructose > maltose=lactose=galactose=glucose, the latter four being very similar to each other, with overlapping values all much less effective than sucrose and fructose.[2]

[2]This order of effectiveness is different from that of the magnitude of whole-nerve summator responses, where fructose gives the largest response. However, there is a second group of primarily salt-sensitive receptors that also respond actively to fructose, but much less to the other sugars. The discharge of these salt receptors adds to that of the sugar receptors, giving the larger summator response when fructose is applied to the tongue.

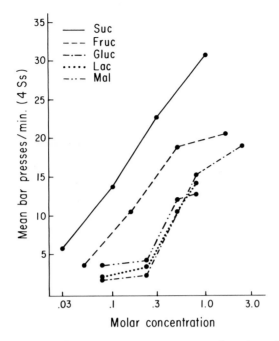

Figure 3-8. Bar pressing to obtain different sugars as a function of concentration. (Fig. 1(b) from Ganchrow & Fisher, 1968, reprinted with permission of the authors and publisher.)

The correspondence between sensory effectiveness measured electrophysiologically and behavioral efficacy indicates a direct relation between sensory input and palatability in this instance. Other stimuli that activate this class of sugar receptors to the same degree will be preferred and accepted (i.e., equally palatable). The association of sensory input with palatability, however, is a contingent one depending on hunger state, past experience, and learning with no change in peripheral sensory function.

Other quite recent evidence with the artificial sweetener aspartame documents further that the turndown in intake at higher concentrations of sugar solutions is due to calories, shown in Figure 3-9 (Kemnitz, Gibber, Lindsay, & Brot, 1981). Eight intact rhesus male monkeys were tested during a 2-hour test period on consecutive days (one test per day). Purina Monkey Chow and tap water were available ad lib during the test period. First, a concentration of sucrose and then the non-caloric sweetener aspartame were prescribed, each in a random order. Maximum intake occurred at .1–.3 M sucrose but decreased with further increases in concentration. Intake of chow was inversely related to amount of sucrose. The noncaloric sweetener intake was asymptotic at concentrations greater than 2.3×10^{-3} M, with no indication of suppression of chow intake.

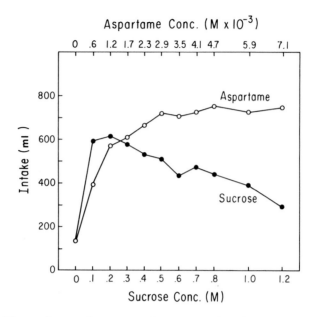

Figure 3-9. The preference for sugar and aspartame (synthetic sweetener) in rhesus males. The higher concentration of sugar shows a reduced volume intake due probably to the increasing caloric value; the relatively weak aspartame solutions show no such effect. (Redrawn with permission from Kemnitz, Gibber, Lindsay, & Brot, 1981.)

Other evidence supporting the view that the turndown in preference for the higher sugar concentrations is caused by postingestive factors comes from studies of the esophagogastrostomized rats (Mook, 1963). This is a double fistulated preparation in which the esophagus is sectioned and attached to a polyethylene discharge tube so that what enters the mouth does not enter the stomach. The proximal stump of the esophagus is fitted with another input tube and fluid pump. Thus the solution being drunk, or a different solution, or no solution can be introduced into the stomach in a controlled sequence. When glucose or sucrose is tasted and tubed into the stomach, a typical peak preference intake curve is obtained. When only water reaches the stomach, the sucrose and glucose curves show only a rising preference function (see Figure 13-1 in Chapter 13 by Stellar). These curves mimic in general form the relative magnitude of the whole-nerve responses of the rat to sucrose and glucose (see Figure 3-10).

Another method of maximizing oral sensory factors controlling intake is the short-term drinking test. Cagan and Maller (1974) trained animals to sample a single-stimulus solution upon presentation in a brief exposure test. Intake of sucrose was greater than of fructose,

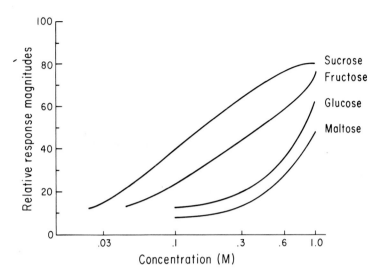

Figure 3-10. Composite curve of the rat's chorda tympani response to sugars. (Based on Tateda & Hidaka, 1966; Hagstrom & Pfaffmann, 1959.)

which was greater than that of glucose. In a control 24-hour test, where ingestion and metabolism ensued, glucose was preferentially ingested over the other two. Davis (1973) utilized a similar method but measured the rat's licking behavior during a short exposure of 3 minutes each of sucrose, fructose, and glucose in order to eliminate negative feedback from postingestive factors. Five male Sprague–Dawley albino rats approximately 200 days old at the start of the experiment were used. Lab pellets available ad lib during the light period of a reversed light–dark schedule were removed at the start of the dark period. Drinkometer tests were begun 8 hours later. Just prior to each test, 30 minutes of access to food were provided. Various postprandial intervals were employed in which testing began either immediately or 30 minutes, 45 minutes, 1.5 hours, or 4.5 hours after having eaten. After 8 hours of deprivation, no food was given.

Although deprivation did have an influence, sugar concentration had by far the most important effect on lick rate. A monotonic growth of lick rate was observed at every level of deprivation in the order of sucrose > fructose > glucose, as shown in Figure 3-11. Response functions practically mimic the order of magnitude of the response function from the chorda tympani preparation shown in Figure 3-10. Not only is this order true for the nerve as a whole, but it is also seen in the relative frequencies of discharge in a sample of single units (Noma et al., 1971). These findings both support the idea that the turndown of sucrose and other sugar intake curves is due to postingestive factors and

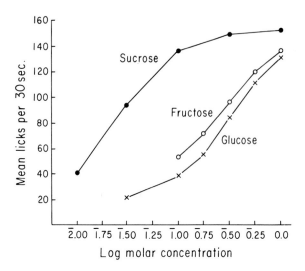

Figure 3-11. Rat's licking rate as a function of concentration of sucrose, fructose, and glucose. (Redrawn from Davis, 1973, with permission of the author and Pergamon Press, Ltd.)

strengthen the correlation of the rising taste function for sugar with the sensory effectiveness of the sugar, what to humans would be degree of sweetness. In the absence of gut filling, the amount of ingestive behaior stimulated by sucrose, fructose, and glucose increases dramatically with concentration.

The Maltose Paradox

Thus far, all is in order and quite understandable. That maltose is less sweet and less reinforcing than sucrose or fructose seems unremarkable. However, Davis and colleagues (Davis, Collins, & Levine, 1975) applied their brief-exposure 3-minute-access drinkometer method to a wider range of sugars in order to elaborate a mathematical model of ingestion (Davis & Levine, 1977). The model assumes that palatable substances activate and drive central nervous system mechanisms controlling rate of ingestion in proportion to palatability. The accumulation of ingested substances in the intestinal tract counteracts excitatory gustatory stimulation, thus inhibiting intake. The model contains a term g representing the effective strength of flavor or taste, which varies with both concentrations and the sensitivity of the gustatory receptors. A weak sucrose solution would be represented by a small value of g, a strong solution by a large value of g. Another term, p (evaluation), can modify the input g according to the significance of the flavor for the organism; for example, in a sodium-depleted animal p is large for sodium compared to its value in an animal in sodium balance. The product *gp* (which is defined as palatability) determines rate of ingestion.

Quite apart from the mathematical theory and determination of its parameters, data obtained with a short-term drinking test give pause for thought. Davis' earlier results (Figure 3-11) showed the expected relation from the electrophysiological data on rat taste receptors; the later results (Figure 3-12), however, are utterly contradictory, for maltose now appears almost as effective as sucrose and surpasses all others in eliciting licking. Why is maltose so effective behaviorally, whereas it is relatively weak as a taste stimulus?

In their early work, Richter and Campbell (1940) showed that in the 24-hour two-bottle preference test, the preference thresholds for the sugars in percentage concentrations were maltose, .060; glucose, 1.03; sucrose, 1.50; fructose, too variable to calculate; galactose, 1.47; and lactose, 4.8. The volume of average daily intake in grams per kilogram was glucose, 31; maltose, 30; sucrose, 24; fructose, 16; galactose, 7; and lactose, 3; an order that Richter correlated with "limits of assimilability" in grams per kilogram of body weight which the animal could metabolize. Since in the 24-hour test procedure, animals are ingesting and metabolizing sugars for calories, postingestive effects are significant. Maltose is a dissaccharide composed of two glucose molecules and is readily metabolized to glucose in the intestinal tract. Its efficacy in a 24-hour ingestion measure is not surprising, but why is it effective in a short-term drinking test?

Under long-term exposure animals can learn that different sweetnesses may not be correlated with different amounts of calories, so that

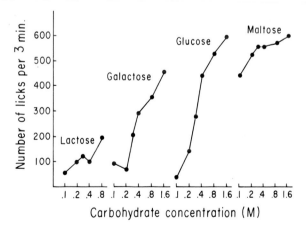

Figure 3-12. The mean number of lick responses elicited by four different sugars at different concentrations. Rats were given daily 3-minute tests to each of the sugars in increasing order of concentration. (Redrawn from Davis et al., 1975.)

they come to be guided by calories regardless of solution sweetness (LeMagnen, 1971). Repeated experience with the noncaloric consequence of a saccharin intake may ultimately lead to the disappearance of its positive palatability. The strength of the saccharin preference increases if paired with caloric intragastric sugar tubing. This is the positive side of the taste aversion learning. If not paired with caloric intubation, the saccharin preference may remain unchanged (Capretta, 1962).

Interestingly enough, it is under an ad-lib regimen that animals regulate and eat for calories; when hungry, however, they eat for sweetness (Jacobs & Sharma, 1969; LeMagnen, 1971). Its intensity apparently serves as an index of presumed caloric content. In a 30-minute drinking test, LeMagnen (1954) showed that food deprivation increased the intake of a nonnutritive saccharin solution moreso than that of a less sweet but nutritious glucose solution. Valenstein (1967) reported that when rats were satiated for food, they switched to a caloric 3% glucose preference over saccharin. However, when food deprived, they gradually switched back to a saccharin preference, which became increasingly greater over the 30-day test period. Valenstein also made the dramatic observation that animals food deprived except for 75 minutes each day developed a large saccharin solution preference and consumed only minimal amounts of glucose when both solutions were available, to such a degree that several animals in the group died of starvation on the saccharin with no tendency to switch to the more nutritious glucose solutions, which would have saved them (Valenstein, cited in Jacobs & Sharma, 1969). Thus, degree of hunger may enhance or synergize the significance of sweetness per se.

Under the conditions of Davis' experiment, 30-minute access to standard lab chow was provided just prior to testing, so that animals were in a postprandial state, presumably not deprived at the time of testing. All sugars were presented in an equivalent postprandial state so that eating for calories rather than sweetness might have prevailed. The maltose paradox may be resolvable as a search for calories.

So far I have emphasized largely the quantitative degree of sweetness or sensory efficacy as the major variable. But the taste of sugar may differ in quality as well. Whereas sucrose is largely sweet to humans, glucose is reported to be sweet plus mildly sour or tart; lactose sweet plus salty; galactose sweet plus a woody flavor (Cameron, 1947). Quite recent psychophysical work in humans (Faurion, Saito, & MacLeod, 1980) has begun to show evidence for different molecular receptor sites for sweetness, a clustering of sensitivities within which thresholds and sensory magnitude judgments tend to covary, but between groups or clusters there is a lesser covariance. Whereas many single-fiber preparations in animals show the order of effectiveness to be sucrose > fructose > glucose > maltose, in some species there are individual-unit preparations where maltose is the best sugar stimulus (Anderson,

Funakoshi, & Zotterman, 1963). It is therefore possible that subquality of sweetness as well as its intensity may be coded in the afferent nerve input.

In the squirrel monkey and hamster, two good sugar-sensing species, we have found all sugars as sensory stimuli to be highly correlated with each other in the cross-fiber correlational measures of similarity. Conditioned-aversion cross-generalization tests in hamsters tend to confirm that all common sugars taste alike and the degree of generalization from each to sucrose is high. This is also true of rats, but in our own studies we did not specifically study maltose until recently. In preliminary results, Nowlis and I found that although an aversion to sucrose produces some aversion to maltose, an aversion conditioned to maltose does not generalize to sucrose. On the other hand, sucrose, glucose, fructose, or even sweet amino acids produce strong cross-generalizations with each other. Maltose may share some sensory qualities with sucrose; it may have some other distinctive qualities as well.

Jakinovich (Note 1) found in another rodent, the gerbil, that a conditioned aversion to .1 M sucrose produced the suppression ratio (an index of similarity) shown in Table 3-1. Although sucrose aversion generalized less to maltose than to the other sugars (including sucrose to itself), the generalization to maltose was significant. More information is needed on how individual-nerve preparations, especially IXth and Xth nerve taste afferents, respond to different sugars.

Maltose, as such, does not occur abundantly in nature, although its occurrence has occasionally been reported (White, Handler, & Smith, 1964). As a disaccharide of two glucose molecules with a glycosidic linkage, it is readily hydrolysed to glucose by the enzyme maltase, which is distributed throughout the length of the mucosa of the small intestine. In a sense, glucose is the major physiological form of sugar in the internal metabolism, and once inside the body is most readily

Table 3-1. Suppression Ratios in Gerbil with Conditioned Aversion to Sugars

Concentration	Sugar	Suppression ratio[a]
.10 M	Sucrose	79
.22 M	Fructose	73
.37 M	Glucose	62
.32 M	Galactose	61
.31 M	Lactose	56
.24 M	Maltose	50

[a]Suppression ratio $= \left(1 - \dfrac{\text{vol. sugar consumed}}{\text{vol. water consumed}}\right) \times 100$.

absorbed and metabolized. The greater taste effectiveness of sucrose, a disaccharide of fructose, plus glucose may appear to be an anomaly from the point of view of biological function. Taste, however, provides the chemical contact with the external world, in which sucrose occurs widely in a variety of fruits, seeds, leaves, flowers, and roots, especially sugar cane and beets, the main commercial sources. There is only a trace of maltose in apple, *Pyrus malus*. Of the total solids in this fruit, 69% is made up of glucose, fructose, and sucrose. In peach, *Prunus persica*, where 71% of the total solid is sugar, less than 1% is maltose. However, in some fruits like grape, *Vitis vinifera*, maltose constitutes 12% of the total solid, sucrose, glucose, and fructose making up the remaining 67% of the total solid. In *Vitis labrus cana* where 97% of the total solid is sugar, maltose constitutes 8% of that total. Sucrose makes up 55% of the total solid in beet, *Beta vulgaris*, 46% in honeydew melon, and 35% in carrot (Shallenberger, 1974). Sucrose, together with its products of hydrolysis, glucose and fructose, is the major carbohydrate of maple syrup, honey, and fruit juices. So there appears to be a functional specialization of taste receptors for those forms of sugar most likely to be encountered in the world around us. The external world and internal world, with their different chemical orders of merit, can be said to meet in the oral cavity.

The CNS and Taste-Motivated Behavior

The anatomical and functional organization of the gustatory and related visceral afferent columns of the medulla, the tractus solitarius (TS) and its nucleus (NTS), is one of the most constant features of the vertebrate nervous system phylogeny. Taste buds, wherever located, send axons into the bilateral V-shaped tract and its nucleus reaching from the obex of the IVth ventricle of the medulla, terminating in the anterior bulbar level. The essential features seen in higher vertebrate brains occur in fish and amphibian brains (Herrick, 1948). Taste afferents in the VIIth, IXth, and a small part of the Xth cranial nerves enter the TS and ascend to the anterior NTS. The major sensory component of the vagus is composed of visceral afferents from the sense organs of the viscera and internal organs and tends to be located caudally in the TS. There is no clear morphological feature of the TS to distinguish taste (sometimes called a special visceral afferent) from the general visceral afferents of the vagus except by electrophysiological, histological tracing methods, or other functional procedures such as selective ablations.

Taste buds are most commonly found in the oral cavity, but in certain fish (carp and catfish and several other species of teleosts) there are enormous numbers of taste buds on the external body surface as well as inside the mouth. The external taste buds are innervated by a sensory branch of the VIIth cranial nerve; the taste buds of the oral cavity and palate, largely by branches of the Xth nerve. Their central primary nuclei in the NTS, visible as distinct enlargements on the dorsal surface of the medulla when dissecting the brain, are called the facial and vagal lobes. The external taste buds function as exteroceptors in searching the aquatic environment for food. In contrast, the taste buds within the mouth and on the palate are more directly related to consummatory swallowing. Atema (1971) selectively ablated the facial lobes of catfish *Ameiurus*, which caused a transitory loss of the turning response toward food when a jet containing dissolved food particles was applied to one of its barbels or the body surface. Ablation of the vagal lobe, on the other hand, caused the transitory loss of swallowing and did not affect the turning response toward the food. In other words, the one lobe primarily functioned for the exteroceptive taste buds on the exterior surface in finding food; the internal taste buds functioned in swallowing and ingestion.

In an electrophysiological study, Biedenbach (1973) found that reactivity to taste in these lobes was intermingled with that for tactile sensitivity of the appropriate body areas, so these neural structures were not exclusively for taste. Electrophysiological recording in the medulla of the rat yields multiunit and single-unit responses to electrical stimulation of the taste nerves or chemical stimulation of the tongue and mouth areas containing taste buds. The anterior tongue innervated by the chorda tympani branch of the VIIth nerve projects to a more rostral area of the NTS than does the posterior tongue, which is innervated by the IXth glossopharyngeal nerve. The chorda tympani area generally gave larger responses to salt and to acid; the posterior tongue area gave larger responses to quinine, in agreement with the relative distribution of these sensitivities in the chorda tympani and IXth nerve of the rat (Frank, 1975; Halpern & Nelson, 1965). The projection of the vagal afferents to the more caudal TS has been studied largely in anatomical rather than physiological preparations.

In the fish and amphibian brain the uncrossed viscerogustatory pathway ascends to a point rostral of the roots of the Vth cranial nerve nucleus. Here the pathway divides, some fibers continuing ventrally to the ventrolateral peduncle, a hypothalamic homologue, others turning dorsally to a secondary gustatory–visceral nucleus. Since this secondary nucleus is very large in the carp and catfish, it is probably largely gustatory in function (see Figure 3-13). From this dorsally located secondary nucleus arises a tertiary viscerogustatory tract which passes ventrally to the hypothalamus (inferior lateral lobe) accompanied by cerebellar fibers of the brachium conjunctivum that pass through the superior secondary nucleus. The dorsal nucleus was thought to be specialized in relation to the somatic musculature involved in feeding, whereas a

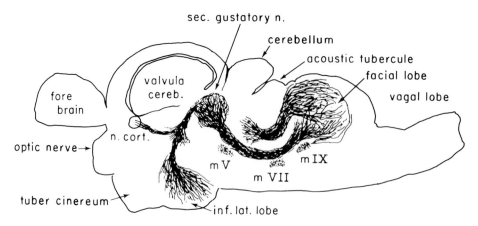

Figure 3-13. Partial tracing of the VIIth-nerve taste pathways of fish brain (based on Herrick, 1905). Afferent taste fibers after entering the brain stem proceed to their first synaptic relay in the facial lobe of the medulla. Second-order fibers ascend to the secondary gustatory nucleus beneath the cerebellum, whence third-order fibers arise, projecting to the ventral diencephalon (mV, mVII, mIX refer to motor nuclei of indicated cranial nerves). (From Pfaffmann, 1977.)

relationship with olfactovisceral function was attributed to the direct ventral pathway to the hypothalamus. Herrick (1948) discussed this organization as follows:

> The swallowing of a morsel of food in response to excitation of taste buds is one of the simplest acts of which the body is capable. This may be done reflexly through the local activation of the bulbar connections of the f. solitarius; but, simultaneously with this local action, nervous impulses may be transmitted to higher centers which are so interconnected as to bring this simple act into relation with any other activities that may be in process in response to internal or external stimuli. The final result of any particular sensory excitation is dependent upon the central excitatory state of the central nervous system as a whole and of every local part of it. (p. 171)

It is only relatively recently that recognition of the existence of a homologous system in the mammalian brain has come to light. The pontine taste area (PTA) originally described in anatomical studies by Norgren and Leonard (1971, 1973) and electrophysiologically by Norgren and Pfaffmann (1975) is located in the parabrachial nucleus (PBN) of the dorsal pons. The PTA is embedded in the brachium conjunctivum such that the descending cerebellar fibers pass through it and parcellate its nuclear mass. In the rat the PTA is clearly a separate nucleus cluster cephalad to and anterior to the NTS. The PTA is a third-order relay sending its fibers not only to the thalamic taste area (TTA) but also ventrally to the subthalamus and far lateral hypothalamus where a number of its fibers terminate. The many resemblances of this system and its connections to the secondary gustatory nucleus described in the fish brain by Herrick should be obvious (see Figure 3-14).

The hypothalamus is known to receive taste afferent information. Norgren (1970) recorded electrophysiological activity aroused by gustatory stimulation of unanesthetized rats from chronically implanted electrodes. Lesions of the ventromedial nucleus cause obesity in rats in which the animals are overreactive to the negative gustatory properties of quinine adulteration on the one hand or the positive stimulus qualities of dextrose on the other (e.g., Teitelbaum, 1955). Rats that have recovered from lateral hypothalamic lesions cannot acquire a taste–illness association, although they can remember a taste aversion acquired before the lesion (Roth, Schwartz, & Teitelbaum, 1973).

Many of the fibers of the ventral pathway continue rostrally to a large terminal field in the substantia innominata and then turn caudally to enter the caudal pole of the central nucleus of the amygdala, which they ultimately fill (Figure 3-14). Some fibers continue from the central nucleus via the stria terminalis to enter its bed nucleus. Schwartzbaum and Morse (1978) have recorded electrophysiological responses in the central nucleus with chronic electrodes in unanesthetized rabbits following taste stimulation. These responses in some instances resembled the discharges seen in primary afferent fibers but more often were more complex, including inhibition and other variants of multimodal activity. From this it is clear that gustatory neurons project to the central nucleus in subprimates.

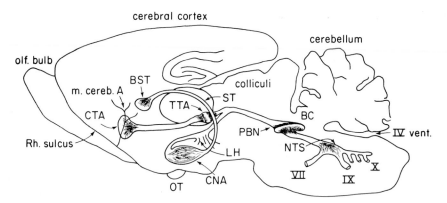

Figure 3-14. Schematic phantom of the medullary pontine thalamocortical and ventral hypothalamic amygdala taste pathways of the rat brain. (BC, brachium conjunctivum; BST, bed nucleus of stria terminalis; CTA, cortical taste area; CNA, central nucleus of the amygdala; LH, lateral hypothalamus; m. cereb A, middle cerebral artery; NTS, nucleus tractus solitarius; OT, optic tract; PBN, parabrachial nucleus; Rh. sulcus, rhinal sulcus; ST, stria terminalis; TTA, thalamic taste area; IV vent, fourth ventricle; VII, IX, X, VIIth, IXth, and Xth cranial nerve afferents.) (Figure by Pfaffmann from Norgren, 1977, with permission.)

Box and Mogenson (1975) reported that lesions of the dorsal aspect of the rat's central nucleus of the amygdala caused a temporary aphagia and adipsia similar to that following lateral hypothalamic lesions. After recovery of food and water intake such animals remained less reactive, showing a lessened preference for sweet solutions, caloric or noncaloric. Kemble and Schwartzbaum (1969) reported similar findings with larger amygdaloid lesions and postulated that the lesions had produced a motivational dysfunction.

Lesions of the amygdala also interfere with learning a conditioned taste aversion; however, most of these studies have involved the baso-lateral nucleus of the amygdala (Nachman & Ashe, 1974). Rats so lesioned did not retain an aversion acquired prior to the lesion. How-ever, they were able to learn after such a lesion, but the learning was not normal and proceeded more slowly. Taste aversion learning depends in part on the neophobia rats show to unfamiliar taste- or food-related stimuli. Such neophobia enhances the learning of taste aversions. Le-sions of the amygdala interfere with the neophobic responses so that all stimuli are treated as familiar. Normal preference–aversion functions to the four basic taste stimuli—saline, sugar, acid, and quinine—are not altered, unlike the case of the central nucleus ablations.

Taste is an important component of the PTA in fish, amphibians, rodents, cats, and ungulates receiving primary ascending chorda tym-pani (CT) fibers as well as secondary afferents from the NTS (Bernard & Nord, 1971; Johnson, 1964; Nageotte, 1906; Rhoton, 1968). The projection of the IXth nerve and the superior laryngeal nerve of X in sheep (Car, Jean, & Roman, 1975) subserving components in the dorsal pontine nucleus that discharge during swallowing (Jean, Car, & Roman, 1975) seems to be an oral sensory system. In primates the parabrachial nucleus does not appear to receive gustatory afferents of the VIIth-nerve chorda tympani. Autoradiographic studies show that the para-brachial area receives a large NTS input primarily from the more caudal, largely vagal, afferent component. Taste afferents in the anterior NTS appear to pass almost exclusively to the thalamic area and thence to the cortex, but the other taste afferents (IX and X) have not been analyzed as yet (Note 2).

The thalamocortical taste system arising from the dorsal pontothala-mic projections has been well studied, especially by Benjamin and his colleagues (reviewed in Burton & Benjamin, 1971). The ventrobasal (VB) group of thalamic nuclei make up its main sensory relay, in which there is a precise somatotopic representation of the limbs and trunk. The face, including the tongue and intraoral structures, projects more medially to the arcuate nucleus. The ventromedial (VM) area, still more medial, and lying below the centrum medianum, is unresponsive to mechanical stimulation, but does respond when taste stimuli are applied to the tongue in its most medial tip and exclusively to taste stimulation. Mechanical and true somatic cold responses of the lingual nerve projection are found surrounding the pure taste area. Lesions of the thalamic taste area (TTA) cause impairment of taste discrimination, as reflected by elevation of quinine aversion thresholds. Electrical stimulation of the TTA via chronically implanted electrodes in unanesthetized animals leads to licking and chewing, gaping, and tongue protrusions characteristic of an aversive pattern (Andersson & Jewell, 1957; Norgren, 1970) with little evidence of responses resembling the positive oral behaviors.

Cortical projections of taste have proven to be multiple, there being a double cortical representation of the chorda tympani nerve when it is stimulated electrically. Most recently, Yamamoto, Matsuo, and Kawamura (1980) have reported that both the chorda tympani (CT) and the lingual nerves project to two separate areas of the rat cortex in a manner resembling the earlier demonstration of a double representation in cat and monkey. In the rat, one area is anterior to the middle cerebral artery (MCA), the other posterior to it. The anterior CT area, just dorsal to the rhinal sulcus, yields electrophysiological responses to taste only, or to both taste and cooling; whereas the cortical units in the posterior CT area respond to taste, cooling, warming, and touch or some combination thereof. The glossopharyngeal (GN) posterior tongue area is a single area and is located posterior to the MCA. Microelectrode single-unit recording of cortical taste cells shows excitatory responses to one or more of the four basic taste stimuli in addition to inhibitory responses to one or more taste stimuli.

Earlier investigations (Benjamin, 1959) have shown that ablations of the general area of the taste cortex in the rat caused only a five-fold transitory elevation of the quinine aversion threshold which soon disappeared and could be prevented by preoperative experience. Lesioning the taste thalamus caused a 13-fold threshold elevation, whereas lesions of the medullary zone raised the quinine threshold 65 times, these two areas showing little recovery of function. Ablation of the cortical taste area does not change the sign of the preference or the aversion responses to taste stimuli; in fact, such lesions may increase the preference for sucrose and weak saline (Braun & Kiefer, 1975; Kiefer & Braun, 1977), as do parabrachial lesions that interrupt the ascending pathways to the cortex and other structures (Nowlis, Braun & Norgren, 1977). In the latter instance it has been suggested that release of cortical inhibitory influences permits greater expression of the unlearned taste preferences intrinsic to the hindbrain mechanisms.

Yamamoto et al. (1980) also reported that conditioned taste aversions (CTAs) acquired prior to cortical ablation were lost when the anterior CT and ventral GN areas were destroyed but were not lost if the other more posterior composite area was ablated. Others (Kiefer & Braun, 1977; Braun, Slick, & Lorden, 1972; Lorden, 1976) previously showed that a CTA is lost after cortical taste ablation but that relearning is possible albeit at a somewhat slower rate. Since discrimination or detectability of taste stimuli is not permanently impaired after neocortical ablation, there is a specific impairment of gustatory learning. Braun (1981) likens this to the different agnosias following cortical damage, depending upon the sensory neocortical area and the modality affected.

In the monkey, one representation of the double area is in the somatosensory face and mouth area; the second is in the buried cortex of the operculum (Benjamin & Burton, 1968), designated TN I and TN II. Selective destruction of TN I or TN II alone did not cause a consistent taste defect nor thalamic retrograde degeneration. A similar double projection occurs in the cat with a somatosensory tongue area and a hidden cortical area of the presylvian area. Relatively little taste aversion learning, however, has been studied relative to the central neuroanatomy and function in species other than the rat.

Figure 3-14 (Pfaffmann in Norgren, 1977) recapitulates the gustatory CNS organization in a phantom schema of the left side of the rat's brain. It shows the major components of the ascending gustatory pathways from the afferent inputs via the sensory branch of cranial nerve VII, via the chorda tympani, and via the taste afferents of IX and X, all of which enter the fasciculus solitarius, proceeding anteriorly to the parabrachial nucleus of the dorsal pons. Here, synaptic connections to the third-order neurons occur, leading to the thalamic, and ultimately the cortical, taste areas. The ventral taste pathway shows its projections to the lateral hypothalamus and ultimately the central nucleus of the amygdala and stria terminalis and its bed nucleus.

In view of the relationship of the ventral taste pathway to the hypothalamic and limbic structures, one is led to suppose that it is this projection that plays a major role in the motivational aspects of taste and food- and fluid-related behaviors. Further studies of these ventral systems should lead to further insights into the potency of certain specific tastes, such as sweetness, which readily serve as potent positive reinforcers for the learning of instrumental responses (viz., bar pressing or other locomotor responses). What distinguishes the normal mechanisms triggered by positive stimuli like sugar or saccharin as compared to the aversions toward quinine is a fundamental and basic question that is far from being understood in terms of its neural underpinnings. What characterizes the changes induced after learning and conditioning in which the sweetness of sugar can be converted to an aversion like that to quinine is another very pertinent and intriguing question. Its answer would begin to reveal how motivational factors not only control or affect learning but are modified by it. The further intriguing question that remains is how the primate taste system carries out such functions, which behaviorally seem very much the same from rat to man.

Acceptance or rejection makes up the final sequence of ingestion behavior, and its reflex components of chewing, licking, and swallowing are functional in decerebrate cats (Sherrington, 1917). After ablation of the cerebral hemispheres, Goltz (1892) had noted that dogs would immediately reject morsels of meat soaked in quinine, and decerebrates similarly reject such stimuli placed in their mouth (Sherrington, 1917; Miller & Sherrington, 1915). Macht (1951), a student of Bard, confirmed these observations in chronic decerebrate cats. Food soaked in either quinine sulfate, acetic acid, or sodium chloride was rejected at essentially the same threshold value as it was by normal cats. Dextrose-soaked food was not rejected by any animal, regardless of concentration. The caudal brain stem, therefore, possesses the reflexological basis of acceptance versus rejection.

This also appears to be true of the gustofacial reflex. Luciani (1917) mentioned that the expressive facial reactions to taste can be considered instinctive reflexes because they were involuntary, having been observed in an anencephalic fetus. Steiner (1973) also examined two anencephalic neonates who survived long enough for such testing. They too showed the characteristic orofacial reactions to taste stimuli. On postmortem, neither had any functional brain tissue above the level of the brain stem. The gustofacial reflex appears to be mediated by (a) the peripheral end organs for taste on the tongue and in the mouth and pharyngeal area; (b) afferent taste fibers in the chorda tympani (VII) and in the IXth and Xth cranial nerves; plus (c) the NTS, which evaluates the incoming signals; and (d) fiber connections to the motor nucleus of the VIIth nerve, by which activation of expressive and orolingual musculature takes place. No cortical components seem involved. A detailed experimental analysis of the behavioral capacities of the hindbrain of the rat follows in the next chapter.

Acknowledgments. The preparation of this manuscript was supported in part by NSF Grant BNS 78-16533.

Reference Notes

1. Jakinovich, W. *Taste perception of sugars by the gerbil.* Manuscript submitted for publication, 1981.
2. Norgren, R. Personal communication, 1981.

References

Andersen, H. T., Funakoshi, M., & Zotterman, Y. Electrophysiological investigation of the gustatory effect of various biological sugars. *Acta Physiol. Scand.*, 1962, *56*, 362-375.

Andersson, B., & Jewell, P. A. Studies on the thalamic relay for taste in the goat. *Journal of Physiology (London)*, 1957, *139*, 191-197.

Atema, J. Structures and functions of the sense of taste in the catfish. *Brain, Behavior and Evolution*, 1971, *4*, 273-294.

Beidler, L. M. Properties of chemoreceptors of tongue of rat. *Journal of Neurophysiology*, 1953, *16*, 595-607.

Benjamin, R. M. Absence of deficits in taste discrimination following cortical lesions as a function of the amount of pre-operative practice. *Journal of Comparative and Physiological Psychology*, 1959, *52*, 255-258.

Benjamin, R. M., & Burton, H. Projection of taste nerve afferents to anterior opercular-insular cortex in squirrel monkey (*Saimiri sciureus*). *Brain Research*, 1968, *7*, 221-231.

Berlyne, D. E. Arousal and reinforcement. In D. Levine (Ed.), *Nebraska Symposium on Motivation* (Vol. 15). Lincoln: University of Nebraska Press, 1967.

Berlyne, D. E. The reward-value of indifferent stimulation. In J. T. Tapp (Ed.), *Reinforcement and behavior*. New York: Academic Press, 1969.

Bernard, R. A., & Nord, S. G. A first-order synaptic relay for taste fibers in the pontine brainstem of the cat. *Brain Research*, 1971, *30*, 349-356.

Bernstein, I. L. Learned taste aversions in children receiving chemotherapy. *Science*, 1978, *200*, 1302-1303.

Biedenbach, M. A. Functional properties and projection area of cutaneous receptors in catfish. *Journal of Comparative Physiology*, 1973, *84*, 227-250.

Boudreau, J. C., & Alev, N. Classification of chemoresponsive tongue units of the cat geniculate ganglion. *Brain Research*, 1973, *54*, 157-175.

Box, B. M., & Mogenson, G. J. Alterations in ingestive behaviors after bilateral lesions of the amygdala in the rat. *Physiology and Behavior*, 1975, *15*, 679-688.

Braun, J. J. Gustatory neocortex: Functional commonalities with other sensory neocortical areas. *Proceedings of the 3rd annual meeting of the association for chemoreceptive sciences*, Sarasota, Fla., 1981.

Braun, J. J., & Kiefer, S. W. Preference-aversion functions for basic taste stimuli in rats lacking gustatory neocortex. *Bulletin of the Psychonomic Society*, 1975, *6*, 438-439.

Braun, J., Slick, T., & Lorden, J. Gustatory neocortex: Involvement in learning taste aversions. *Physiology and Behavior*, 1972, *9*, 637-641.

Burton, H., & Benjamin, R. M. Central projections of the gustatory system. In L. M. Beidler (Ed.), *Handbook of Sensory Physiology*, Vol. 4, *Chemical Senses, 2: Taste*. New York: Springer-Verlag, 1971.

Cabanac, M. Physiological role of pleasure. *Science*, 1971, *173*, 1103-1107.

Cabanac, M. Sensory pleasure. *Quarterly Review of Biology*, 1979, *54*, 1-29.

Cagan, R. H., & Maller, O. Taste of sugars: Brief exposure single-stimulus behavioral method. *Journal of Comparative and Physiological Psychology*, 1974, *87*, 47-55.

Cameron, A. T. The taste sense and the relative sweetness of sugars and other sweet substances. *Scientific report series 9*. New York: Sugar Research Foundation, 1947.

Capretta, P. J. Saccharin consumption under varied conditions of hunger drive. *Journal of Comparative and Physiological Psychology*, 1962, *55*, 656-660.

Car, A., Jean, A., & Roman, C. A pontine primary relay for ascending projections of the superior laryngeal nerve. *Experimental Brain Research*, 1975, *22*, 197-210.

Carpenter, J. A. Species differences in taste preferences. *Journal of Comparative and Physiological Psychology*, 1956, *49*, 139-144.

Davis, J. D. The effectiveness of some sugars in stimulating licking behavior in the rat. *Physiology and Behavior*, 1973, *11*, 39-45.

Davis, J. D., Collins, B. J., & Levine, M. W. Peripheral control of meal size: Interaction of gustatory stimulation and postingestional feedback. In D. Novin, W. Wyricka, & G. Bray (Eds.), *Hunger: Basic mechanisms and clinical implications*. New York: Raven Press, 1975.

Davis, J. D., & Levine, M. W. A model for the control of ingestion. *Psychological Review*, 1977, *84*, 379-412.

Desor, J. A., Maller, O., & Greene, L. S. Preference for sweet in humans: Infants, children and adults. In J. M. Weiffenbach (Ed.), *Taste and development, the genesis of sweet preference* (NIH Publication No. 77-1068). Bethesda, Md.: USDHEW, National Institute of Health, 1977.

Diamant, H., & Zotterman, Y. Has water a specific taste? *Nature*, 1959, *183*, 191-192.

Dua-Sharma, S., & Smutz, E. R. Taste acceptance in squirrel monkeys (*Saimiri sciureus*). *Chemical Senses and Flavor*, 1977, *2*, 341-352.

Faurion, A., Saito, S., & MacLeod, P. Sweet taste involves several distinct receptor mechanisms. *Chemical Senses and Flavor*, 1980, *5*, 107-121.

Frank, M. Response patterns of rat glossopharyngeal taste neurons. In D. A. Denton & J. P. Coghlan (Eds.), *Olfaction and taste, V*. New York: Academic Press, 1975.

Ganchrow, J., & Fisher, G. L. Two behavioral measures of the squirrel monkey's (*Saimiri sciureus*) taste for four concentrations of five sugars. *Psychological Reports*, 1968, *22*, 503-511.

Garcia, J. Tilting at the paper mills of academe. *American Psychologist*, 1981, *36*, 149-158.

Garcia, J., Hankins, W. G., & Rusiniak, K. W. Behavioral regulation of the milieu interne in man and rat. *Science*, 1974, *185*, 824-831.

Goltz, F. Der Hund ohne Grosshirm. *Pflügers Archiv*, 1892, *51*, 570.

Guttman, N. Operant conditioning, extinction and periodic reinforcement in relation to concentration of sucrose used as a reinforcing agent. *Journal of Experimental Psychology*, 1953, *46*, 213-224.

Hagstrom, E. C., & Pfaffmann, C. The relative taste effectiveness of different sugars for the rat. *Journal of Comparative and Physiological Psychology*, 1959, *52*, 259-261.

Halpern, B. P., & Nelson, L. M. Bulbar gustatory responses to anterior and to posterior tongue stimulation in the rat. *American Journal of Physiology*, 1965, *209*, 105-110.

Herrick, C. J. The central gustatory paths in the brains of bony fishes. *Journal of Comparative Neurology and Psychology*, 1905, *15*, 375-456.

Herrick, C. J. The brain of the tiger salamander, *Ambystoma tigrinum*. Chicago: University of Chicago Press, 1948.

Hulse, S. H. Licking behavior in rats in relation to saccharin concentration and shifts in fixed-ratio reinforcement. *Journal of Comparative and Physiological Psychology*, 1967, *64*, 478-484.

Jacobs, H. L., & Sharma, K. N. Taste versus calories: Sensory and metabolic signals in the control of food intake. *Annals of the New York Academy of Sciences*, 1969, *157*, 1084-1125.

Jakinovich, W. Stimulation of the gerbil's gustatory receptors by disaccharides. *Brain Research*, 1976, *110*, 481-490. (a)

Jakinovich, W. Stimulation of the gerbil's gustatory receptors by monosaccharides. *Brain Research*, 1976, *110*, 491-504. (b)

Jean, A., Car, A., & Roman, C. Comparison of activity in pontine versus medullary neurones during swallowing. *Experimental Brain Research*, 1975, *22*, 211-220.

Johnson, F. H. The secondary visceral-gustatory tract in the cat. *Anatomical Record*, 1964, *148*, 295.

Kemble, E. D., & Schwartzbaum, J. S. Reactivity to taste properties of solutions following amygdaloid lesions. *Physiology and Behavior*, 1969, *4*, 981-985.

Kemnitz, J. W., Gibber, J. R., Lindsay, K. A., & Brot, M. D. Preference for sweet and the regulation of caloric intake by *Macaca mulatta. American Society of Primatologists Abstracts*, 1981.

Kiefer, S., & Braun, J. Absence of differential associative responses to novel and familiar taste stimuli in rats lacking gustatory neocortex. *Journal of Comparative and Physiological Psychology*, 1977, *91*, 498-507.

LeMagnen, J. Le processus de discrimination par le rat blanc des stimuli sucres alimentaires et non alimentaires. *Journal de Physiologie (Paris)*, 1954, *46*, 414-418.

LeMagnen, J. Habits and food intake. In C. F. Code (Ed.), *Handbook of physiology*, Section 6: *Alimentary canal* (Vol. 1, *Control of food and water intake*). Washington, D.C.: American Physiological Society, 1967.

LeMagnen, J. Advances in studies of physiological control and regulation of food intake. In E. Stellar & J. M. Sprague (Eds.), *Progress in physiological psychology* (Vol. 4). New York: Academic Press, 1971.

Lorden, J. Effects of lesions of the gustatory neocortex on taste aversion learning in the rat. *Journal of Comparative and Physiological Psychology*, 1976, *90*, 665-679.

Luciani, L. *Human physiology: The sense organs* (Vol. 4, G. M. Holmes, Ed.; F. A. Welby, trans.). London: Macmillan, 1917.

Lucretius. *De rerum natura.* In W. J. Oates (Ed. and trans.), *The Stoic and Epicurian philosophers: The complete extant writings of Epicurus, Epictetus, Lucretius and Marcus Aurelius.* New York: Random House, 1940.

Macht, M. B. Subcortical localization of certain taste responses in the cat. *Federation Proceedings*, 1951, *10*, 88.

McMurray, T. M., & Snowdon, C. T. Sodium preferences and responses to sodium deficiency in rhesus monkeys. *Physiological Psychology*, 1977, *5*, 477-482.

Meiselman, H. L. The role of sweetness in the food preferences of young adults. In J. M. Weiffenbach (Ed.), *Taste and development: The genesis of sweet preference.* (NIH Publication No. 77-1068). Bethesda, Md.: USDHEW, National Institutes of Health, 1977.

Miller, F. R., & Sherrington, C. S. Some observations on the bucco-pharyngeal stage of reflex deglutition in the cat. *Quarterly Journal of Experimental Physiology*, 1915, *9*, 147-186.

Mook, D. G. Oral and postingestional determinants of the intake of various solutions in rats with esophageal fistulas. *Journal of Comparative and Physiological Psychology*, 1963, *56*, 645-659.

Morrison, S. D. Origins of anorexia in neoplastic disease. *American Journal of Clinical Nutrition*, 1978, *31*, 1104-1107.

Moskowitz, H. R. The psychology of sweetness. In H. L. Sipple & K. W. McNutt (Eds.), *Sugars in nutrition.* New York: Academic Press, 1974.

Moskowitz, H. R. Sensations, measurement and pleasantness: Confessions of a latent introspectionist. In J. M. Weiffenbach (Ed.), *Taste and development: The genesis of sweet preference.* (NIH Publication No. 77-1068). Bethesda, Md.: USDHEW, National Institutes of Health, 1977.

Moskowitz, H. W., Kumaraiah, V., Sharma, K. N., Jacobs, H. L., & Sharma, S. D. Cross-cultural differences in simple taste preferences. *Science,* 1975, *190,* 1217-1218.

Nachman, M., & Ashe, J. H. Effects of basolateral amygdala lesions on neophobia, learned taste aversions, and sodium appetite in rats. *Journal of Comparative and Physiological Psychology,* 1974, *87,* 622-643.

Nageotte, J. The pars intermedia or nervus intermedius of Wrisberg, and the bulbo-pontine gustatory nucleus in man. *Review of Neurology and Psychiatry,* 1906, *4,* 472-488.

Noma, A., Goto, J., & Sato, M. The relative taste effectiveness of sugars and sugar alcohols for the rat. *Kumamoto Medical Journal,* 1971, *24,* 1-9.

Norgren, R. Gustatory responses in the hypothalamus. *Brain Research,* 1970, *21,* 63-77.

Norgren, R. On the anatomical substrate for flavor. In D. Muller-Schwarze & M. M. Mozell (Eds.), *Chemical signals in vertebrates.* New York: Plenum Press, 1977.

Norgren, R., & Leonard, C. M. Taste pathways in rat brainstem. *Science,* 1971, *173,* 1136-1139.

Norgren, R., & Leonard, C. M. Ascending central gustatory pathways. *Journal of Comparative Neurology,* 1973, *150,* 217-238.

Norgren, R., & Pfaffmann, C. The pontine taste area in the rat. *Brain Research,* 1975, *91,* 99-117.

Nowlis, G. H., Braun, J. J., & Norgren, R. The central gustatory system: Ingestion and rejection functions after lesions. *Abstracts of the 6th International Conference of Physiology of Food and Fluid Intake,* 1977.

Nowlis, G. H., & Kessen, W. Human newborns differentiate differing concentrations of sucrose and glucose. *Science,* 1976, *191,* 865-866.

Pangborn, R. M. Individual variations in affective responses to taste stimuli. *Psychonomic Science,* 1970, *21,* 125-126.

Pfaffmann, C. Gustatory afferent impulses. *Journal of Cellular and Comparative Physiology,* 1941, *17,* 243-258.

Pfaffmann, C. The pleasures of sensation. *Psychological Review,* 1960, *67,* 253-268.

Pfaffmann, C. The sensory and motivating properties of the sense of taste. In M. R. Jones (Ed.), *Nebraska Symposium on Motivation* (Vol. 9). Lincoln: University of Nebraska Press, 1961.

Pfaffmann, C. de Gustibus. *American Psychologist,* 1965, *20,* 21-31.

Pfaffmann, C. de Gustibus. *Rockefeller University Review,* 1966, *4,* 12-20.

Pfaffmann, C. Phylogenetic origins of sweet sensitivity. In D. A. Denton & J. P. Coghlan (Eds.), *Olfaction and taste,* Vol. 5. New York: Academic Press, 1975.

Pfaffmann, C. Biological and behavioral substrates of the sweet tooth. In J. M. Weiffenbach (Ed.), *Taste and development: The genesis of sweet preference.* (NIH Publication No. 77-1068). Bethesda, Md.: USDHEW, National Institutes of Health, 1977.

Pfaffmann, C. Wundt's schema of sensory affect in the light of research on gustatory preferences. *Psychological Research*, 1980, *42*, 165-174.

Rhoton, A. L. Afferent connections of the facial nerve. *Journal of Comparative Neurology*, 1968, *133*, 89-100.

Richter, C. P. Total self-regulatory functions in animals and human beings. *Harvey Lectures*, 1942, *38*, 63-103.

Richter, C. P., & Campbell, K. H. Taste thresholds and taste preferences of rats for five common sugars. *Journal of Nutrition*, 1940, *20*, 31-46.

Ross, G. R. T. (Ed. and trans.), *Aristotle: De sensu and de memoria.* Cambridge, England: Cambridge University Press, 1906. (Originally published ca. 330 B.C.)

Roth, S. R., Schwartz, M., & Teitelbaum, P. Failure of recovered lateral hypothalamic rats to learn specific food aversions. *Journal of Comparative and Physiological Psychology*, 1973, *83*, 184-197.

Rozin, P. The use of characteristic flavorings in human culinary practice. In C. M. Apt (Ed.), *Flavor: Its chemical, behavioral and commercial aspects.* Boulder: Westview Press, 1978.

Salber, P., & Zucker, I. Absence of salt appetite in adrenalectomized and DOCA-treated hamsters. *Behavioral Biology*, 1974, *10*, 295-311.

Sato, M., Ogawa, H., & Yamashita, S. Response properties of macaque monkey chorda tympani fibers. *Journal of General Physiology*, 1975, *66*, 781-810.

Schneirla, T. C. A theoretical consideration of the basis for approach-withdrawal adjustments in behavior. *Psychological Bulletin*, 1939, *37*, 501-502.

Schneirla, T. C. An evolutionary and developmental theory of biphasic processes underlying approach and withdrawal. In M. R. Jones (Ed.), *Nebraska Symposium on Motivation* (Vol. 9). Lincoln: University of Nebraska Press, 1959.

Schneirla, T. C. Aspects of stimulation and organization in approach/withdrawal processes underlying vertebrate behavioral development. *Advances in Studies of Behavior*, 1965, *1*, 1-74.

Schwartzbaum, J. S., & Morse, J. Taste responsivity of amygdaloid units in behaving rabbit: A methodological report. *Brain Research Bulletin*, 1978, *3*, 131-141.

Schallenberger, R. S. Occurrence of various sugars in foods. In H. L. Sipple (Ed.), *Sugars in nutrition.* New York: Academic Press, 1974.

Sherrington, C. S. Reflexes elicitable in the cat from pinna vibrissae and jaws. *Journal of Physiology (London)*, 1917, *51*, 404-431.

Steiner, J. E. The gusto-facial response: Observation on normal and anencephalic newborn infants. In J. F. Bosmas (Ed.), *4th Symposium on oral sensation and perception.* Washington, D.C.: U.S. Government Printing Office, 1973.

Tateda, H., & Hidaka, I. Taste responses to sweet substances in rat. *Memoirs of the Faculty of Science, Kyushu University*, Series E, 1966, *4*, 137-149.

Teitelbaum, P. Sensory control of hypothalamic hyperphagia. *Journal of Comparative and Physiological Psychology*, 1955, *48*, 156-163.

Valenstein, E. S. Selection of nutritive and nonnutritive solutions under different conditions of need. *Journal of Comparative and Physiological Psychology*, 1967, *63*, 429-433.

White, A., Handler, P., & Smith, E. *Principles of biochemistry* (3rd ed.). New York: McGraw-Hill, 1964.

Wundt, W. *Grundzüge der physiologischen psychologie.* Leipzig: Englemann, 1874.

Yamamoto, T., Matsuo, R., & Kawamura, Y. Localization of cortical gustatory area in rats and its role in taste discrimination. *Journal of Neurophysiology*, 1980, *44*, 440-455.

Young, P. T. Food seeking, drive, affective process, and learning. *Psychological Review*, 1949, *56*, 98–121.

Young, P. T. The role of hedonic processes in motivation. In M. R. Jones (Ed.), *Nebraska Symposium on Motivation* (Vol. 3). Lincoln: University of Nebraska Press, 1955.

Young, P. T. Hedonic organization and regulation of behavior. *Psychological Review*, 1966, *73*, 59–86.

Zotterman, Y. The recording of the electrical response from human taste nerves. In L. M. Beidler (Ed.), *Handbook of Sensory Physiology, Vol. 4, Chemical Senses, 2: Taste*. New York: Springer-Verlag, 1971.

Chapter 4

Brain-Stem Control
of Ingestive Behavior

RALPH NORGREN and HARVEY GRILL

Hunger is a psychological construct, usually operationally defined as being directly proportional to hours of food deprivation (Silverstone, 1976), but assumed to be a neurophysiological reality. As with most psychological constructs, however, the neural substrates representing hunger have yielded slowly to neurophysiological analysis. This resistance to reductionistic assaults stems from oversimplifying the problem in the first place, and then trying to locate the oversimplification within the brain. Although neither oversimplification has been eliminated, both are now recognized, and this recognition has diverted scientific energy from the frontal assault on the hypothalamus initiated in Ranson's laboratory and led by John Brobeck and his colleagues almost 40 years ago (Brobeck, Tepperman, & Long, 1943; Anand & Brobeck, 1951; Hetherington & Ranson, 1940) into subsidiary investigations aimed at deciphering hunger variables and integrating psychological concepts into neurophysiological analysis.

Eating is just one facet, albeit an essential one, of a continuous physiological process of regulating energy balance. Most aspects of energy balance regulation consist of controlling the body's use and distribution of its energy stores. These functions involve the endocrine and autonomic nervous systems, and their separation from other homeostatic mechanisms such as water and electrolyte balance or thermoregulation reflects more the interests and convenience of physiologists than the logic of physiology. Behavior plays a relatively minor role in these processes, although the behaviors associated with hibernation and hoarding are obvious adaptations for conserving energy. Where behavior becomes essential in the energy balance equation is in adding new resources. Even when an organism exists in a limitless food supply, such as a rat in a grain elevator or a laboratory animal colony, for that matter, it must ingest food in appropriate amounts in order to remain healthy. For the vast majority of animals, of course, food is not in constant supply, but must be discovered periodically and often competed for. Within this context, the motivation to eat, hunger, becomes a heuristic, perhaps unavoidable, adjuvant in accounting for energy balance.

Most of the processes required for a regulated physiological system, particularly a homeostatic one such as energy balance, can be conceived in reflex terminology if a reference value or two is admitted. Indeed, many aspects of feeding behavior could be accounted for by a sequence of predetermined stimulus–response relationships. Conceptually, the sequence of events that falls under the rubric of hunger is not complex. First, the organism must detect a food (energy) deficit. Next, it must organize and sustain behavior that increases the likelihood of contacting food. Once the substance is contacted, it must be assessed to determine its suitability as a foodstuff. If it is satisfactory, it must be ingested. Finally, if a surplus of food is available, the organism must detect repletion and cease ingestion. Although the process is conceptually simple, it must be pointed out that none of the steps in the sequence can be reconstructed at the neurophysiological level and several are poorly elaborated at the behavioral level. For instance, rats given a choice between relatively pure sources of amino acids, carbohydrates, and fats will select them in proportions that provide a balanced diet (Richter, 1943; Richter, Holt, & Barelare, 1938; Rozin, 1968). Even for a rat, food has several dimensions.

In addition, this homeostatic model does not integrate such supraordinate initiating conditions as habits, circadiam rhythms, food availability, or incentives, which do not arise from metabolic signals (LeMagnen, 1967; Fitzsimons, 1972; Mogenson & Phillips, 1976; Pfaffmann, Chapter 3, this volume). Given a surfeit, some or all of these conditions result in eating in anticipation of need. These nonregulatory initiating events must be sensitive to metabolic feedback, lest the animal become obese, but the time course of the feedback could be on the order of days (body weight or long-term regulation) rather than minutes or hours (meal-to-meal or short-term regulation). Some role for nonregulatory factors in the initiation of feeding or drinking cannot be denied, but their importance vis-à-vis deficit signals continues to be debated (Toates, 1979). In the discussion that follows it is assumed, although not without trepidation, that the later stages of the hunger process—identification, ingestion, and satiation—are subserved by the same neural mechanisms regardless of the provenience of the initiating events. This is not to say that the initiating events do not influence subsequent aspects—a rotten apple discarded by a midnight nosher might well be consumed after a 48-hour fast (Norgren, 1978). The nature of the initiating events probably influences food-seeking behavior even more. In some circumstances, nonregulatory initiating events and food-seeking behavior might not be distinguishable. An animal patrolling its home range will attend to cues related to a variety of life processes. It is not necessarily just hunting or defending territory or seeking a mate (McFarland, 1977).

By embedding hunger in the homeostatic process of energy balance, we temporarily circumvent these intimations of complexity. Only sustained food-seeking behavior appears to require neural mechanisms that differ from the reflex model. Even here some psychologists maintain that a reflex model can be invoked to account for sustained behavior unless the behavior can be experimentally disconnected from any direct relationship with food seeking (Teitelbaum, 1977). The usual criterion for this condition is the interpolation of an operant response rewarded by access to food, but otherwise unrelated to food-seeking behavior. This is a restrictive criterion because it denies motivation to animals that cannot learn an operant. It also emphasizes food-finding behavior, the most varied and most variable aspect of the sequence, at the expense of the other aspects—deficit detection, identification, ingestion, and satiation—which do not vary as much within and between species (Craig, 1918).

The neural substrates of hunger, however, cannot be separated easily from neural mechanisms controlling other aspects of the process of feeding behavior or from the remainder of the energy balance system. For 20 years or more, the hypothalamus was considered to contain the neural substrates for hunger and satiety; the former in the lateral hypothalamic area, the latter in the ventromedial nucleus (Grossman, 1975; Stellar, 1954). Initially it was assumed that the effects of hypothalamic lesions and stimulation on feeding behavior represented secondary sequelae of direct disruption of the hypothalamopituitary axis or the autonomic nervous system. Subsequently this concept was set aside, first because the removal of the pituitary did not block the effects (Hetherington & Ranson, 1942) and later because the effects of lateral hypothalamic stimulation fit the psychological definition of hunger— satiated animals would work to obtain food under the influence of electrical stimulation of the lateral hypothalamus (Coons, 1964; Coons, Levak, & Miller, 1965; Miller, 1957). Research focused upon the interrelations between the hypothalamic feeding centers, their relation to reward systems, and the existence and possible function of intrahypothalamic receptors for glucose and free fatty acids in the detection of energy deficits (Anand, Chhina, Sharma, Dua, & Singh, 1964; Hoebel, 1969; Hoebel & Teitelbaum, 1962; LeMagnen, Devos, Guadilliere, Louis-Sylvestre, & Tallon, 1973; Margules & Olds, 1962; Oomura,

1976; Oomura, Ooyama, Yamamoto, & Naka, 1967). Little attention was afforded the interaction of behavioral, endocrine, and autonomic systems in the hypothalamus, or to the involvement of the remainder of the brain in the regulation of energy balance. If not theoretically, at least functionally, the hypothalamus was considered the neural focus of all facets of the hunger-feeding process. This viewpoint can be summarized as the single integrator hypothesis (Grill, 1980).

The hegemony of the hypothalamus over the control of feeding behavior was broken by two seemingly disparate developments. First came the discovery of the long ascending catecholaminergic systems that pass through the hypothalamus and innervate not only large areas of the limbic system, but also the basal ganglia and the neocortex (Fuxe, 1965; Lindvall & Bjorklund, 1974; Ungerstedt, 1971a). The demonstration by Ungerstedt (1971b) that the destruction of the dopaminergic system arising from the substantia nigra and the ventral tegmental area reproduced the behavioral deficits of the lateral hypothalamic syndrome without damage to the hypothalamus led to a substantial reassessment of the role of intrinsic hypothalamic mechanisms in the control of feeding behavior and energy balance. At approximately the same time, hypothalamic lesions that eliminate eating also were shown to induce profound neglect of sensory stimuli in a number of modalities (Marshall, Levitan, & Stricker, 1976; Marshall, Turner, & Teitelbaum, 1971; Marshall & Teitelbaum, 1974). Subsequently, pharmacological lesions of the dopaminergic systems in the midbrain reproduced not only the deficits in feeding behavior characteristic of the lateral hypothalamic syndrome, but the sensory neglect as well. These observations implied that some aspects of the apparent hypothalamic control over feeding behavior resulted from secondary effects on processing of sensory information that depends upon neural systems ramifying throughout the forebrain.

At the same time, however, a series of theoretical and experimental developments were beginning to provide the outlines of an explanation for the hypothalamic control of consummatory behavior based upon descending rather than ascending neural systems. Drawing upon ethological theories and classical hierarchical concepts of Jacksonian neurology, Glickman and Schiff (1967) proposed a mechanism for biological reward that consisted of descending hypothalamic activity selectively facilitating subunits preprogrammed in the lower brain stem and spinal cord. At about the same time, Flynn and his colleagues began publishing a series of studies demonstrating that electrical stimulation of the hypothalamus that elicited attack behavior from cats did, in fact, facilitate reflex-like behaviors that were an integral part of the attack sequence (Flynn, 1972; Flynn, Edwards, & Bandler, 1971). In addition, a peripheral nerve, the vagus—the major parasympathetic conduit to the thoracic and abdominal viscera—was implicated in the elaboration of hypothalamic control over feeding behavior. After sectioning of the cervical vagus, stimulation at lateral hypothalamic sites that elicited feeding behavior ceased to have that effect and would no longer support intracranial self-stimulation (Ball, 1974). Section of the subdiaphragmatic vagus blocked the hyperphagia that is commonly observed after bilateral lesions of the hypothalamic ventromedial nucleus (Powley & Opshal, 1974). Beginning with these observations, Powley recently assembled a variety of evidence to support an explanation of hypothalamic hyperphagia as the result of an exaggeration of normal gastrointestinal reflexes, particularly the neurally mediated release of insulin (Powley, 1977).

These separate sets of discoveries—ascending catecholaminergic systems and the descending influence of the hypothalamus—changed accepted ideas about the neural basis of hunger and motivated behavior in general. First, they permitted a more realistic estimate of the complexity of the neural mechanisms required to integrate even comparatively simple behavioral sequences. Second, they raised the distinct possibility that some of the peculiar phenomena resulting from lesions or stimulation in the hypothalamus might be the fortuitous result of contiguous neural systems that are not necessarily functionally related. Third, some aspects of the hypothalamic control over behavior relevant to regulatory physiology may result from the normal response of other areas of the brain to the altered autonomic or endocrine status of the organism. The autonomic and endocrine functions of the hypothalamus and limbic system, if not fully understood, remain intact. The behavioral functions previously ascribed to the hypothalamus, on the other hand, clearly required the participation of many other neural areas as well. This third point in particular seemed implicit in Hess' interpretation of his own hypothalamic stimulation studies (Hess, 1958), but was overlooked in the ensuing infatuation with motivational centers in the brain.

Without the hypothalamus as a theoretical focus, research concerned with the neural control of feeding behavior dealt less with identifying substrates for hunger per se and more with the separate aspects of the process. The metabolic indices of an energy deficit are being cataloged and documented with emphasis on peripheral rather than central receptors (Friedman & Stricker, 1976; Novin & Oomura, 1980). At the other end of the process, putative satiety signals also have increased in number and complexity (Smith, Chapter 5, this volume). Our own work has dealt with identifying the neural systems that mediate the intermediate steps in the hunger process, the identification and ingestion or rejection of food. By tacit agreement, the neural systems that sustain, direct, and coordinate the appetitive phase of food seeking, between energy deficit and food identification, with its requirements for mnemonic, cognitive, and perceptual activity, await more complete analysis of those aspects of the process that are more directly related to afferent and efferent neural mechanisms and thus may be more accessible with the present neuroscience armamentarium.

Ingestive Behavior

In studying feeding behavior, psychologists most often concern themselves with the beginning and end of the cycle—the factors that initiate feeding and those that terminate it. The actual ingestion process usually is inferred by measuring the amount of food consumed. In some cases the inference of ingestion becomes twice removed; the animal is simply weighed before and after an ingestion test or, if an operant response is required to obtain access to food, only the number of responses is counted. Some components of ingestion, primarily mastication and swallowing, have been examined electromyographically and neurophysiologically (Chase & McGinty, 1970; Doty, 1968; Hiiemae & Ardran, 1968; Lund & Dellow, 1973; Sessle & Hannam, 1976, Sessle & Kenny, 1973; Storey, 1968a, 1968b; Weijs & Dantuma, 1975), but usually as mechanical processes without functional context. In addition to inferring ingestion based on some index of consumption, virtually all investigators defined satiation as the cessation of consumption and used similar indices. This implies the inhibition of ingestion, but during the process of consuming food, the animal has another option—active rejection of the contents of the oral cavity.

We became interested in the behavior that constitutes ingestion and rejection of stimuli already within the oral cavity, because these sequences represent the final behavioral steps not only in the process of obtaining food (restoring energy balance), but also in the process of obtaining water and electrolytes (restoring hydromineral balance). The same behaviors serve several regulatory systems, and thus must be influenced by a variety of hormonal and neural signals germane to these homeostatic systems. Indeed, some change in these internal monitors of homeostasis reliably reverses the behavioral response to the same stimulus from avid ingestion to active rejection or vice versa. For example, after a few days on a diet lacking sodium, rats will consume many milliliters of a strong NaCl solution (.5–1.0 M) that they normally reject after one or a few licks. The analysis of these behavioral end points of motivation and their neural substrates represents a requisite step in comprehending the physiology of hunger.

For both practical and theoretical considerations, gustatory stimuli provide a useful probe for investigating ingestive behavior. Although gustatory afferent activity is not necessary to elicit feeding behavior, it is sufficient. Three easily specifiable stimuli—water, sucrose in water, and quinine in water—provide rudimentary control over ingestion and rejection behavior that responds to standard manipulations of water and energy balance regulation. If NaCl is added, you obtain sensory control of electrolyte balance as well. As long as extremes of deprivation or stimulus concentration are avoided, the behavioral effects of these stimuli are quite reliable. If water deprived, an animal will choose water in preference to sucrose; if food deprived, sucrose to water. In either case, quinine will be avoided. Water, of course, is the only adequate stimulus to correct dehydration. While not an adequate long-term diet, in the absence of other sensory cues, rats respond to sucrose as a food (Mook, 1974).

Not only are gustatory stimuli chemically specified in a behaviorally active form, but also the neuroanatomical basis for this afferent information has been defined, at least in the brain stem (Norgren, 1977). To a degree, the gustatory afferent system is separable from the bulk of the trigeminal system, which in conjunction with the olfactory system provides the intraoral sensory information that characterizes more complex foods. Gustatory afferent axons travel in the VIIth, IXth, and Xth cranial nerves and synapse in the rostral one third of the nucleus of the solitary tract. A relatively small contingent of trigeminal somatosensory axons also reaches the solitary nucleus, though not exclusively in the gustatory zone; but the vast majority, of course, terminate in the principal and spinal trigeminal nuclei (Astrom, 1953; Beckstead & Norgren, 1979; Torvik, 1956). Gustatory information relates almost exclusively to ingestion or to the regulatory systems within which ingestive behavior is embedded. In rodents, at least, trigeminal sensory information functions in a variety of behaviors, such as grooming, exploration, and care of the young, in addition to its role in monitoring the quality of food. A degree of anatomical separation between the two systems affords an opportunity to analyze afferent neural systems intimately related to the one behavioral function, the decision whether to ingest or reject the contents of the oral cavity.

The practical considerations for using gustatory stimulation for examining ingestive behavior involve stimulus delivery and removal. We wanted to examine ingestive behavior in a situation that did not require any appetitive or food-seeking behavior from the preparation. First, an animal that must seek food can also avoid it. We wanted to examine both ingestion and rejection. Second, an animal that will not seek food may nevertheless ingest it when it is placed in the mouth. Shortly after large bilateral lesions of the lateral hypothalamus, rats actively reject food placed in their mouths. Recent observations indicate that the rejection responses of first-stage lateral hypothalamic rats can be ameliorated by deprivation (Grill & Fluharty, 1981). Somewhat later, as the recovery process begins, they still do not voluntarily seek food, but ingest it once it is in their mouth (Teitelbaum & Epstein, 1962; Norgren, Note 1). Chronically decerebrate cats are completely aphagic and adipsic, but Bard and Macht (1958; Macht, 1951) reported main-taining such preparations for many months by placing small cubes of liver in their mouths. Even acute decerebrate cats exhibit elements of ingestion and rejection (Miller & Sherrington, 1916).

Using chronically implanted cheek catheters (Figure 4-1), it is pos-sible to deliver calibrated amounts of a fluid stimulus into the oral cavity, and subsequently dilute it away, without active participation by the animal. The version of this system used in our experiments em-ployed two intraoral catheters, one in either cheek, positioned just rostral to the first maxillary molar with the other end anchored to the top of the skull. Polyethylene tubes extend from the catheters to a swivel in the roof of the circular cage. These tubes serve as guides for the stimulus delivery tubes, which are designed to protrude approxi-mately 1 mm beyond the intraoral opening of the catheters. In this way the stimulus delivery tubes can be changed in a matter of seconds without disturbing the animal. Normally, one catheter is used for sapid stimuli, the other for water rinse. Stimuli can be delivered at any rate that does not overwhelm the animal's ability to respond, but we have limited ourselves to three paradigms—discrete trials of .05 ml each, continuous infusion of 1.0 ml over 1 minute, and continuous infusion at the same rate but with the volume determined by the animal. During a test, the orofacial responses of the animal to the fluid stimuli are videotaped via a mirror mounted beneath the plexiglas floor of the observation cage (Figure 4-2). Subsequent frame-by-frame analysis (16.7 msec/frame) of the behavior permits a detailed description of the

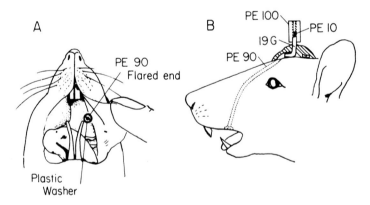

Figure 4-1. Diagram of the intraoral catheter. The intraoral end is placed just rostral to the first maxillary molar. The tubing is led out subcutaneously to the skull and secured to a short piece of 19-gauge (19 G) stainless steel tubing with dental acrylic. PE 10, 90, and 100 are standard sizes of medical grade polyethylene tubing. (A) Ventral view. (B) Lateral view. (Reprinted with permission from Phillips & Norgren, 1970.)

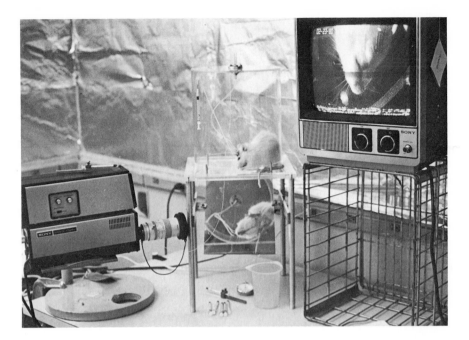

Figure 4-2. Apparatus for videotaping orofacial responses to sapid stimuli injected into the mouth via chronic intraoral catheters. Because a rat's mouth is located on the ventral side of its head, taping is done from a mirror located beneath the plexi-glass floor of the cage. The view thus obtained is demonstrated on the video moni-tor in the upper right-hand corner of the figure.

response components and their duration, frequency, magnitude, and sequencing.

In our initial experiments (Grill & Norgren, 1978c), we examined the responses of normal rats to discrete infusions of four different concentrations of sucrose, sodium chloride, HCl, and quinine HCl, plus water. Each stimulus trial was preceded and followed by two water rinses. Within an ascending concentration series, individual infusions of stimulus or rinse occurred 30–45 sec after the cessation of the previous response. At the end of a concentration series, the catheters were flushed with air and 10 minutes elapsed prior to beginning the next series. The responses elicited by sapid stimuli were constructed from stereotyped orofacial and whole-body response components that were highly consistent within and between rats. The response to water, on the other hand, varied considerably from trial to trial and from rat to rat. In about one third of the trials, .05 ml of water evoked no noticeable response. After a few such trials, water could be seen pooled up between the lips and eventually several drops might fall to the cage floor.

In the remainder of the trials, water evoked brief irregular bouts consisting of one or two components of the ingestion sequence.

The Ingestion Sequence

Sucrose, sodium, and hydrochloric acid each elicited an orofacial response made up of three distinct components: mouth movements, tongue protrusions, and lateral tongue movements. The magnitude and duration of the lateral tongue movements following Na and HCl were greater than those following sucrose, but otherwise the responses to the different chemicals did not differ in form or sequence. For this reason we will describe only the response to sucrose in detail. The initial behavioral responses to an intraoral infusion of sucrose are rhythmic low-amplitude movements of the mandible occurring at a rate of approximately 6.6 per second (Figure 4-3). The mouth opens maximally within one video frame (<17 msec), remains open one more frame, then remains closed for approximately 116 msec before starting the cycle again. Following the rhythmic mouth movement, tongue protrusions begin at a rate of 8.8 per second. The tongue protrudes to

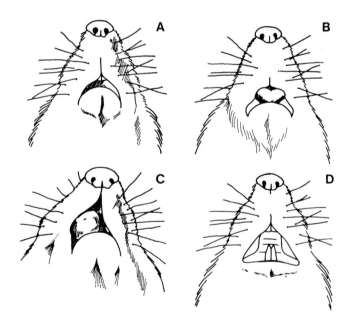

Figure 4-3. The lexicon of four orofacial response components elicited by sapid stimuli injected directly into the oral cavity. The figures are traced from single video frames and represent the maximal amplitude of each of the components. (A) Mouth movement. (B) Tongue protrusion. (C) Lateral tongue movement. (D) Gape. (Reprinted with permission from Grill & Norgren, 1978c.)

cover the upper incisors, but remains centered on the midline. Protrusion and retraction requires 50 msec, after which the jaw remains closed for an additional 65 msec (Figure 4-3). The tongue protrusion is not merely added onto a normal mouth movement, because the total period for a tongue protrusion (116 msec) is less than that of a mouth movement, and the timing of the individual subcomponents also differs. When the response continues beyond an initial bout of mouth movement and tongue protrusions, the next behavior usually is one or several lateral tongue movements. As the tongue emerges, it pushes the upper lip laterally, then retracts closer to the angle of the mouth (Figure 4-3). Lateral tongue movements occur singly on either side of the mouth with a variable duration (85–215 msec) or in pairs of equal duration. The second lateral movement of a pair always occurs on the opposite side of the mouth after a delay of 80–90 sec. The initial sequence of mouth movements, tongue protrusions, and lateral tongue movements is almost invariant. The concentration of the stimulus has relatively little influence on the duration of the initial mouth movement and tongue protrusion bouts, but the lateral tongue protrusions and total duration of the response increase with increasing stimulus concentration. After the initial fixed sequence, the three components reoccur in no apparent order until the response ceases. In virtually all trials, the animal remains quiet throughout the response, which then ceases abruptly and does not reappear. Within this restricted testing environment, we consider this highly stereotypic response to be an ingestion sequence. As long as these components constitute the behavior elicited by an intraoral fluid stimulus, many milliliters (we stop testing at 20) can be infused without any fluid wetting the lips, much less dripping on the cage floor. Nevertheless, an electromyographic analysis is necessary to establish the relation between these response components and swallowing. Such an analysis currently is in progress (Travers & Norgren, Note 2).

The Rejection Response

If the responses to sucrose, sodium, and hydrochloric acid are remarkably similar to each other, the responses elicited by quinine could not be more different. At lower concentrations (3×10^{-6} and 3×10^{-5} M QHCl) some elements of the ingestive response occur, but beginning at 3×10^{-5} M and more dramatically at higher concentrations, the response changes form. An orofacial component, the gape, initiates the response to quinine at higher concentration (Figure 4-3). The mandible drops rapidly (1 frame) revealing lower incisors. Concomitantly the angle of the lips is retracted and the upper lip elevated, producing a large triangular opening that can be held for as long as 83 msec. Gapes occur in bursts of 2–6 with intergape intervals of 83–115 msec. It should be noted that gapes differ in appearance, frequency, and duration from yawns.

The other major difference between the response to the ingestion stimuli and to quinine is movement. Aside from the orofacial activity, rats exhibit no consistent movement in response to intraoral sucrose, sodium, or hydrochloric acid. After a 50-μl infusion of strong quinine, however, rats gape a few times and then engage in a stereotyped sequence of whole-body responses (Figure 4-4). After the initial gapes, rats first chin rub on the substrate with a forward motion, then shake their head by rapidly rotating it around the long axis of the body. Next they wash their vibrassae and perioral region with their front paws, then rapidly flail their paws beside their heads, and finally rub their paws backward and forward on the substrate. At lower concentrations (3×10^{-5} M), usually only gaping occurs, but at higher concentrations, the full sequence appears and always in the same order. We consider this sequence of behaviors to be a rejection response because after only a few trials the animal's muzzle and paws are wet and the cage floor covered with drops of fluid. Nevertheless, it will be interesting to determine whether any swallowing occurs in conjunction with these behaviors, and if so, whether any of the sapid stimuli reaches the gut.

Given these admittedly contrived circumstances—fluid stimuli and the absence of food-seeking behavior—ingestion and rejection behavior are constructed from a lexicon of stereotypic subcomponents. Although they vary somewhat in duration and amplitude, the form of the sub-

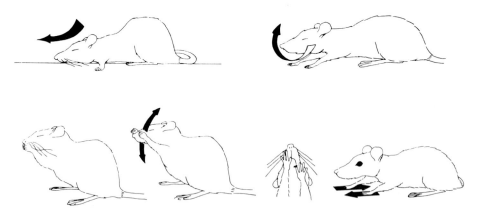

Figure 4-4. The whole-body lexicon following gapes after an intraoral injection of a strong quinine solution. Beginning at the top left, the rat first rubs its muzzle on the substrate, then shakes its head rapidly by rotating it from side to side around the long axis of the body. Subsequently it rears on its hind legs, washes the perioral region with its paws, then rapidly shakes its paws beside the head. Finally, it returns to a quadrupedal posture and rubs its forepaws back and forth on the substrate.

components and their sequencing remains the same regardless of the eliciting stimulus. This can be demonstrated graphically by using a taste aversion paradigm. Using a standard consumption test, a water-deprived animal is presented with a normally preferred, but relatively novel, sapid stimulus. After consuming it for a while, the animal is subjected to any of a variety of conditions (drug injection, irradiation, rotation) designed to induce visceral malaise, to make it "sick." In many instances, one such pairing of taste and "sickness" is sufficient to eliminate consumption of that sapid stimulus when it is offered subsequently, but leaves water intake and intake of other sapid chemicals nearly normal (Ashe & Nachman, 1980). When this paradigm—a single intraperitoneal injection of LiCl after a few trials of .05 ml of .3 M sucrose solution— was used with intraoral infusions, the normal ingestive sequence elicited by sapid sucrose was converted into a virtual replica of the response elicited by strong quinine (Grill, 1975). In other words, the component lexicon may be inflexible, and the sequencing of components largely predetermined, but the eliciting stimulus need not be fixed.

Our observations of the components of ingestion and rejection behavior in the rats recall the more extensive behavioral component lexicons derived from field observations by ethologists (Hinde, 1970; Tinbergen, 1951). At least in their earlier formulations, however, ethologists felt that these irreducible behavior components could be sequenced in different orders for use in a variety of behavioral circumstances, in much the same way that letters of the alphabet (or perhaps more appropriately, syllables) are used to construct words. In our experimental situation, the number of degrees of freedom available for sequencing elements seemed much more limited. Although limits probably do exist governing the possible combinations of behavior elements, some recent observations indicate that the testing procedure restricts these boundaries even further.

In our standard "taste reactivity test" (discrete infusions of .05 ml each), sucrose, sodium, and HCl elicit nearly identical responses. In standard consumption tests, however, sucrose and weak sodium are preferred to water, whereas strong salt (>.5 M) and all concentrations of HCl are avoided when possible. We cite this finding as an indication that preference and aversion are not synonymous with ingestion and rejection. Since we first documented the lexicon of ingestion and rejection, we have also altered the taste reactivity test to increase the scope of behavioral situations to which it is applicable and reduce time spent in data analysis (Berridge, Grill, & Norgren, 1981). One major change has been to substitute continuous infusion for discrete trials. Typically, 1 ml of a stimulus is infused over 1 minute during continuous videotaping. With frame-by-frame analysis, this method would vastly increase data analysis, but because we now know the lexicon, the behavioral components can be scored while viewing the tape in slow motion. In

these circumstances, the responses to sapid stimuli begin to differentiate (Figure 4-5). Glucose elicits a standard ingestion sequence (the
chemicals vary from previous standards because the objective of the

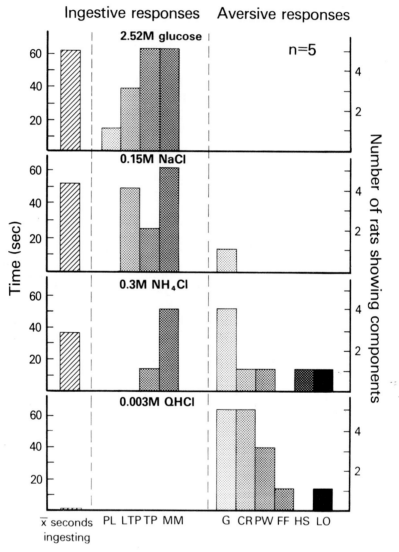

Figure 4-5. Response components observed from slow motion videotapes during
continuous infusions of different sapid stimuli (1.0 ml in 1.0 minute). Response
categories: PW, paw licking; LTP, lateral tongue protrusion; TP, tongue protrusion;
MM, mouth movements; G, gape; CR, chin rub; PW, paw wipes; FF, forelimb flailing; HS, head shakes; LO, locomotion. Ingestion time is the total seconds of stimulus consumption. (Reprinted with permission from Berridge, Grill, & Norgren,
1981.)

experiment is quite different), but NaCl elicits an occasional gape and NH₄Cl quite a few. The form of the behavioral components remained the same, but in a somewhat more realistic test situation—rats often drink at least 1 ml in a single bout—the sequencing of the components may be more flexible (Berridge et al., 1981).

Chronic Decerebrate and Thalamic Rats

This analysis of the responses elicited by sapid stimuli obviously does not exhaust the behavioral possibilities for ingestion or rejection, even in the rat. Lapping, gnawing, nibbling, and mastication serve similar functions and presumably are constructed from a lexicon of subcomponents as well. The intent of this analysis was to examine one form of ingestion and rejection behavior that mimics the final sequences of the process of obtaining food. Since these behaviors are the end point of the process, all the other aspects must influence this final common path. By isolating the neural substrates for these consummatory behaviors, we have a point to begin connecting to the neural systems subserving other aspects of the hunger process.

Although hunger was invested in the hypothalamus, or more recently, perhaps in the limbic forebrain, serious investigators never proposed that the motor components of ingestion were located in the diencephalon. Most sensory information relevant to eating enters the brain through cranial nerves terminating in the medulla and pons. All of the motor neurons necessary for ingestion are located in the same two areas. The forebrain hunger system functioned to assess energy deficits, organize food-seeking behavior, and decide whether to ingest or reject food and to terminate ingestion once it had started. Except for Flynn's analysis of the mechanisms controlling attack behavior in cats, the process of translating all these forebrain hunger functions into actual behavior generated by the hindbrain usually was left vague. Even Flynn's hypothesis of hypothalamic facilitation of hindbrain patterned reflexes maintained the control of the behavior in the forebrain (Flynn, 1972).

Because the taste reactivity test does not presuppose appetitive behavior, it can be used to test the hypothesis that forebrain mechanisms orchestrate the ingestive behavior generated by the hindbrain. In addition to neurologically normal rats, the first series of investigations utilized two chronic preparations with gross transections of the neuraxis. The thalamic rat has virtually all telencephalic tissue removed in a one-stage aspiration, leaving the diencephalon relatively intact (Figure 4-6). Hypothalamic and, in most cases, some preoptic connections to and from the hindbrain are not disturbed. The decerebrate preparation has a transection beginning just rostral to the superior colliculus and ending in the anterior half of the interpeduncular fossa just posterior to the

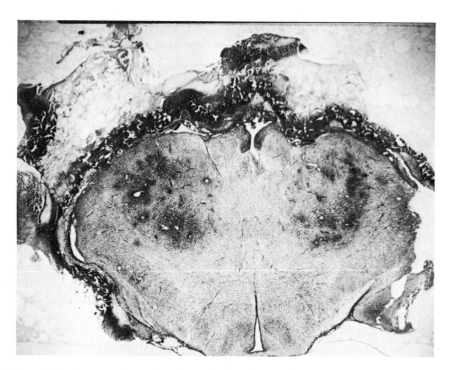

Figure 4-6. A coronal section through the brain of a thalamic rat preparation (Cresylecht violet stain). Neocortex, hippocampus, amygdala, and the basal ganglia were removed by aspiration 20 days prior to sacrifice. Note the extensive retrograde degeneration in the ventrobasal complex of the dorsal thalamus. The hypothalamus, on the other hand, appears grossly normal. (Reprinted with permission from Grill & Norgren, 1978d.)

mammillary bodies (Figure 4-7). This procedure also can be performed in a single stage, but the survival rate improves markedly (up to 80%) by performing lateral hemisections at 2-week intervals (Grill & Norgren, 1978d). With adequate nursing care, both of these preparations survive for several months, or until the experiment is completed.

Although neither preparation spontaneously eats or drinks, on other behavioral measures they differ substantially from one another, as well as from normal animals (Grill & Norgren, 1978b). Relatively simple response sequences, such as righting, hind-limb stepping, and paw placing, do not differ noticeably from the responses of intact animals, nor does grooming elicited by water on the fur or orientation to sound. The chronic decerebrate rat responds sluggishly if at all in situations that require sustained muscle tonus, such as hanging on a vertical wire mesh or from their forepaws. Thalamic preparations have nearly normal muscle tonus, rhythmic vibrissae movement, and responses to noxious stimulation (tail pinch) (Figure 4-8). Thalamic animals are more active

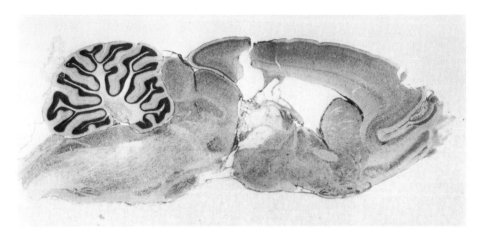

Figure 4-7. A sagittal section through the brain of a representative decerebrate rat preparation (Cresylecht violet stain). This animal survived 37 days after the second stage of the decerebration. The plane of section was highly similar in all rats. The tissue posterior to the transection appeared normal in the light microscope. In many preparations the space normally occupied by the thalamus and hippocampus was replaced by a fluid-filled cyst. (Reprinted with permission from Grill & Norgren, 1978d.)

than normal rats both in an open field and in their home cages. Decerebrate preparations, on the other hand, remain virtually motionless unless stimulated. When they do respond to stimulation, the behavior is appropriate and well coordinated, but usually ceases abruptly shortly after the stimulation (Figure 4-9). For example, a decerebrate rat suddenly sprayed with water (to reduce hypothermia) might leap from its cage and run away in an apparently normal manner, but stop in its tracks within a second or two and initiate no further locomotion unless prodded. Decerebrate rats exhibit one "spontaneous" behavioral sequence—grooming. The behavior is effective (they maintain clean fur) and grossly normal, in that they begin with their head, then clean down one side, switch to the other side, and end with the tail. A videotape analysis, however, did reveal differences in the execution of some subcomponents (Freed & Grill, 1979). The thalamic rat, grossly normal in so many ways, exhibits completely ineffective grooming behavior. The movements are relatively normal, but misdirected such that the paws and teeth seldom contact the fur.

Thalamic rats also are abnormal in the tast reactivity test. They are utterly aphagic and adipsic, and—at least after tube feeding—they actively reject any fluid entering the oral cavity. Except for its duration, the response to water or weak sucrose is identical to that for the strongest quinine. The components of the response are a subset of those in

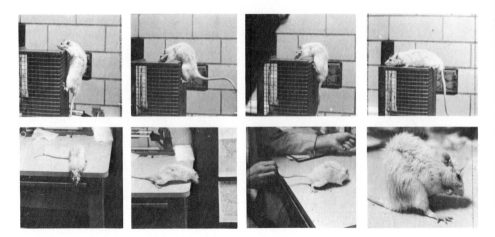

Figure 4-8. Behavioral capacity of the chronic thalamic rat preparation. Cage climbing is brisk and well coordinated (upper panel). Tactile stimulation from the snout and vibrissae provides sufficient information to prevent walking off a table edge (first and second frame, lower panel). Tail pinch elicits forward motion. Grooming is spontaneous but misdirected. During grooming the head of a thalamic preparation is held lower than it is by either a normal or decerebrate preparation. (Reprinted with permission from Grill & Norgren, 1978b.)

the normal rejection response, but the sequencing is different and more variable (Figure 4-10). Initially the animal gapes while rearing to a bipedal posture. While still on its hind legs, it will wipe at its muzzle with a paw or begin washing its face. After washing its muzzle, the thalamic rat chin rubs several times, then paw pushes. Unlike the response in normal or decerebrate preparations, however, the order of these last two components can vary. With stimuli of increasing concentration, the entire sequence may be repeated up to four or five times, and the individual components displayed for increasing periods. Components of the ingestion sequence never occur.

From the viewpoint of analyzing feeding behavior, the thalamic preparation is far from promising. If an animal will not ingest, further investigation of the hunger process must falter. Nevertheless, one characteristic of its behavior is of interest with regard to feeding. On most of the tests that we used, chronic thalamic preparations were less debilitated than chronic decerebrate rats, and were in fact similar to normal animals. The two situations in which thalamic animals exhibited gross disturbances, grooming and ingestion, both involve stimuli contacting oral or perioral receptors. In addition, whereas both normal animals and chronic decerebrate preparations quickly adapt to gavage via an infant feeding tube, thalamic animals in the same situation never cease to struggle. These behavioral abnormalities resembled the major

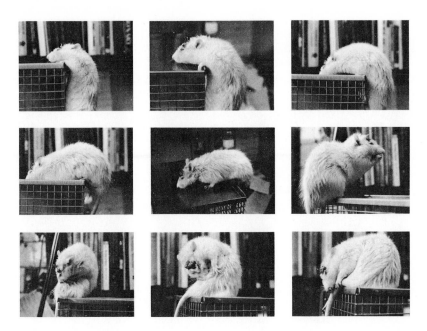

Figure 4-9. The behavior of a chronic decerebrate rat preparation. Unlike a normal or a thalamic rat, the chronic decerebrate rat will hang on the edge of a cage or gradually slide off. If its tail is pinched lightly, however, it will execute a well-coordinated cage climb (top two panels). The decerebrate rat displays good balance and spontaneous grooming (third frame, second panel and bottom panel). (Reprinted with permission from Grill & Norgren, 1978b.)

symptoms of the first stage of the lateral hypothalamic syndrome (Teitelbaum & Epstein, 1962), adding another instance to the now almost commonplace observation that eliciting the symptoms of that syndrome does not require direct intervention in the hypothalamus. The difference between the two preparations lies in recovery. In virtually all lateral hypothalamic preparations, time ameliorates the symptoms, whereas chronic thalamic animals never improve. The chronic thalamic rat behaves as if peri- or intraoral stimulation is unredeemedly aversive.

Despite their poor muscle tonus and lack of spontaneity, chronically decerebrate rats display nearly normal ingestion and rejection sequences in response to fluid stimuli. Sucrose, NaCl, and HCl elicit mouth movements, tongue protrusions, and lateral tongue movements at the same concentrations and in the same order as in normal rats. The only differences are in the frequency of the individual components, the magnitude of the tongue component, and the length of the bouts. Decerebrate rats perform the component movements somewhat more slowly, but

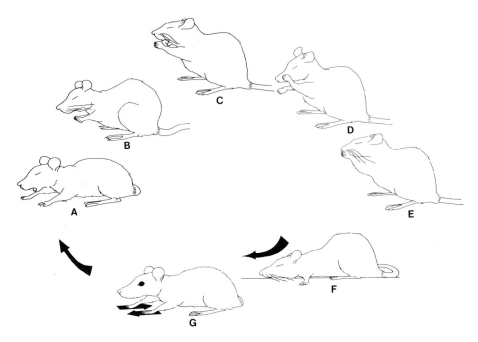

Figure 4-10. The response of a chronic thalamic preparation to intraoral fluid stimuli. The response began with gaping (A), which was coincident with rearing (A–C) and assuming bipedal posture. Additional gapes were followed by paw wiping (D) and face washing (E). The thalamic rat then resumed the initial quadrupedal posture and performed chin rubbing (F) and paw pushing (G). The entire response sequence was repeated up to four times as a function of stimulus concentration and category. Eyes were closed and facial muscles were tightly contracted during all components except paw pushing. (Reprinted with permission from Grill & Norgren, 1978d.)

often produce more repetitions per bout than do normal animals. Both these differences might be attributable to the same defect that lowers muscle tonus. The responses to quinine also closely mimic the rejection sequence of normal animals, although two components are dropped and a few new ones appear. The threshold for gaping is the same in chronic decerebrate and normal rats—3×10^{-5} M quinine HCl. The execution, timing, and number of gapes is identical in the two preparations. The whole-body sequelae of gapes also appear in decerebrates in the same order as in the normal rejection response—chin rubbing, head shaking, and face washing—but only at the highest concentration tested. The last two components of the sequence—forelimb flailing and paw pushing—do not occur, but three novel components—brusking, head elevation, and paw wipes—do. Brusking (grinding of the incisors) occurs in normal rats, but is not observed in response to intraoral sapid stimuli.

In the decerebrate rat, when brusking occurs it terminates the response sequence. Head elevation occurs while gaping takes place. Paw wipes consist of contact of one paw with the perioral region while the opposite paw remains in contact with the substrate. This is also a component of the thalamic rat's response to fluid stimuli and does appear in the repertoire of the normal rat responding to continuous infusions of fluids, but not during discrete trials.

If the taste reactivity test can be taken as an index, one aspect of the hunger process, the decision to ingest or reject food that is in the mouth, requires no forebrain whatsoever, and indeed can be seriously disrupted by adding part of it. For all intents and purposes, the ingestion and rejection responses of normal rats are completely integrated within the hindbrain. In our test circumstances, at least, whatever goes on in the forebrain cancels itself out. Although neither thalamic nor decerebrate preparations ever seek food, the observations on the capacity of the chronic decerebrate rat to accurately respond to fluid stimuli prompted us to examine this preparation further.

Control of Ingestive Behavior in the Chronically Decerebrate Rat

As mentioned earlier, the processes from which hunger is inferred include detection of an energy deficit, organization of food-finding behavior, discrimination of food from nonfood, ingestion, and satiation. If one stage in the process can be demonstrated to function, then the subsequent stages remain available for analysis. For example, the chronic decerebrate preparation never initiates food-seeking behavior, but if the experimenter circumvents this deficit by directly placing food stimuli in the animal's mouth, the decerebrate preparation discriminates between substances that a normal rat ingests or rejects. Thus, it is feasible to study the influence of events subsequent to ingestion. The processes prior to ingestion present more of a challenge because they are more diverse, less directly determined by external events, and probably involve more neural circuits.

The decerebrate rat not only fails to initiate food-seeking behavior, it fails to initiate any behavior except grooming unless goaded by relatively intense auditory or somatosensory stimulation. The stimuli that initiate grooming may be present in the fur. Internal stimuli also are present, however, but fail to provoke any behavior. The difference may be in the availability of an appropriate consummatory or goal stimulus. The consummatory stimulus for grooming, the animal's body, is available constantly, but for behaviors elicited by internal stimuli the consummatory stimuli must be sought out. Chronic thalamic rats do initiate behavior—they are active—but fail to respond to consummatory stimuli.

Failure to initiate food-seeking behavior may indicate an inability to detect the need for food, an inability to translate the need into organized activity, or an inability to use sensory or mnemonic information necessary to guide the behavior effectively, or some combination of these incapacities. At present it is difficult to weigh these possible explanations for the lack of spontaneous feeding behavior in decerebrate preparations because the internal stimuli that signal an energy deficit cannot be specified with certainty. One venerable candidate is lowered blood glucose, or in a somewhat updated version, lowered glucose utilization rate detected by specific glucoreceptor neurons allegedly concentrated in the hypothalamus (Mayer & Arees, 1968; Mayer, 1953). Although we have not tested the effects of glucoprivation on ingestive behavior in decerebrate rats, another regulatory response to lowered glucose utilization, the sympathoadrenal mobilization of glycogen stores, occurs normally in these preparations (DiRocco & Grill, 1979). Because this response is neurally mediated (transecting the spinal cord abolishes it) and the forebrain including the hypothalamus has been disconnected, some capacity to detect and respond to glucose utilization rates exists in the mid- or hindbrain or in the peripheral afferent neurons that synapse there. This hardly constitutes proof that the energy deficit detectors for the hunger process report to the hindbrain, because the glucose utilization rate may not be the appropriate signal, and even if it is, the sympathoadrenal response to glucoprivation may represent a crisis control activity rather than a normal aspect of energy balance regulation.

The two other regulatory functions that utilize ingestive behavior as a source of supply, water and electrolyte balance, apparently require a forebrain connection before deficits can influence the behavior. If they are water sated, normal rats subjected to a continuous intraoral infusion of water will ingest a few milliliters, then begin either passively or actively to reject the fluid. When deprived or otherwise challenged with extracellular or intracellular dehydration, however, these animals will ingest many milliliters of water. When subjected to the same hydrational challenges, chronic decerebrate preparations never alter the amount of water they ingest (Grill & Miselis, 1981). Similarly, salt deprivation drastically increases the amount of strong NaCl solution a normal rat will ingest, but has little if any influence on the salt ingestion of the decerebrate rat (Grill, Note 3). Electrophysiological evidence exists that neurons in the hindbrain or afferent neurons that synapse there are sensitive to a variety of metabolic variables that could signal energy, water, or electrolyte deficits (Clemente, Sutin, & Silverstone, 1957; Haberich, 1968; Rogers, Novin, & Butcher, 1979). The caudal brain stem also contains the neural mechanisms necessary to generate behavior appropriate for redressing the deficits. The forebrain may contain additional deficit detectors, but in any event it seems to be required for linking the deficit signals with the initiating of ingestive resupply.

The available evidence indicates that discrimination of sapid stimuli, and by inference of other foods, as well as ingestion or rejection behavior, can be accomplished by the neural apparatus of the caudal brain stem. Some aspects of the antecedent processes of hunger apparently require a forebrain connection for their expression. What about the processes subsequent to ingestion? Satiation is an active process (see Chapter 5 in this volume). In addition to the short-term consequences, longer term consequences of ingestion substantially influence subsequent food choices. The most dramatic example of a long-term consequence of ingestive behavior is taste aversion learning, but an analogous process occurs in the establishment of some forms of specific hunger (Rozin & Kalat, 1971) and may have a role in developing the idiosyncratic food preferences of individuals.

As described earlier, in a normal rat a single intraperitoneal dose of LiCl after the ingestion of sucrose, or of any other sapid stimulus for that matter, transforms the ingestion sequence elicited by the paired stimulus into a replica of the rejection responses elicited by quinine. This effect is remarkably resistant to extinction and even more persistent. After a single pairing of sucrose with a LiCl injection, a rat exposed to sucrose for the second time several months later will reject it vigorously (Grill, 1975; Norgren & Grill, Note 4). The taste aversion paradigm not only alters the orofacial response, but also changes at least one nonbehavioral response to sapid stimuli. A number of food stimuli, but most notably sugars, elicit a vagally mediated preabsorptive release of insulin from the pancreas. Normally rejected stimuli and some that are ingested (NaCl) do not trigger insulin release. An injection of LiCl following an intraoral infusion of glucose changes subsequent orofacial responses to glucose to the rejection pattern and inhibits the preabsorptive insulin release to that moiety, but not to others (Berridge et al., 1981).

In chronically decerebrate preparations, the identical taste aversion paradigm never alters subsequent orofacial responses to sapid stimuli. The usual taste aversion paradigm employs one pairing of taste and malaise per day (24-hour intertrial interval). In the chronic decerebrate rat, up to 12 such trials failed to influence the ingestion response, even after exogenous "activation" of the preparations with tail pinches or amphetamine (Grill & Norgren, 1978a). Subsequently, we reasoned that a decerebrate rat might be capable of associating taste with malaise, but incapable of remembering the association for 24 hours. Pilot tests indicated that normal rats exhibit altered taste reactivity as soon as 1 hour after the pairing of a sapid stimulus with a LiCl ingestion. Although no data exist on the issue, it seems plausible that at this short an interval the animal still suffers from the effects of the LiCl ingestion. Nevertheless, chronic decerebrate rats tested 1 hour after a sucrose–LiCl pairing exhibit normal ingestive sequences to sucrose (Norgren & Grill, Note 4).

Two other conceivable explanations for the failure of decerebrate preparations to make this association came to mind. First, the LiCl may not induce the same degree of malaise in decerebrate rats as it does in normal animals. Second, the LiCl may induce similar symptoms in both preparations, but the decerebrate may not be capable of detecting the symptoms. The physiological nature of "visceral malaise" has not been determined, and given the variety of agents that can serve as an unconditioned stimulus (UCS) in this paradigm, it seems unlikely that any single parameter will be crucial (see Ashe & Nachman, 1980, for a review). Whatever the effect, if anything, chronic decerebrate rats are more susceptible to the debilitating effects of LiCl than are normal rats. Repeated injections of a standard dose of LiCl (3.0 meq/kg of body weight) never have been lethal in normal rats (Nachman & Ashe, 1973); in our initial tests with the chronic decerebrate preparations, a single injection at this dose killed three of the five animals.

Less anecdotal evidence militates against the second rationale, that chronic decerebrate rats get sick, but cannot detect it. Intragastric copper sulfate serves as an effective USC for the taste aversion paradigm, but its effects are mitigated substantially by section of the subdiaphragmatic vagi (Coil, Rogers, Garcia, & Novin, 1978; Coil & Norgren, 1979). The afferent axons in the vagus nerve synapse in the hindbrain, and vagal efferent neurons originate there. Intraperitoneal or intravenous injections, of course, distribute throughout the body, and predictably vagal section does not reduce the effectiveness of either $CuSO_4$ or LiCl administered via these routes. Extirpation of the area postrema, a circumventricular organ associated with the nucleus of the solitary tract in the medulla, however, does vitiate the effectiveness of both intravenous $CuSO_4$ and intraperitoneal LiCl as taste aversion UCSs (Coil & Norgren, 1981; Ritter, McGlone, & Kelley, 1980). This leaves the failure of decerebrate rats to associate taste with subsequent illness in a situation analogous to their failure to initiate food-seeking behavior. The hindbrain receives the requisite information—that is, gustatory and visceral afferent axons synapse in the medulla and blood-borne toxins can be detected there at low concentrations—and possesses the neural apparatus to generate the appropriate responses. Apparently, neural systems in the hindbrain either cannot associate one set of sensory signals with the other, or if they can, cannot exhibit that association by switching responses. As the final set of experiments will demonstrate, in some circumstances the chronic decerebrate rat can respond to the same intraoral stimulus with different behaviors.

The rats in these studies of ingestive behavior are fed by gavage; the thalamic and decerebrate preparations because they do not eat spontaneously and the normal rats for control purposes. A test for the influence of satiation consists of infusing a weak sucrose solution (.03 M) either after a 24-hour fast or an hour after their morning feeding (i.e., 1-hour vs. 24-hour deprivation). After feeding, normal rats ingest a few milliliters of sucrose, then either actively reject the fluid or merely stop responding so that it dribbles out of their mouth. Prior to tube feeding, they always ingest more weak sucrose than they do afterward. Chronically decerebrate rats behave in an identical manner (Figure 4-11) (Grill & Norgren, 1978a; Grill, 1980). The deprivation effect probably does not reflect arousal because water intake does not change (Grill & Miselis, 1981). The relatively small amounts ingested after tube feeding cannot be attributed to inanition because, in many instances, both normal and decerebrate rats actively reject the weak sucrose by gaping, chin rubbing, and face washing. The stimulus elicits more, not less, activity in the sated condition. In addition, other sapid stimuli (NaCl and 1.0 M sucrose) continue to elicit the ingestion sequence in both preparations. The satiation effect has been evident in every chronic decerebrate tested to date (N=36), and the only differences among

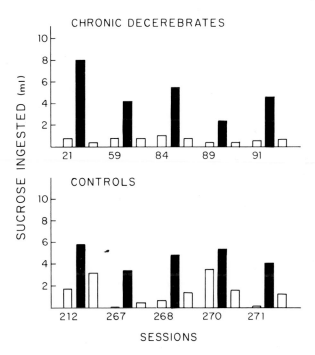

Figure 4-11. The effect of deprivation on ingestion during continuous infusion of a weak sucrose solution (.03 M) for chronic decerebrate preparations ($N = 5$) and neurologically normal rats ($N = 5$). Open bars represent the amount of sucrose consumed in the just-fed condition; dark bars, the amount consumed after a 24-hour fast. (Reprinted with permission from Grill, 1980.)

them can be attributed to differences in the infusion paradigm. In the early experiments, ingestion was measured by repeating .05-ml discrete trials until the preparation ceased to ingest. In subsequent tests, continuous infusion has been used, which results in more rapid ingestion and smaller differences between deprived and sated totals for both normal and decerebrate preparations. At least in our test situation, satiation affects ingestion via neural systems that are complete within the caudal brain stem. One of the cardinal indices of the hunger process, a change in response to the same stimulus from ingestion to rejection or vice versa, requires only the neurons caudal to the diencephalon.

Constructing Hunger in the Brain

Motivation supplies the intervening variable used by psychologists to account for differing behavior in similar external circumstances, or conversely, the same behavior in differing circumstances. This absence of predictable stimulus control and the concomitant variability in behavior differentiate motivational from reflex systems, but also obfuscate research directed at establishing the neural basis for motivation. At the neural level, the differences between motivational and reflex systems seem analogous to the differences between humans and other primates —analysis tends to transform qualitative chasms into quantitative clefts (Teitelbaum, Schallert, de Ryck, Whishaw, & Golani, 1980).

Most research into the neural basis of hunger relies upon physiological or pharmacological lesions or stimulation, and analysis of subsequent behavioral deficits. The logical inferences that can be based on lesion data, however, involve not what is missing (deficits), but what remains. If a function remains intact after a lesion, it seems reasonable to conclude that the neural systems damaged do not contribute significantly to that function. If the function is disrupted, the converse inference is not necessarily justified, because the disruption could result from indirect interference with the systems in question. A lesion can prevent function without damaging its anatomical basis. A neural lesion might reduce muscle tonus, and thus prevent walking, without impinging upon the neural systems that organize or execute that behavior. More to the point, lesions in the medial hypothalamus frequently are followed by a period of overeating with subsequent obesity. On the basis of this observation, the medial hypothalamus was first dubbed the satiety center and later the area controlling the set point for body weight. As mentioned earlier, it now appears that the effects of medial hypothalamic lesions on feeding behavior may be the indirect result of increased resting and reflex insulin release. Perhaps more important is that the basic phenomenon of satiety occurs in a decerebrate rat when the entire hypothalamus is disconnected from the midbrain.

Although the caudal brain stem supports several aspects of the hunger process—discrimination, ingestion or rejection, and satiation—one might assert that the hunger motivation neurons exist elsewhere because food-seeking behavior, which many psychologists consider the *sine qua non* of hunger, remains absent in decerebrate preparations. Indeed, food seeking also is absent in thalamic rats, so using a similar inference, one could exclude the thalamus and hypothalamus as components critical for hunger motivation.

Although restricted ablations of anterior neocortex or the amygdala disrupt feeding behavior in a manner reminscent of hypothalamic damage, the severity and duration of the changes usually are less pronounced (Braun, 1975; Cole, 1974; Fonberg, 1974; Kaada, 1972; Kolb & Nonneman, 1975; Kolb, Whishaw, & Schallert, 1977; Mabry & Campbell, 1975). In a laboratory environment, rats with complete ablations of neocortex and hippocampal formation eventually eat, drink, and maintain energy and hydromineral balance (Schwartz & Kling, 1964; Sorenson & Ellison, 1970; Vanderwolf, Kolb, & Cooley, 1978). Indeed, a neodecorticate rat is able not only to respond to deficit signals (salt deprivation), it can also utilize learned information to redress the deficit (Wirsig & Grill, in press). Nevertheless, although data are scarce, a functioning cerebral cortex probably is crucial in an environment requiring foraging for food.

Sorenson and Ellison (1970) reported that spontaneous feeding behavior became progressively disrupted as ablations encroached upon the corpus striatum or its outflow. Spontaneous feeding behavior in cats also depends on the integrity of the caudate nuclei (Wang & Akert, 1962). These observations paralleled evidence that lesions of the globus pallidus or ansa lenticularis abolished feeding behavior (Morgane, 1961). More recently these effects have been attributed to interference with dopaminergic innervation of the forebrain arising from the substantia nigra in the midbrain (Ungerstedt, 1971a). In his original analysis, however, Ungerstedt did not burden the nigrostriatal system with specific responsibility for organizing feeding and drinking behavior, but assumed that these salient deficits reflected more general disabilities in arousal or attention. In fact, many of the functions lost to dopamine depletion can be restored with exogenous activation (Marshall, Levitan, & Stricker, 1976).

Even when defined by food seeking, hunger cannot be localized to a gross division of the brain, much less a specific subset of neurons. Hunger is a psychological construct, related to, even embedded in, a physiological construct, energy balance regulation. A construct is an explanatory abstraction. Its physical reality may be desired fondly, but it is not required by the logic that created it. Neurophysiological systems supporting the final steps of the hunger process exist in the caudal brain stem. Some of the important energy deficit detectors may reside or report there as well. In the normal animal, the hunger process cannot be completed without food-finding behavior, which (even when highly stereotyped, as in cats) requires perceptual, cognitive, and mnemonic processes that are not inherently related to the food-finding behavior. These aspects of the hunger processes require the forebrain for their expression, but do not necessarily require the concept of hunger for their explanation (Teitelbaum et al., 1980).

Acknowledgments. The authors' work summarized in this chapter was supported by NIH Grants NS-10150 and AM-21397.

Reference Notes

1. Norgren, R. Personal observations, 1965.
2. Travers, J., & Norgren, R. Electromyographic analysis of ingestion and rejection sequence in rats, in preparation.
3. Grill, H. Personal observations, 1981.
4. Norgren, R., & Grill, H. Personal observations, 1980.

References

Anand, B. K., & Brobeck, J. R. Hypothalamic control of food intake in rats and cats. *Yale Journal of Biology and Medicine*, 1951, *24*, 123-140.
Anand, B. K., Chhina, G. S., Sharma, K. N., Dua, S., & Singh, B. Activity of single neurons in the hypothalamic feeding centers: Effect of glucose. *American Journal of Physiology*, 1964, *207*, 1146-1154.
Ashe, J. H., & Nachman, M. Neural mechanisms in taste aversion learning. In E. Stellar & A. Epstein (Eds.), *Progress in psychobiology and physiological psychology* (Vol. 9). New York: Academic Press, 1980.
Astrom, K. E. On the central course of afferent fibers in the trigeminal, facial, glossopharyngeal, and vagal nerves in their nuclei in the house. *Acta Physiologica Scandinavica*, 1953, *29*, 206-320 (Supp. 106).
Ball, G. Vagotomy: Effect on electrically elicited eating and self-stimulation in the lateral hypothalamus. *Science*, 1974, *184*, 484-485.
Bard, P., & Macht, M. B. The behavior of chronically decerebrate cats. In *Ciba Foundation symposium on the neurological bases of behavior*. London: Churchill, 1958.
Beckstead, R., & Norgren, R. An autoradiographic examination of the central distribution of the trigeminal, facial, glossopharyngeal, and vagal nerves in the monkey. *Journal of Comparative Neurology*, 1979, *184*, 455-472.
Berridge, K., Grill, H. J., & Norgren, R. The relation of consummatory responses and preabsorptive insulin release to palatability and learned taste aversions. *Journal of Comparative and Physiological Psychology*, 1981, *95*, 363-382.

Braun, J. J. Neocortex and feeding behavior in the rat. *Journal of Comparative and Physiological Psychology*, 1975, *89*, 507-522.

Brobeck, J. R., Tepperman, J., & Long, C. N. H. Experimental hypothalamic hyperphagic in the albino rat. *Yale Journal of Biology and Medicine*, 1943, *15*, 831-853.

Chase, M. H., & McGinty, D. J. Modulation of spontaneous reflex activity of the jaw musculature by orbital cortical stimulation in the freely-moving cat. *Brain Research*, 1970, *19*, 117-126.

Clemente, C. D., Sutin, J., & Silverstone, J. T. Changes in electrical activity of the medulla on the intravenous injection of hypertonic solutions. *American Journal of Physiology*, 1957, *188*, 193-198.

Coil, J., & Norgren, R. Cells of origin of motor axons in the subdiaphragmatic vagus of the rat. *Journal of the Autonomic Nervous System*, 1979, *1*, 203-210.

Coil, J. D., & Norgren, R. Taste aversions conditioned with intravenous copper sulfate: Attenuation by ablation of the area postrema. *Brain Research*, 1981, *212*, 425-433.

Coil, J. D., Rogers, R., Garcia, J., & Novin, D. Conditioned taste aversions: Vagal and circulatory mediation of the toxic US. *Behavioral Biology*, 1978, *24*, 509-519.

Cole, S. O. Changes in the feeding behavior of rats after amygdala lesions. *Behavioral Biology*, 1974, *12*, 265-270.

Coons, E. E. *Motivational correlates of eating elicited by electrical stimulation in the lateral hypothalamic feeding areas.* Unpublished doctoral dissertation, Yale University, 1964.

Coons, E. E., Levak, M., & Miller, N. E. Lateral hypothalamus: Learning of food-seeking response motivated by electrical stimulation. *Science*, 1965, *150*, 1320-1321.

Craig, W. Appetites and aversions as constituents of instincts. *Biological Bulletin*, 1918, *34*, 91-107.

DiRocco, R. J., & Grill, H. J. The forebrain is not essential for sympathoadrenal hyperglycemic response to glucoprivation. *Science*, 1979, *204*, 1112-1114.

Doty, R. W. Neural organization of deglutition. In C. F. Code & C. L. Prosser (Eds.), *Handbook of physiology*, Section 6: *Alimentary canal* (Vol. 4). Washington, D.C.: American Physiological Society, 1968.

Fitzsimons, J. Thirst. *Physiological Reviews*, 1972, *52*, 468-561.

Fluharty, S. J. & Grill, H. J. Taste reactivity of lateral hypothalamic lesioned rats: Effects of deprivation and tube feeding. *Society for Neuroscience Abstracts*, 1981, *7*, 28.

Flynn, J. P. Patterning mechanisms, patterned reflexes, and attack behavior in cats. In J. K. Cole & D. D. Jensen (Eds.), *Nebraska Symposium on Motivation* (Vol. 20). Lincoln: University of Nebraska Press, 1972.

Flynn, J. P., Edwards, S. B., & Bandler, R. J., Jr. Changes in sensory and motor systems during centrally elicited attack. *Behavioral Sciences*, 1971, *16*, 1-19.

Fonberg, E. Amygdala functions within the alimentary system. *Acta Neurobiologiae Experimentalis*, 1974, *34*, 435-466.

Friedman, M., & Stricker, E. The physiological psychology of hunger: A physiological perspective. *Psychological Review*, 1976, *83*, 409-431.

Fuxe, K. Evidence for the existence of monoamine neurons in the central nervous system, IV: Distribution of monoamine nerve terminals in the central nervous system. *Acta Physiologica Scandinavica*, 1965, *64*, 37-85.

Freed, E. K., & Grill, H. J. Levels of function in rat grooming behavior. *Society for Neuroscience Abstracts*, 1979, *5*, 468.

Glickman, E., & Schiff, B. B. A biological theory of reinforcement. *Psychological Review*, 1967, *74*, 81-109.

Grill, H. J. Sucrose as an aversive stimulus. *Society for Neuroscience Abstracts*, 1975, *1*, 525.

Grill, H. J. Production and regulation of ingestive consummatory behavior in the chronic decerebrate rat. *Brain Research Bulletin*, 1980, *5*, 79-87.

Grill, H. J., & Miselis, R. R. Lack of ingestive compensation to osmotic stimuli in chronic decerebrate rats. *American Journal of Physiology*, 1981, *240*, R81-86.

Grill, H. J., & Norgren, R. Chronic decerebrate rats demonstrate satiation, but not baitshyness. *Science*, 1978, *201*, 267-269. (a)

Grill, H. J., & Norgren, R. Neurological tests and behavioral deficits in chronic thalamic and chronic decerebrate rats. *Brain Research*, 1978, *143*, 299-312. (b)

Grill, H. J., & Norgren, R. The taste reactivity test, I: Mimetic responses to gustatory stimuli in neurologically normal rats. *Brain Research*, 1978, *143*, 263-279. (c)

Grill, H. J., & Norgren, R. The taste reactivity test, II: Mimetic responses to gustatory stimuli in chronic thalamic and chronic decerebrate rats. *Brain Research*, 1978, *143*, 281-297. (d)

Grossman, S. Role of the hypothalamus in the regulation of food and water intake. *Psychological Review*, 1975, *82*, 200-224.

Haberich, F. Osmoreception in the portal circulation. *Federation Proceedings*, 1968, *27*, 1137-1141.

Hess, W. R. *The functional organization of the diencephalon*. New York: Grune & Stratton, 1958.

Hetherington, A. W., & Ranson, S. W. Hypothalamic lesions and adiposity in the rat. *Anatomical Record*, 1940, *78*, 149-172.

Hetherington, A., & Ranson, S. Effect of early hypophysectomy on hypothalamic obesity. *Endocrinology*, 1942, *31*, 30-34.

Hiiemae, K., & Ardran, G. A cinefluorographic study of mandibular movement during feeding in the rat (*Rattus norvegicus*). *Journal of Zoology (London)*, 1968, *154*, 139-154.

Hinde, R. A. *Animal behaviour: A synthesis of ethology and comparative psychology* (2nd ed.). New York: McGraw-Hill, 1970.

Hoebel, B. G. Feeding and self-stimulation. *Annals of the New York Academy of Sciences*, 1969, *157*, 758-778.

Hoebel, B. G., & Teitelbaum, P. Hypothalamic control of feeding and self-stimulation. *Science*, 1962, *135*, 375-377.

Kaada, B. R. Stimulation and regional ablation of the amygdaloid complex with reference to functional representations. In B. E. Eleftheriou (Ed.), *The neurobiology of the amygdala*. New York: Plenum Press, 1972.

Kolb, B., & Nonneman, A. Prefrontal cortex and the regulation of food intake in the rat. *Journal of Comparative and Physiological Psychology*, 1975, *88*, 806-815.

Kolb, B., Whishaw, I. Q., & Schallert, T. Aphagia, behavior sequencing and body weight set point following orbital frontal lesions in rats. *Physiology and Behavior*, 1977, *19*, 93-103.

LeMagnen, J. Habits and food intake. In C. F. Code (Ed.), *Handbook of physiology*, Section 6: *Alimentary canal* (Vol. 1, *Control of food and water intake*). Washington, D.C.: American Physiological Society, 1967.

LeMagnen, J., Devos, M., Gaudilliere, J.-P., Louis-Sylvestre, J., & Tallon, S. Role of a lipostatic mechanism in regulation by feeding of energy balance in rats. *Journal of Comparative and Physiological Psychology*, 1973, *84*, 1-23.

Lindvall, O., & Bjorklund, A. The organization of the ascending catecholamine neuron systems in the rat brain as revealed by the glyoxylic acid fluorescence method. *Acta Physiologica Scandinavica*, 1974, 1-48 (Suppl. 412).

Lund, J. P., & Dellow, P. G. Rhythmical masticatory activity of hypoglossal motoneurons responding to an oral stimulus. *Experimental Neurology*, 1973, *40*, 243-246.

Mabry, P. D., & Campbell, B. A. Food-deprivation-induced behavioral arousal: Mediation by hypothalamus and amygdala. *Journal of Comparative and Physiological Psychology*, 1975, *89*, 19-38.

Macht, M. B. Subcortical localization of certain "taste" responses in the cat. *Federation Proceedings*, 1951, *10*, 88.

Margules, D., & Olds, J. Identical "feeding" and "reward" systems in the lateral hypothalamus of rats. *Science*, 1962, *135*, 374-375.

Marshall, J., Levitan, D., & Stricker, E. Activation-induced restoration of sensorimotor functions in rats with dopamine-depleting brain lesions. *Journal of Comparative and Physiological Psychology*, 1976, *90*, 536-546.

Marshall, J., & Teitelbaum, P. Further analysis of sensory inattention following lateral hypothalamic damage in rats. *Journal of Comparative and Physiological Psychology*, 1974, *86*, 375-395.

Marshall, J. F., Turner, B. H., & Teitelbaum, P. Sensory neglect produced by lateral hypothalamic damage. *Science*, 1971, *174*, 523-525.

Mayer, J. Glucostatic mechanism of regulation of food intake. *New England Journal of Medicine*, 1953, *249*, 13-16.

Mayer, J., & Arees, E. A. Ventromedial glucoreceptor system. *Federation Proceedings*, 1968, *27*, 1345-1348.

McFarland, D. J. Decision making in animals. *Nature*, 1977, *269*, 15-21.

Miller, F. R., & Sherrington, C. S. Some observations on the bucco-pharyngeal stage of reflex deglutition in the cat. *Quarterly Journal of Experimental Physiology*, 1916, *9*, 147-186.

Miller, N. E. Experiments on Motivation: Studies combining psychological, physiological, and pharmacological techniques. *Science*, 1957, *126*, 1271-1278.

Mogenson, G. J., & Phillips, A. G. Motivation: A psychological construct in search of a physiological substrate. *Progress in Psychobiology and Physiological Psychology*, 1976, *6*, 189-243.

Mook, D. G. Saccharin preference in the rat: Some unpalatable findings. *Psychological Review*, 1974, *81*, 475-490.

Morgane, P. J. Alterations in feeding and drinking behavior of rats with lesions in globi pallidi. *American Journal of Physiology*, 1961, *201*, 420-428.

Nachman, M., & Ashe, J. H. Learned taste aversions in rats as a function of dosage, concentration, and route of administration of LiCl. *Physiology and Behavior*, 1973, *10*, 73-78.

Norgren, R. A synopsis of gustatory neuroanatomy. In J. LeMagnen and P. MacLeod (Eds.), *Olfaction and taste, VI*. London: Information Retrieval Ltd., 1977.

Norgren, R. Flavor and the neural organization of feeding behavior. In C. M. Apt

(Ed.), *Flavor: Its chemical, behavioral, and commercial aspects.* Boulder: Westview Press, 1978.

Novin, D., & Oomura, Y. (Eds.). Integration of central and peripheral receptors in hunger and energy metabolism. *Brain Research Bulletin*, 1980, 5 (Suppl. 4).

Oomura, Y. Significance of glucose, insulin and free fatty acid on the hypothalamic feeding and satiety neurons. In D. Novin, W. Wyrwicka, & G. Bray (Eds.), *Hunger: Basic mechansims and clinical implications.* New York: Raven Press, 1976.

Oomura, Y., Ooyama, H., Yamamoto, T., & Naka, F. Reciprocal relationship of the lateral and ventromedial hypothalamus in the regulation of food intake. *Physiology and Behavior*, 1967, 2, 97-115.

Phillips, M. I., & Norgren, R. A rapid method for permanent implantation of an intraoral fistula in rats. *Behavioral Research Methods and Instrumentation*, 1970, 2, 124.

Powley, T. The ventromedial hypothalamic syndrome, satiety and a cephalic phase hypothesis. *Psychological Review*, 1977, 84, 89-126.

Powley, T., & Opshal, C. Ventromedial hypothalamic obesity abolished by subdiaphragmatic vagotomy. *American Journal of Physiology*, 1974, 226, 25-33.

Richter, C. P. Total self-regulatory functions in animals and human beings. *Harvey Lectures*, 1943, 38, 63-103.

Richter, C. P., Holt, L. E., & Barlare, B. Nutritional requirements for normal growth and reproduction in rats studied by the self-selection method. *American Journal of Physiology*, 1938, 122, 734-744.

Ritter, S., McGlone, J. J., & Kelley, K. W. Absence of lithium-induced taste aversion after area postrema lesion. *Brain Research*, 1980, 201, 501-506.

Rogers, R., Novin, D., & Butcher, L. Electrophysiological and neuroanatomical studies of hepatic portal osmo- and sodium-receptive afferent projections within the brain. *Journal of the Autonomic Nervous System*, 1979, 1, 183-202.

Rozin, P. Are carbohydrate and protein intakes separately regulated? *Journal of Comparative and Physiological Psychology*, 1968, 65, 23-29.

Rozin, P., & Kalat, J. W. Specific hungers and poison avoidance as adaptive specializations of learning. *Psychological Review*, 1971, 78, 459-486.

Schwartz, N., & Kling, A. The effect of amygdaloid lesions on feeding, grooming, and reproduction in rats. *Acta Neuroregulation*, 1964, 26, 12-34.

Sessle, B. J., & Hannam, A. G. (Eds.). *Mastication and swallowing: Biological and clinical correlates.* Toronto: University of Toronto Press, 1976.

Sessle, B. J., & Kenny, D. J. Control of tongue and facial motility: Neural mechanisms that may contribute to movements such as swallowing and sucking. In J. F. Bosma (Ed.), *Fourth symposium on oral sensation and perception.* Bethesda, Md.: USDHEW, National Institutes of Health, 1973.

Silverstone, J. T. The CNS and feeding: Group report. In *Dahlem workshop on appetite and food intake.* Berlin: Abakon Verlagsgesellschaft, 1976.

Sorenson, C. A., & Ellison, G. D. Striatal organization of feeding behavior in the decorticate rat. *Experimental Neurology*, 1970, 29, 162-179.

Stellar, E. The physiology of motivation. *Psychological Review*, 1954, 61, 5-22.

Storey, A. B. Laryngeal initiation of swallowing. *Experimental Neurology*, 1968, 20, 359-365. (a)

Storey, A. B. A functional analysis of sensory units innervating epiglottis and larynx. *Experimental Neurology*, 1968, 20, 366-383. (b)

Teitelbaum, P. Levels of integration of the operant. In W. K. Honig & J. E. R. Staddon (Eds.), *Handbook of operant behavior*. Englewood Cliffs, N. J.: Prentice-Hall, 1977.

Teitelbaum, P., & Epstein, A. N. The lateral hypothalamic syndrome: Recovery of feeding and drinking after lateral hypothalamic lesions. *Psychological Review*, 1962, *69*, 74-90.

Teitelbaum, P., Schallert, T., de Ryck, M., Whishaw, I. Q., & Golani, I. Motor subsystems in motivated behavior. In R. F. Thompson, L. H. Hicks, & V. B. Shvyrokov (Eds.), *Neural mechanisms of goal-directed behavior and learning*. New York: Academic Press, 1980.

Tinbergen, N. *The study of instinct*. Oxford, England: Clarendon Press, 1951.

Toates, F. M. Homeostasis and drinking. *Behavioral and Brain Sciences*, 1979, *2*, 95-139.

Torvik, A. Afferent connections to the sensory trigeminal nuclei, the nucleus of the solitary tract and adjacent structures: An experimental study in the rat. *Journal of Comparative Neurology*, 1956, *106*, 51-141.

Ungerstedt, U. Adipsia and aphagia after 6-hydroxydopamine induced degeneration of the nigro-striatal dopamine system. *Acta Physiologica Scandinavica*, 1971, *82* (Suppl. 367). (a)

Ungerstedt, U. Stereotaxic mapping of the monoamine pathways in the rat brain. *Acta Physiologica Scandinavica*, 1971, *82*, 1-48 (Suppl. 367). (b)

Vanderwolf, C. H., Kolb, B., & Cooley, R. Behavior of the rat after removal of neocortex and hippocampus formation. *Journal of Comparative and Physiological Psychology*, 1978, *92*, 156-175.

Wang, G. H., & Akert, K. Behavior and reflexes of chronic striatal cats. *Archives Italiennes de Biologie*, 1962, *100*, 48-85.

Weijs, W. A., & Dantuma, R. Electromyography and mechanics of mastication in the albino rat. *Journal of Morphology*, 1975, *146*, 1-34.

Wirsig, C. R. & Grill, H. J. The contribution of the rat's neocortex to ingestive control: I. Latent learning for the taste of sodium chloride. *Journal of Comparative and Physiological Psychology*, 1982, *in press*.

Chapter 5

Satiety and the Problem of Motivation

GERARD P. SMITH

> But neither is the reflex an abstraction, and in this respect Sherrington is mistaken: The reflex exists; it represents a very special case of behavior, observable under certain determined conditions. But it is not the principal object of physiology, it is not by means of it that the remainder can be understood. (Merleau-Ponty, 1963, p. 46)

Motivation is a word for a category of problems that emerges from a functional analysis of behavior. This places motivation in a conceptual realm that transcends movement and posture. It is the realm in which we view animals and humans as agents (Mischel, 1976). I believe the use of motivation to talk about and investigate these behavioral problems should be judged pragmatically. By this criterion, motivation gets mixed reviews. Its critics point to how often motivation is used as an explanation (*He ate more because he was hungrier.*) or as a thing (*Are there motivational neurons in the lateral hypothalamus?*). But these are the kinds of mistakes Whitehead called "misplaced concreteness." They are particularly easy to make in physiological psychology, where the work requires that psychological phenomena be related to physiological measurements within the limits of biological meaning. If you want to know how physiological mechanisms are articulated to produce the behavioral sequences that achieve biological meaning, then the problems that motivation refers to must be solved.

There is a tendency to accept this argument, but to ignore it by going straight to the brain. This strategy is a variant of Sutton's Law (1980). Its logic is simple: If motivation refers to problems of behavior, and if behavior depends on neural mechanisms, then motivation will be solved by studying neural mechanisms. (But this move is too neat because it is a logical reduction of psychology to neurophysiology.) Such a logical reduction assumes that we know the rules for reducing psychological problems into neurophysiological events. We don't. This is just what we seek in physiological psychology—the mysterious relationship(s) of the functions and forms (Merleau-Ponty, 1963) of behavior to the membranes and metabolic movements of the nervous system. The reduction, when we do it, will be empirical, not logical. To go straight to the brain is to study the brain. But a complete description of the structure, chemistry, and membranous movements of the brain will not reveal motivation, because motivation is not a thing in the brain but a relationship that involves the brain.

Motivation and Feeding Behavior

The problems motivation refers to are revealed by a consideration of an appetitive behavior, such as feeding. Consider the laboratory rat living in its cage with constant access to food. The rat approaches food, eats a meal, then does not feed for a period of time. This cycle repeats about a dozen times in 24 hours (Richter, 1922). Since the relationship between the rat and food changes intermittently when external conditions are apparently held constant, the changes in the relationship must reflect changes in the rat. But what kind of change in the rat could account for the rat's approaching food and eating it? This internal change, whatever it is, has remarkable access to the sensorimotor system because the rat will perform diverse movements to obtain food. This is what is elusive about motivation: It is embodied in movements and postures, but it transcends them. Motivation is never a single movement or posture except when we constrain the rat's behavior in an instrumental situation so that an arbitrary movement or posture is used to index the motivational relationship (Teitelbaum, 1966).

It has been traditional to postulate antecedent metabolic events, such as a decrease in glucose utilization (LeMagnen, 1980; Mayer, 1955) to account for the initiation of the movements that lead to feeding. There is no question that an abrupt and major decrease in glucose utilization elicits feeding (for a review, see Smith, in press-a), but the occurrence of small decreases in plasma glucose prior to a meal and the relevance of such decrements to the initiation of that meal are controversial. LeMagnen considers his most recent data to establish the glucostatic mechanism as the metabolic signal to eat (Louis-Sylvestre & LeMagnen, 1980; LeMagnen, 1980). His data don't move me (Smith, 1976, in press-a).

If the glucostatic hypothesis is not proven, then what other change should we consider? Having rejected gastric contractions (Penick, Smith, Wieneke, Jr., & Hinkle, 1963; Smith, 1979) and other suggested metabolic changes (Smith, 1976, in press-a), one is left with the weak experimental position of total empiricism. Thus, at this time, experimental attempts to detect the antecedent *internal* change that initiates feeding are limited to obtaining decisive evidence for the glucostatic hypothesis or to guessing. But I believe there is an indirect approach to this problem that has been neglected. That approach is through an analysis of postprandial satiety.

The suggestion seems odd. How can the analysis of the termination of feeding help us learn about the mechanisms that initiate the behavioral sequence that leads to eating? The answer is that this approach to hunger through satiety retraces the path of the functional relationship. Recall that motivation emerges from a functional analysis of behavior. A functional analysis is retrospective—it goes from the goal object, such as food, back along the behavioral stream of eating movements (consummatory phase) to the diverse movements that preceded feeding (appetitive phase). Since the ingestion of food is what the antecedent behavior and its physiological mechanisms are for, then the neurophysiological effects of food that terminate this sequence must have an intimate and relevant relationship to the neurophysiological mechanisms that underlie the entire appetitive sequence. The promise of such an approach is that it will lead us to the neurophysiological schema for feeding. This schema could then be used as the dependent variable with which to evaluate metabolic and other internal changes that are suggested to be sufficient for the arousal of the motivation to feed.

Satiety

What are the advantages of approaching hunger through satiety? They are not conceptual because such an indirect approach does not lend itself to the kind of compelling and elegant simplicity that characterizes good theory. On the other hand, we could accept the awkwardness of an indirect approach if it led to explicit description and semantic rigor because the clear and the rigorous would carry us beyond our current theories, which are either too simple or too vague.

I believe there are five experimental advantages to approaching hunger through satiety (Table 5-1). The fundamental experimental advantage is that we know food is the adequate stimulus for satiety. This is a major difference from hunger, where the adequate stimulus has not been identified. Since it is axiomatic that the success of behavioral analysis is a function of stimulus control, the ability to decompose food

Table 5-1. Experimental Advantages of Satiety

---

1. Its adequate stimulus is food.
2. It is present at birth.
3. It has a short time course.
4. It causes a large change of behavior.
5. It has characteristics of a negative feedback control.

---

into its constituent chemical and mechanical components and to vary these chemical and mechanical stimuli quantitatively gives experiments on satiety great potential analytic power.

The second advantage is that food elicits satiety in the newborn, so a sufficient number of physiological mechanisms are innate and "hard wired." Satiety operates as soon as hunger does and could play as large a theoretical part as hunger in the drama of development (Dowling, 1977).

The third advantage is that food elicits satiety in a matter of minutes. Satiety occurs while we watch. This temporal aspect of the stimulus–response relationship facilitates simple experiments and a "causal" analysis (Merleau-Ponty, 1963). This is the kind of situation in which the current tools of physiological psychology are sharpest.

The fourth advantage is that when food elicits satiety, there is a large change of behavior. Feeding stops; a short period of nonfeeding activities, such as grooming, sniffing, locomotion, and rearing, occurs; and then the animals rests or sleeps (Antin et al., 1975). Such a fixed sequence of behaviors is easily measured.

The fifth advantage is that feeding has the characteristics of a control system with a negative feedback loop (Booth, 1978). The activation of this negative feedback loop by ingested food produces satiety. The presence of a negative feedback loop in a physiological control system is a promise of progress because wherever a negative feedback loop has been brought under experimental control, the physiological analysis has been successful (Yamamoto & Brobeck, 1965). Examples of such success include cellular metabolic pathways, regulation of body temperature, the anterior pituitary gland and its target gland tissues, and the contribution of muscle sense to the control of movement.

The Neglect of Satiety

If satiety offers such experimental advantages, why has it not been pursued to the same extent that hunger has been? It is always hazardous to attempt to explain failures of development, but I think a sociological, an experimental, and a theoretical factor have slowed the study of satiety, and that it is instructive to consider them.

The sociological factor was probably the most important. Up until the last decade, we thought we knew the adequate stimuli (glucostatic and gastromechanic) for hunger and we busied ourselves with demonstrating how these stimuli worked. Only when a number of investigators became disillusioned with this effort were we willing to consider an alternative. As Kuhn (1970) would have it, the guiding paradigm was no longer adequate. Although I believe giving up the earlier paradigm was necessary and urged it repeatedly in the last 10 years (Smith, 1976, 1979, in press-a; Smith, Gibbs, Strohmayer, & Stokes, 1972), the fact that we are between paradigms makes for acute intellectual discomfort and difficult communication. Only patient experimentation and intelligence will yield a new paradigm. This is one of the reasons why I believe the approach to hunger through satiety should be tried.

The experimental factor that slowed the study of satiety was that the inhibition of behavior is more difficult to analyze than the production of behavior. In the case of feeding, the inhibition of food intake could be due to the satiating effects of ingested food, or to competing behaviors elicited by external stimuli (e.g., fleeing, fighting, or exploring), or to anorectic drugs, or to bad taste (quinine adulteration), or to incapacity produced by neurological damage (lateral hypothalamic syndrome), or to drug action (large doses of dopamine antagonists). Such an ambiguous measure does not invite experiments.

In addition to the sociological and experimental factors, I believe the analysis of satiety has been neglected because it has not been emphaed in theoretical writings about motivation in general or about feeding in particular (Bolles, 1975; Hinde, 1970; Hull, 1952; LeMagnen, 1971; Miller, 1957). Stellar is the exception to this rule (Smith, in press-b). His classic paper of 1954 (Stellar, 1954) gave satiety parity with hunger and he urged its study with characteristic enthusiasm.

This combination of a mostly silent theoretical literature, the difficulties of interpreting the inhibition of feeding behavior, and the reluctance to give up a paradigm delayed the analysis of satiety. But with the study of hunger at an experimental impasse for the physiological psychologist, satiety became more attractive and the outlines of its structure have emerged in the past decade.

The Structure of Satiety

The study of satiety has been stimulated by four contributions in the past 10 years. First, Booth (1972) stipulated that a satiety treatment should act in the terminal part of a meal, but not in the initial part of a meal. If a treatment affected the initial part of a meal, then it was probably aversive rather than satiating.

Second, Antin et al. (1975) described a sequence of behaviors that characterized spontaneous postprandial satiety. Since this behavioral sequence did not always occur when food intake was inhibited (e.g., amphetamine administration or quinine adulteration inhibited feeding, but did not elicit the satiety sequence), requiring a satiety treatment to inhibit food intake and elicit the satiety sequence reduced the ambiguity of the measure of satiety. Note that the logical relationship between the behavioral sequence and the internal state is assymetrical: When the sequence occurs, it is evidence that satiety is present, but the absence of the sequence is not evidence that satiety is not present. This means that the presence of the sequence is a conservative criterion for satiety.

The third contribution was the use of the sham-feeding technique in the rat (Davis & Campbell, 1973; Young, Gibbs, Antin, Holt, & Smith, 1974). The observation that when rats sham feed after 17 hours of food deprivation, they eat almost continually and never display the satiety sequence was particularly important (Young et al., 1974; Antin et al., 1975). This made the sham-feeding rat a reliable behavioral assay system to evaluate treatments for satiety effects because the absence of spontaneous satiety made the production of satiety by a treatment a significant effect. It is this combination of an assay that has no spontaneous incidence of satiety and the double requirement of any putative satiety treatment that it inhibit food intake and elicit the behavioral sequence of satiety that has enabled the investigation of satiety to go forward in a more rigorous and cumulative way in the past decade.

The fourth contribution came from gut endocrinologists (Bloom, 1978). Over the past 20 years, they have discovered a number of peptide hormones that have significant effects on gut organs and other tissues. Their presence in the gut and the fact that they are released by food stimuli make them candidates for mediating negative feedback information, that is, to be short-term satiety signals. Their ready availability has led to numerous studies of such a possibility.

Stimulated by these four contributions, the analysis of satiety has been guided by the search for answers to five questions (Table 5-2). These questions are listed in the order of experimental difficulty. The order reflects a necessary sequence: Answers to the first question must be available for the investigation of the second question, and so on. The work of the past decade has taken up the first two questions in some detail, has touched on the third question, and has not reached the fourth or fifth questions. Present knowledge about postprandial satiety can be summarized easily (Smith & Gibbs, 1979). Satiety can be elicited by food stimuli acting preabsorptively and postabsorptively. Preabsorptive sites have been identified in the mouth, the stomach, and the small

Table 5-2. Questions About Satiety

1. Where do food stimuli act to elicit satiety?
2. What neural and/or endocrine mechanisms mediate the effect?
3. Where are the central nervous mechanisms that process the physiological information contained in the neuroendocrine effects of food stimuli?
4. What kind of processing is performed by these central neural mechanisms?
5. How do the central neural mechanisms produce the changes in behavior that characterize postprandial satiety?

intestine. The postabsorptive sites have not been identified with the same precision. The most likely postabsorptive sites are the liver, pancreatic islets, fat tissue, and brain.

None of the mechanisms activated by food stimuli at these sites have been rigorously demonstrated. The possible mechanisms for which there is suggestive evidence appear in Table 5-3. Gastric and intestinal mechanisms may interact so that the inhibition of gastric emptying and of feeding are closely coordinated (McHugh, 1979). In addition to these presumably unconditioned mechanisms, Booth (1972) has demonstrated that satiety can be conditioned to oropharyngeal stimuli.

The structure of satiety revealed by this recent work has two aspects that are surprising. One is the prominence of preabsorptive sites. The

Table 5-3. Possible Mechanisms of Postprandial Satiety

Site	Mechanism
Preabsorptive	
Mouth	Cranial nerves 7, 9, and 10
Stomach	Cranial nerve 10
	Bombesin
Small intestine	Cholecystokinin
	Bombesin
Postabsorptive	
Liver	Glycogenolysis—Cranial nerve 10
Pancreatic islet	Glucagon
	Insulin
	Pancreatic polypeptide
	Somatostatin
Fat	?
Brain	Cholecystokinin, bombesin

Note. For details and individual references, see the reviews by Smith and Gibbs (1979, 1981).

second is the number of gut peptide hormones that are considered as possible mediating mechanisms. The fact that some of these hormones (e.g., cholecystokinin) have satiety effects after central or peripheral administration may be an example of how the brain and the gut synthesize, store, and release the same peptide hormone to produce an identical behavioral effect from action at receptors in the brain (Della-Fera & Baile, 1979) and in the gut (Smith, Jerome, Simansky, Eterno, & Cushin, 1981), respectively.

The experimental approaches to the third question have produced a theoretical revision. The revision has concerned the role of the ventromedial hypothalamus as the primary central mechanism for integrating food-contingent satiety signals. It is generally admitted that there is no strong evidence for this traditional view, which originated from the early analysis of the hyperphagic syndrome produced by bilateral VMH lesions. The VMH syndrome is now a problem to be explained and not an insight to be used (Smith, 1979).

This is all we know of the structure of satiety at this time. Although this is a modest achievement, the orderly accumulation of evidence and the increasing experimental power that the evaluation of peripheral sites and mechanisms has provided impresses me. The promise of this approach is that central mechanisms can be analyzed by using specific peripheral neural and/or endocrine mechanisms activated by ingested food.

Summary and Speculation

I have attempted to persuade the reader of the experimental usefulness of approaching hunger through satiety. I have reviewed the work of the last decade based on this idea and argued that this experimental approach is productive. The question arises whether such an approach might be useful beyond the example of feeding behavior. I think so. In fact, it seems plausible to consider using satiety in the analysis of any appetitive behavior because of its experimental and theoretical advantages. The experimental advantages have been emphasized in this chapter: accessibility, stimulus control, and a short time course.

The theoretical advantages are less obvious, but I think they are equally important. The study of satiety would free us from the mechanical idea of animals and humans as machines whose main mystery for us is what starts them and what drives them. Attempting to understand what physiological information stops the consummatory phase of an appetitive behavioral sequence is no less interesting, and it is *the* physiological basis of the biological adaptations that animals and humans act for.

This leads to the final point. Interest in what stops a behavioral sequence carries our consideration of satiety into the law of effect. The relations between satiety and reward have received little attention (for a review, see Smith, in press-a). Successful analysis of satiety will permit us to investigate that important issue. Since both of these processes occur as a consequence of behavior, and since consequences organize behavior, the analysis of satiety appears to be central to the analysis of motivated behavior and its satisfactions.

Acknowledgments. I thank Dr. James Gibbs for helping me hammer out these ideas over the last 10 years and for his helpful suggestions about this paper.

I thank Ms. Nina Di Filippo and Mrs. Marion Jacobson for typing the manuscript. I wrote it during the tenure of Career Development Award MH 00149.

References

Antin, J., Gibbs, J., Holt, J., Young, R. C., & Smith, G. P. Cholecystokinin elicits the complete behavioral sequence of satiety in rats. *Journal of Comparative and Physiological Psychology*, 1975, *89*, 784–790.

Bloom, S. R. (Ed.). *Gut hormones.* New York: Churchill Livingstone, 1978.

Bolles, R. C. *Theory of motivation* (2nd ed.). New York: Harper & Row, 1975.

Booth, D. A. Conditioned satiety in the rat. *Journal of Comparative and Physiological Psychology*, 1972, *81*, 457–471.

Booth, D. A. (Ed.). *Models of hunger.* New York: Academic Press, 1978.

Davis, J. D., & Campbell, C. S. Peripheral control of meal size in the rat: Effect of sham feeding on meal size and drinking rate. *Journal of Comparative and Physiological Psychology*, 1973, *83*, 379–387.

Della-Fera, M. A., & Baile, C. A. Cholecystokinin octapeptide: Continuous picomole injections into the cerebral ventricles of sheep suppress feeding. *Science*, 1979, *206*, 471–473.

Dowling, S. Seven infants with esophageal atresia: A developmental study. In R. S. Eissler, A. Freud, M. Kris, P. B. Neubauer, & A. J. Solnit (Eds.), *The psychoanalytic study of the child* (Vol. 32). New Haven: Yale University Press, 1977.

Hinde, R. A. *Animal behaviour* (2nd ed.). New York: McGraw-Hill, 1970.

Hull, C. L. *A behavior system.* New Haven: Yale University Press, 1952.

Kuhn, T. S. The structure of scientific revolutions. *International encyclopedia of unified science* (2nd ed., Vol. 2, No. 2). Chicago: University of Chicago Press, 1970.

LeMagnen, J. Advances in studies on the physiological control and regulation of food intake. In E. Stellar & J. M. Sprague (Eds.), *Progress in physiological psychology* (Vol. 4). New York: Academic Press, 1971.

LeMagnen, J. The body energy regulation: The role of three brain responses to glucopenia. *Neuroscience and Biobehavioral Review*, 1980, *4*, Suppl. 1, 65–72.

Louis-Sylvestre, J., & LeMagnen, J. A fall in blood glucose levels precedes meal onset in free feeding rats. *Neuroscience and Biobehavioral Reviews*, 1980, *4*, Suppl. 1, 13-15.

Mayer, J. Regulation of energy intake and the body weight: The glucostatic theory and the lipostatic hypothesis. *Annals of the New York Academy of Science*, 1955, *63*, 5-43.

McHugh, P. R. Aspects of the control of feeding: Application of quantitation in psychobiology. *Johns Hopkins Medical Journal*, 1979, *144*, 147-155.

Merleau-Ponty, M. *The structure of behavior.* Boston: Beacon Press, 1963. (Originally published in French under the title *La Structure du comportement* by Presses Universitaires de France, 1942.)

Miller, N. E. Experiments in motivation: Studies combining psychological, physiological, and pharmacological techniques. *Science*, 1957, *126*, 1271-1278.

Mischel, T. Psychological explanations and their vicissitudes. In W. J. Arnold (Ed.), *Nebraska Symposium on Motivation, 1975*, Vol. 23. Lincoln: University of Nebraska Press, 1976, pp. 133-204.

Penick, S. B., Smith, G. P., Wieneke, K., Jr., & Hinkle, L. E., Jr. An experimental evaluation of the relationship between hunger and gastric motility. *American Journal of Physiology*, 1963, *205*, 421-426.

Richter, C. A behavioristic study of the activity of the rat. *Comparative Psychology Monographs*, 1922, *1* (No. 2).

Smith, G. P. Humoral hypotheses for the control of food intake. In G. Bray (Ed.), *Obesity in perspective* (Vol. 2, Pt. 2). Bethesda, Md.: National Institutes of Health, 1976, pp. 349-355.

Smith, G. P. The control of food intake. In J. R. Brobeck (Ed.), *Best & Taylor's physiological basis of medical practice* (10th ed.). Baltimore: Williams & Wilkins, 1979.

Smith, G. P. The physiology of the meal. In T. Silverstone (Ed.), *Drugs and appetite.* New York: Academic Press, in press. (a)

Smith, G. P. Eliot Stellar and the physiological psychology of satiety. In A. R. Morrison & P. L. Strick (Eds.), *Changing concepts of the nervous system.* New York: Academic Press, in press. (b)

Smith, G. P., & Gibbs, J. Postprandial satiety. In J. M. Sprague & A. N. Epstein (Eds.), *Progress in psychobiology and physiological psychology* (Vol. 8). New York: Academic Press, 1979.

Smith, G. P., & Gibbs, J. Brain-gut peptides and the control of food intake. In J. B. Martin, S. Reichlin, & K. L. Bick (Eds.), *Neurosecretion and brain peptides.* New York: Raven Press, 1981.

Smith, G. P., Gibbs, J., Strohmayer, A. J., & Stokes, P. E. Threshold doses of 2-deoxy-D-glucose for hyperglycemia and feeding in rats and monkeys. *American Journal of Physiology*, 1972, *222*, 77-81.

Smith, G. P., Jerome, C., Cushin, B. J., Eterno, R., & Simansky, K. J. Abdominal vagotomy blocks the satiety effect of cholecystokinin in the rat. *Science*, 1981, *213*, 1036-1037.

Stellar, E. The physiology of motivation. *Psychological Reviews*, 1954, *61*, 5-22.

Sutton, W. When asked why he robbed banks, Sutton replied "Because that's where the money is." This is Sutton's Law. *New York Times* Obituary, p. 38, National Edition. Nov. 18, 1980.

Teitelbaum, P. The use of operant methods in the assessment and control of motivational states. In W. K. Honig (Ed.), *Operant behavior, areas of research and application.* New York: Appleton-Century-Crofts, 1966.

Yamamoto, W. S., & Brobeck, J. R. (Eds.). *Physiological controls and regulations.* Philadelphia: W. B. Saunders, 1965.

Young, R. C., Gibbs, J., Antin, J., Holt, J., & Smith, G. P. Absence of satiety during sham feeding in the rat. *Journal of Comparative and Physiological Psychology,* 1974, *87,* 795–800.

Chapter 6

Physiological and Behavioral Basis of Human Obesity

Joel A. Grinker

Obesity is a state in which the abnormality is clearly evident and easily measurable—an excess of adipose tissue relative to lean body mass. Obesity reflects the long-term imbalance of energy intake and expenditure. The potential reasons for this imbalance are many and range from simple overeating or underactivity to defects in adipose cell metabolism. The known metabolic correlates of this condition, such as hyperinsulinemia or elevated free fatty acids are, in the main, secondary consequences. This limited understanding of the pathogenesis of obesity has resulted in therapeutic interventions largely limited to the intake side of this relation. The uniformly simple and effective treatment, reduction of caloric intake through dieting, is always effective if followed carefully and for a long enough period of time. However, many studies suggest that permanent maintenance of the reduced body weight is often difficult or impossible (see Krotkiewski, Sjostrom, Bjorntorp, Calgren, Garrelik, & Smith, 1977; Stunkard & McLaren-Hume, 1959). Thus, the view of both clinician and nonclinician has been that the obese subject is perverse, uncooperative, or the victim of some psychological imbalance. Only recently has serious attention been paid to this disorder. Obesity has ceased to be considered a trivial biological problem and is now considered a complex disorder of physiological as well as psychological importance.

The following discussion will summarize current theoretical approaches to the etiology and maintenance of the obese state. Radically different but provocative hypotheses of the etiology and maintenance of the obese state are included in the discussion that follows. One is a theory of active regulation of the elevated body weight and emphasizes the role of adipose tissue—the target organ in obesity. Another is a theory of failure to regulate and of overeating through reliance on external or sensory factors. Other recent theoretical approaches postulate deficiencies in learned satiation or hunger or in the thermogenic response to feeding.

Motivational concepts are represented in theories of the regulation of body weight/fat. "Set point" theory presupposes a regulated degree of adipose tissue as a direct consequence of either positive feedback or passive regulation (Booth, 1978). Drive theory is represented by theories of increased food intake through increased hunger or impaired satiety (e.g., more frequent meals or larger, more sustained meals). Output theory focuses on disorders that occur in the process of energy expenditure, such as impaired thermogenesis, increased metabolic efficiency, or underactivity. Current usage substitutes the word "palatability" for "incentive value" and "learned satiation" for "reinforcement." Finally, psychological theories focus on learned impairments in appetite and satiety. At this time, no one theory provides a complete explanation; purely psychological or purely physiological–biochemical theories can offer only partial insights into the nature of these disturbances in energy balance.

Definitions

Overweight and obesity are defined in terms of normative values that depend on culturally accepted standards and vary with the age as well as the sex of the individual. Aesthetic standards change and thus a normal or attractive weight for a woman in a Rubens or Renoir painting would be considered obese today. Normative values typically depend on measured weights rather than measured fatness; tables such as those of the Metropolitan Life Insurance Company list a range of weights separately for women and men of differing physiques. Obesity is usually defined as greater than 20% overweight by these tables. Other more exact methods for assessing overweight include underwater weighing, body potassium content, skinfold thickness, or estimates of body fatness such as body mass index $\left(\dfrac{\text{weight}}{\text{height}^2}\right)$.

Obesity as a Disorder of Weight Regulation

The hypothesis that obesity represents a disorder of weight regulation arises from the persistent failures of treatment. In normal human beings, a complex series of integrated systems control food intake and energy production to assure that a fixed proportion of body weight (15% or one month's supply of calories) will be stored in adipose tissue. The evidence for active regulation of body weight comes primarily from three sources: epidemiological studies of body weight stability in adults, overfeeding and starvation experiments in humans, and similar experimental studies in animals.

Several studies report relative constancy in body weight over long periods of time. The weight of white males from the highest income group increased from 73 kg at age 21 to only 77 kg at age 30 and remained constant to age 60 (USDHEW Ten State Nutrition Survey, 1972). Lower socioeconomic groups showed similar patterns. White females showed a rise from 60 kg at age 21 to 63 kg at age 30 and 66 kg at age 40 with no change to age 70. A similar stability of weight in adult years occurred among black males and females and across different socioeconomic groups. Another study reported that relative body weight established in childhood was maintained in adult years (Abraham, Collins, & Nordsieck, 1971). Retrospective studies of obese adults show a strong relationship between adult obesity and childhood or infant obesity (Charney, Goodman, McBride, Lyon, & Pratt, 1976). Figure 6-1

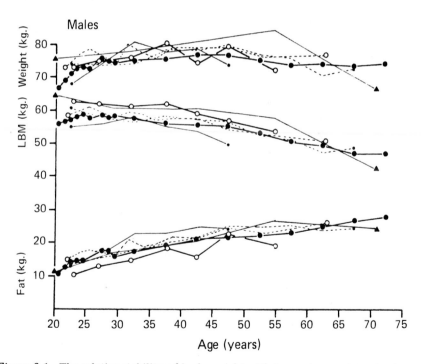

Figure 6-1. The relative stability of body weight with increasing age in males (cross-sectional measurement from several studies) and changes in body composition are shown. Note the rise in percentage of body fat and decline in percentage of lean body mass (LBM). (From Forbes & Reina, 1970.)

shows changes in body composition and stability in weight during adult years; lean body mass declined while fat content increased.

Even when human volunteers are subjected to experimental semi-starvation or overfeeding, body weight returns to normal levels when the experimental manipulations are ended. In one study (Sims & Horton, 1968; Sims et al., 1973) body weight increased 25% in the period of voluntary overeating. However, when the experimental over-feeding ended, the subjects spontaneously restricted food intake and body weight returned to its original levels. Similar results have been reported with force-fed (Cohn & Joseph, 1962) or starved adult rats (McCance & Widdowson, 1962). Figure 6-2 graphically demonstrates this "regulation" of body weight. The best evidence of the constancy of body weight comes from our own studies of obese individuals in the hospital. Figure 6-3 shows an actual graph of one patient's weight changes during and after repeated hospitalizations. Weight is lost in the hospital, but when the patient is released from the hospital, weight is invariably regained.

These observations have led to the suggestion that adipose mass is

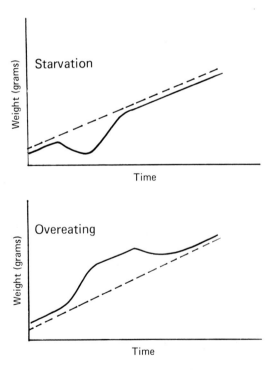

Figure 6-2. Graphic illustration of the "regulation" of body weight/fat in the rat. Once over- or underfeeding is discontinued, the rat changes food intake–energy ex-penditure appropriately and its weight returns to prior baseline levels.

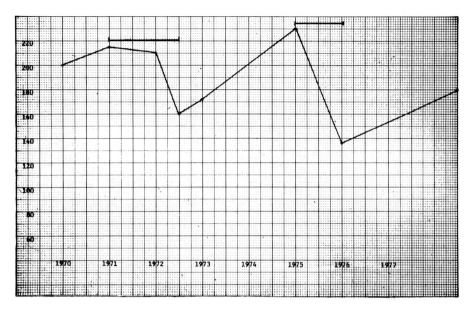

Figure 6-3. Sequential weight history of a male adult during repeated hospitalizations for weight reduction. The reduced weight is only briefly maintained and a new plateau of obesity is reached soon after. (Time is shown in years, weight in kilograms, and hospitalizations by the two heavy lines at the top.)

actively regulated via "lipostatic" sensors that control food intake or energy expenditure to maintain a fixed level of fat storage (Hirsch, 1972; Kennedy, 1953). At various times, plasma levels of insulin, glucose, glycerol, free fatty acids, amino acids, growth hormone, corticosteroids, thyroxine, or some combination of these factors have been suggested as potential long-term controllers of adipose storage. Unfortunately, abnormalities in levels or metabolism of these substances that have been found in obese subjects either disappear after weight reduction or can be shown to occur when experimental animals or humans are force fed. Thus, hyperinsulinemia or reduced glucose tolerance or elevated free fatty acids, while often reported in the obese state, are all reduced or restored to near normal levels following weight reduction. These results suggest that most abnormalities are consequences of the obese state and thus not relevant to the etiology of the disorder.

Set Point Theory

Set point theory hypothesizes that there are physiological mechanisms that control energy intake and output (Keesey, 1980; Mrosovsky & Powley, 1977) to maintain a stable weight or body composition. Feeding is considered a regulatory behavior serving to stabilize body fat. Keesey has suggested an active monitoring of internal states in the service of maintaining body fat and consequently weight at some pre-determined level. Both reductions and elevations in set point are as-sumed to exist and are defended in certain animal models (e.g., the lateral hypothalamic-lesioned rat [Keesey, Boyle, & Storlien, 1978] and the genetically obese Zucker rat). In both, the deviation from stable body weight is accompanied by appropriate increases in energy expen-diture or food intake to maintain the new body weight.

Other investigators, however, have argued strongly against the con-cept of active regulation and have suggested that body fat or total body energy can be maintained at some relatively constant level solely through simple negative feedback processes (Booth, 1978, 1980; Gar-row, 1978). While set point can serve as a valuable conceptual device, these investigators feel that the existence of set points has often been overstated and that set points do not necessarily possess a physiological or structural existence.

Growth and Development of Adipose Tissue

Studies of Human Adipose Tissue

The hypothesis that adipose tissue itself could be directly involved in regulation is partly supported by studies of adipose tissue morphology in obese man and animals and by studies of weight reduction and surgi-cal removal of adipose tissue. The original work by Hirsch and Knittle (1970) documented the occurrence of hyperplasia (increases in adipose cell number) as well as hypertrophy (increases in adipose cell size) in the adipose depots of severely obese humans. Normal weight individuals have an average of 25×10^9 cells with an average size of .665 μg of lipid per cell, whereas obese individuals have an average of 65×10^9 cells and a cell size of .94 μg. Cellularity patterns are often correlated with age of onset of obesity, hyperplastic obesity being most often associated with the early onset of obesity. Knittle (1977) has reported that differences in the adipose cell morphology of obese and non-obese children can occur as early as 2 years of age. The stability of adipose cell number in adult life is demonstrated in obese individuals following weight reduction. The obese individual cannot change the number of adipose cells through dieting. The individual with a large number of adipose cells may thus be programmed for a higher level of adipose storage. The application of external forces to reduce weight would be in conflict with internal forces that maintain the obese weight. Bjorntorp and associates (Krotkiewski et al., 1977) have shown that weight loss is usually terminated when an individual reaches a plateau of normal cell size (see Figure 6-4).

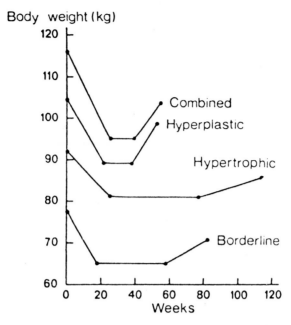

Figure 6-4. Schematic summary of the average results of treatment for four obese groups with differing adipose cell morphologies. The plateau in weight reduction occurs when adipose cell size approaches normal levels. (From Krotkiewski et al., 1977.)

Studies of Rat Adipose Tissue

It is possible to perform experimental manipulations on animals (such as the creation of obese or stunted animals and the testing of genetic strains) that would be impossible to perform with human subjects. Through such experiments, it is possible to demonstrate that adipose tissue cellularity and the quantity of body fat are to a large extent determined early in development. However, adult rats fed high-fat or high-carbohydrate diets over a long term show significant enhancement of adipose cell number (Faust, Johnson, Stern, & Hirsch, 1978). Nutritional manipulations (rearing in artificially large litters) prior to weaning produces permanent stunting of adult rats with a reduction in adipose cell number (Knittle & Hirsch, 1968). These rats, however, do respond to high-fat feeding later in life and show the normal increase in body fat and adipose cell number (Faust, Johnson, & Hirsch, 1980). But it appears difficult if not impossible to reduce the adult cell number of the genetically obese Zucker rat by early food restriction (Cleary, Vasselli, & Greenwood, 1980). Zucker obese rats raised in large litters and pair fed to the level of lean controls showed reduction in lean body mass and brain weight but no reduction in total amount of body fat at 33 weeks of age.

Lipectomy in Investigations of Adipose Mass Regulation

The hypothesis that body weight regulation is achieved via a signal from adipose tissue is highly speculative. If adipose tissue morphology is involved in the regulation of body weight or body fat, then there are only three possibilities as to what could be regulated—fat cell number, fat cell size, or the mass of fat itself. Fat cell number would appear to be an unlikely choice, since cell number can be increased during the later stages of growth and development by chronic long-term manipulations (Faust et al., 1978). Temporarily overfed and underfed animals restore normal fat mass, without changes in fat cell number, when the animals are returned to ad-libitum feeding. Adipose cell size appears the most likely candidate. By surgical removal of a portion of adipose tissue mass, it is possible to distinguish between the theoretical possibilities of regulation via adipose mass or adipose cell size. The mass of the tissue is reduced by the surgical removal of some cells, but cell size is unaltered. By following the animal's body weight and food intake for a long period of time, it is possible to test different hypotheses. In one experiment (Faust, Johnson, & Hirsch, 1977), following lipectomy at 23 days of age, Osborne-Mendel rats and sham-operated controls were fed a high-fat diet. Both the lipectomized rats (with 25% fewer adipocytes) and the sham controls overate for several weeks. Then the lipectomized rats reduced their food intake and consequently by the end of 9 weeks had accumulated less fat than sham-operated controls. Their adipose cell size, however, remained equal to the size of the adipose cells of the controls. This was the first demonstration of a direct relationship between adipocyte size and food intake.

Brown Adipose Tissue

The most recent metabolic defect postulated to be important in the development of rodent obesity is that of a malfunctioning of brown adipose tissue. Brown adipose tissue is found in mammals at multiple sites. It is innervated by sympathetic fibers and its fat stores are preferentially utilized for heat production. Dietary-induced thermogenesis generally refers to the rise in heat produced following a meal (the former 'specific dynamic action'). It is a metabolic response modulating the effects of fluctuations in food intake. Rothwell and Stock (1978) reported that this form of thermogenesis also involved stimulation of brown adipose tissue. During voluntary overeating in rats, both resting oxygen consumption and intrascapular brown fat increased. Brown adipose tissue has therefore been hypothesized to be related to the resistance to obesity.

Recent studies have shown a thermoregulatory defect in several genetically determined strains of rodents, for example, the ob/ob mouse (Trayhurn & James, 1978) and the db/db mouse (Trayhurn, Thurlby, & Woods, in press). These obese animals have a reduced metabolic activity of brown adipose tissue. At present, the extrapolation of these results to larger animals such as man is unjustified. Although man possesses brown adipose tissue in small amounts, the possible significance of brown adipose tissue in the genesis of human obesity remains speculative.

Epidemiological Studies: Prevalence and Dietary Preference

Epidemiological studies indicate that 25–45% of adult American men and women suffer from overweight or obesity, making obesity one of the most prevalent nutritional disorders in the United States. Obesity can lead to both severe psychological disability and increased risk to physical health, including hypertension, diabetes, and coronary heart disease.

The accompanying table (see Table 6-1) shows normative data taken from various U.S. Government studies over the past 70 years. The actual weights for the reference men or women of standard height over the decades have been increasing. Not only has the American population been increasing in fatness, but men and women have shown persistent tendencies to become heavier as they get older. The prevalance of obesity and overweight is inversely related to socioeconomic levels

Table 6-1. Changes in Average Weights (lb.) Corrected by Age and Height from 1912 to 1974 (U.S.) (see Scala, 1978)

Group	Age	1912[a]	1940[b]	1959[c]	1960-1962[d]	1971-1974[e]
Men 5 ft. 8 in. tall						
	25	149	152	153	156	159
	35	155	159	161	166	170
	45	160	164	165	169	174
Women 5 ft. 4 in. tall						
	25	128	123	125	129	135
	35	134	129	132	138	142
	45	141	141	140	145	152

[a]From a Medico-actuarial Study, 1912.
[b]From an Equitable Life Study, 1940.
[c]From a Build and Blood Pressure Study, Society of Actuaries, 1959.
[d]From an HES Survey, 1960-1962.
[e]From the Hanes Survey, 1971-1974.

(Stunkard, 1975a; Silverstone, Gordon, & Stunkard, 1969). Among most socioeconomic groups, overweight and obesity are more prevalent in females (Heald, 1972).

The increased prevalence of obesity has been associated with dramatic changes in the American diet since the early 1900s. Consumption of meat, refined sugars, and especially fats has increased, whereas the consumption of potatoes, grains, or other complex carbohydrates has decreased. Total caloric consumption has remained nearly constant, although activity levels have assuredly declined. Table 6-2 shows the estimated daily caloric intakes and the percentages of calories deriving from protein, fat, and carbohydrate for the years 1909–1979. This shift toward richer and calorically denser foods is partly the result of changes in the technology of food production, and partly the result of the increased availability of processed and refined foods containing fats and a wide variety of nutritive and nonnutritive sweeteners.

Epidemiological studies, however, fail to support the view that excessive carbohydrate or sweet intake or an increased number of meals produces obesity (Keen, Thomas, Jarret, & Fuller, 1979; Kaufmann, Poznanski, & Guggenheim, 1975; Fabry & Tepperman, 1970). Food choices and consumption of carbohydrates, sugar, and sweets were inversely related to body weight in two separate studies of London workers and Israeli teenagers. Those workers with higher skinfold thicknesses, an index of greater body fatness, reported lower intakes of sucrose. Similar findings were obtained in studies of Israeli adolescent girls and boys. As body weight increased, sugar intake and the con-

Table 6-2. Food Energy Available for Consumption and Distribution (%) Among the Three Major Food Groups

Year	Food energy (cal)	Percentage of calories as		
		Protein %	Fat %	Carbohydrate %
1909–1913	3480	11.7	32.1	56.2
1935–1939	3260	10.9	36.1	53.0
1947–1949	3230	11.7	38.7	49.6
1957–1959	3140	12.0	40.6	47.4
1965	3150	12.1	40.9	47.0
1970	3300	12.0	42.2	45.7
1975	3220	12.2	42.2	45.6
1976	3300	12.2	42.5	45.3
1979*	3500	11.8	42.9	45.4

Note. Data from USDA Agr. Econ. Rept. No. 138 and from USDA Bulletin CNC (Adm.)-299-14, June 1980.
*Preliminary.

sumption of desserts decreased. Frequency of snacking and number of meals per day also declined with increasing body weight. Fabry et al. have also reported that heavier adult males were more likely to eat three or fewer meals per day, whereas lighter individuals ate five or more meals. These studies are based on self-reports and are therefore subject to intentional as well as unintentional errors.

One study in which the frequency of consumption of carbohydrates (snacks, sweets, and desserts) can actually be estimated shows no positive correlation between body fatness and carbohydrate consumption (Keene, Sklair, & Hoerman, 1973). A group of naval recruits free from dental caries was actually fatter (but not taller) than a group with an excessive number of caries. The cavity-free group presumably consumed fewer carbohydrates (sweets and snacks) than those with the higher incidence of dental caries. Further, the caries-free group appeared somewhat fatter than a control population. These studies fail to provide support for a theory of obesity based on a desire to consume highly palatable foods, a psychological aberration that overrides biological regulation.

Psychological theories of hyperphagia, or eating in response to inappropriate signals, in obese individuals have been prominent in the last decades. These theories have included psychosomatic theories of anxiety or tension reduction following eating as well as social-psychological explanations of inappropriate learned responses. The data base for these theories has generally been laboratory studies rather than naturalistic observations.

Externality Theory

Experimental social psychologists have advanced a theory known as the "externality–internality" hypothesis which characterizes the feeding responses of obese people as different from those of normal weight individuals. This research was originally promulgated by an experimental social psychologist, Stanley Schachter (1968). This theory of human obesity suggested that the eating behavior of obese humans was under the control of external or sensory factors rather than internal or physiological factors. Obese individuals were reported to be less influenced by physiological deprivation states or hunger than normal weight subjects and to overeat because of external cognitive or perceptual factors (Schachter & Rodin, 1974). Relative overeating by moderately obese subjects occurred when food was freely available and attractive (e.g., prominently displayed shelled nuts, particularly good-tasting ice cream); and relative undereating occurred when food was unattractive or when effort was required to obtain the food (e.g., food out of sight—in the refrigerator, unshelled nuts, or ice cream adulterated with quinine).

Experimental Illustrations

In a typical experiment, subjects were not informed that their eating behavior was being recorded. Instead, subjects were told that some other behavior, rating crackers or vitamin tablets, was being studied. In one early study comparing the eating behavior of normal weight and overweight subjects (from 15 to 60% overweight by Metropolitan Life Insurance standards), Schachter and his associates directly manipulated the subjects' degree of deprivation by requiring the subjects to refrain from eating for several hours prior to the experiment (Schachter, Goldman, & Gordon, 1968). Half of the subjects were then given a sandwich lunch and all subjects were asked to "taste" a variety of crackers and rate them on a number of dimensions, such as saltiness and cheesiness. Normal weight subjects ate more crackers in the tasting session when they were deprived than when they had just eaten the sandwiches, whereas overweight subjects ate slightly more crackers after eating the sandwiches than when they had not eaten for several hours. However, obese subjects did not eat more than the normal weight subjects.

In contrast to their apparent unresponsiveness to internal cues, the obese subjects in Schachter's subsequent experiments were affected by manipulations of external food-related signals, such as the passage of time and the taste and sight of food (Nisbett, 1968). Overweight subjects ate more when they were persuaded that it was their dinner time by means of a rigged clock than when they thought it was somewhat earlier, whereas the opposite was true for normal weight subjects. Additionally, overweight subjects ate considerably more of good-tasting food (French vanilla ice cream) than of bad-tasting food (ice cream adulterated with quinine), whereas normal and underweight subjects were less responsive to the different tastes. Again, in many of these studies (see Table 6-3) obese subjects failed to eat more than the normal weight subjects.

These studies can also be interpreted as supporting the notion of generalized heightened responsiveness. This interpretation stimulated an additional line of research (Rodin, 1976) in which eating behavior was assumed to be a special case of a broader phenomenon of generalized stimulus sensitivity. Studies of shock avoidance behavior, emotional responsiveness, and reaction-time studies supported this interpretation (Rodin, 1976). When subjects listened to neutral or emotionally disturbing tape recordings obese subjects reported being more upset than normal weight subjects.

Theoretical Issues

Many experiments over the past decade have failed to confirm these hypotheses. Not all obese individuals behave in an external manner. Furthermore, the experimental results of many of Schachter's experiments have been interpreted in alternative ways. Obese individuals could have strong internal drives for food which they continuously deny and therefore disregard internal signals; or the obese could be concerned with or ashamed of their obesity and consequently have attemped to control eating by responding only to stimuli that are socially appropriate. The obese subjects would therefore eat the amounts implicitly designated in the experiment. The "external" behavior of the obese can then be seen as a correlate of the obesity rather than a causal factor.

Other experiments suggest that cognitive cues can influence the amount eaten by both obese and normal weight individuals. When cognitive and perceptual cues were carefully controlled by requiring subjects to drink from a tube attached to a hidden reservoir, both obese and normal weight subjects responded primarily to cognitive information about preload caloric value rather than to actual caloric value (Jordan, Stellar, & Duggan, 1968). Even when subjects were instructed to attend to and interpret the metabolic cues associated with meals, their intake and hunger ratings were highly related to initial belief about caloric values and unrelated to actual caloric value (Wooley, 1972; Wooley, Wooley, & Dunham, 1972).

Another theoretical issue lies in the unstated assumption that obese individuals consume more food in certain conditions than do normal weight individuals. The theory has attempted to document these conditions. However, the verdict must be that the majority of experiments fail to support the theory (see Rodin, 1978, 1980).

Table 6-3 compares the food intake of obese and normal weight subjects in field studies and laboratory studies. The major discrepancies among studies, such as types of foods, degree of overweight, and the

Table 6-3. Reported Differences in Food Intake Between Obese and Normal Weight Subjects

	Obese > normal weight	Obese = normal weight
Laboratory		
Snacks	$N = 7$	$N = 14$
Sandwiches	$N = 1$	$N = 4$
Meals	$N = 1$	$N = 1$
Observation		
Cafeteria		
restaurant	$N = 3$	$N = 1$

Note. N = number of studies; these results are based on a survey of studies, made from 1968 to 1979 and published in behavioral journals, that directly tested some aspect of externality theory. Representative studies include those of Nisbett (1968), Nisbett and Storms (1975), Price and Grinker (1973), Ross (1974), Schachter and Gross (1968), Schachter, Goldman, and Gordon (1968), and Wooley (1972).

subjects' perception of the experimental demands, can be ignored. In the majority of the laboratory studies, the obese subjects failed to eat more than the normal weight subjects. Thus, a critical assumption of the theory has failed to be substantiated. It is therefore difficult to conclude that the obese subjects' response to the quality, the availability, or the packaging of foods is critical in situations in which obese subjects fail to eat more than normal weight subjects. Table 6-4 shows the results of experiments by many investigators testing another aspect of the externality model, namely, that obese subjects fail to respond appropriately to internal physiological cues of hunger or satiety and consequently when "preloaded" fail to decrease food intake appropriately. Again, it is clear that the majority of studies over the years have failed to confirm this hypothesis.

Finally, Table 6-5 shows the results of many investigators' tests of the externality aspects of the hypothesis, for example, that obese subjects respond more to social or cognitive cues than do normal weight subjects. These cues have variously included the salience of food items, the attractiveness of the food items, the place or the location, and even the palatability. Again, with the exception of palatability, the data fail to confirm the hypothesis. Price and Grinker (1973) reported that neither obese nor normal weight subjects were responsive to preloads, but that there were differences in response to palatability. These results suggest that current concerns with dietary-induced obesity in the rat and the factors promoting variability or susceptibility to an obesity-producing diet may be of critical importance in understanding human variation.

These provocative studies, while now undergoing reinterpretation (Rodin, 1980), have been influential in directing attention to the way in which obese individuals overeat and in focusing attention on developmental factors. From a basis of clinical practice, Bruch (1969) has ad-

Table 6-4. Effect of Preloading on Subsequent Food Intake by Obese and Normal Weight Subjects

Response to preload	
Obese < normal weight	Obese = normal weight
$N = 4$	$N = 8$

Note. N = number of studies. Results are based on a survey of studies published in behavioral journals and directly testing this apsect of externality theory. Representative studies include those of Pliner (1973), Price and Grinker (1973), Schachter, Goldman, and Gordon (1968), and Wooley and Wooley (1973).

Table 6-5. Effect of Cognitive or Social Cues[a] on
Food Intake of Obese and Normal Weight Subjects

Obese > normal weight	Obese = normal weight
$N = 7$	$N = 5$

Effect of palatability or taste factors on food intake
of obese and normal weight subjects

Obese > normal weight	Obese = normal weight
$N = 5$	$N = 1$

[a]Salience, perceived caloric value, self-consciousness.
Based on survey of studies published in behavioral
journals and directly testing this aspect of externality
theory. Representative studies include those of
McKenna (1972), Nisbett (1968), Nisbett and Storms,
(1975), Price and Grinker (1973), Ross (1974), and
Schachter and Gross (1968).

vanced a similar hypothesis that severely obese individuals suffered
from a learning deficiency: Internal cues for food intake or satiety were
never appropriately integrated in early childhood. Studies of learned
satiety provide a basis for these hypotheses.

Conditioned Responses: Hunger and Satiety

Several investigators (Booth, 1977, 1980; LeMagnen, 1955; Stunkard,
1975) have suggested that satiety is a conditioned or learned phenomenon. LeMagnen and Stunkard suggest that absorption occurring by the
end of a meal is not sufficient to explain the cessation of feeding.
Therefore, satiety must be a conditioned response, the conditioning
arising from the delayed aftereffects of eating the food on earlier occa-
sions. LeMagnen demonstrated that the amount consumed in successive
portions of a meal decreased but that differently flavored forms of the
same diet could induce a hypermeal. Thus, the learned meal size would
be disinhibited by novelty or variety.

   Booth (1972) made a further distinction between aversion and
satiety: Aversion affects the initiation or early part of a meal and satiation affects the termination of the meal. Booth has demonstrated
experimentally that the volume of food consumed depends on postingestional or metabolic consequences and that a relative aversion occurs
in the later stages of a meal in rats (Booth, 1972), monkeys (Booth &
Grinker, unpublished), and human subjects (Booth, Lee, & McAleavey,

1976). During early exposure to different diets, rats will consume substantial amounts of different flavors (a dilute diet or a concentrated diet). With repeated exposure, however, when rats are presented with the flavor of the concentrated diet, they learn to take smaller meals and, equivalently, when presented with the flavor of a diluted diet, they learn to take larger meals. Thus, learning can involve increasing the intake of a dilute diet as well as decreasing the intake of a concentrated diet. These experiments of Booth further show that in the early part of a single meal rats will choose the flavor that has been associated with a calorically rich diet (40% starch) rather than the flavor of a dilute carbohydrate diet (5% starch). Toward the end of the same meal, however, the rats will reverse their preferences and will prefer the flavor of the dilute diet. The control of meal size is therefore conditioned, as is the process of satiation within a meal. Booth has recently suggested (1980) that the ability to learn the satiating values of foods may be related to resistance to obesity. "Externality," while not a trait of all obese individuals, was associated with poor conditioning and thus may bear some relation to susceptibility to obesity-producing foods.

Dietary-Induced Obesity

Dietary-induced obesity is critically dependent on an initial hyperphagia, and the behavioral response is an essential component of the obese state. Obesity can be induced in many normal rat and mouse strains by manipulating the composition and the palatability of the diet. High-fat diets (Schemmel, Mickelsen, & Gill, 1970), sweet sucrose solutions (Kanarek & Hirsch, 1977), and a supermarket diet consisting of sweetened condensed milk, cookies, and candies in addition to laboratory chow (Sclafani & Springer, 1976) have all been employed to promote obesity in rodents. The severity of the obesity produced varies considerably according to rat strain, duration of dietary treatment, and the age at which the diet is introduced (Faust, Johnson, Stern, & Hirsch, 1978). When the rats are returned to the standard laboratory diet, some elevation in body weight persists (Faust et al., 1978; Rolls, Rowe, & Turner, in press).

Differences in behavioral responsiveness are seen among various strains of rats and among individual animals. Osborne-Mendel rats are extremely responsive to high-fat feeding; Sprague-Dawley rats are not. Some Sprague-Dawley rats actually fail to become obese on a high-fat diet, gaining no more weight during the experimental period than chow-fed controls. The factors that determine the degree of responsiveness to dietary manipulation in rats of a single strain have so far received little experimental attention.

Summary

Human obesity is possibly best considered as an end product of a succession of risk factors, rather than simply as a result of one metabolic or behavioral abnormality. Although this discussion of physiological and behavioral factors in the etiology of obesity has focused primarily on theories of regulation and on theories of external responsivity to external or dietary cues, there are other genetic, metabolic, behavioral, and environmental factors involved.

The assumptions behind these various theories have been extremely different. The theory of metabolic regulation suggests that the increase in food intake is secondary or in the service of regulation via adipose tissue or adipose cell size. The externality theory, however, suggests that increased food intake occurs because of sensory or external factors and that the increased adiposity is merely a secondary consequence. Recent investigators of dietary obesity are now examining individual differences in responsivity. Both theories have revolutionized the study of obesity. Previously no mechanism or explanation for the increased food intake of obesity was available. In spite of theoretical limitations, these theories represent the first step toward understanding an intractable and incurable disease.

References

Abraham, S., Collins, G., & Nordsieck, M. Relationship of childhood weight status to morbidity in adults. *H.S.M.H.A. Health Reports*, 1971, *86*, 273-284.

Booth, D. A. Conditioned satiety in the rat. *Journal of Comparative and Physiological Psychology*, 1972, *81*, 457-471.

Booth, D. A. Appetite and satiety as metabolic expectancies. In Y. Katsuki, M. Sato, S. F. Takagi, & Y. Oomura (Eds.), *Food intake and chemical senses.* Japan Scientific Societies Press, 1977.

Booth, D. A. Prediction of feeding behavior from energy flows in the rat. In D. A. Booth (Ed.), *Hunger models: Computable theory of feeding control.* London: Academic Press, 1978.

Booth, D. A. Acquired behavior controlling energy intake and output. In A. J. Stunkard (Ed.), *Obesity.* Philadelphia: W. B. Saunders, 1980, pp. 101-143.

Booth, D. A., Lee, M., & McAleavey, C. Acquired sensory control of satiation in man. *British Journal of Psychology*, 1976, *67* (2), 137-147.

Bruch, H. Hunger and instinct. *Journal of Nervous and Mental Diseases*, 1969, *149*, 91-114.

Charney, E., Goodman, H. C., McBride, M., Lyon, B., & Pratt, R. Childhood antecedents of adult obesity: Do chubby infants become obese adults? *New England Journal of Medicine*, 1976, *295* (1), 6-9.

Cleary, M. P., Vasselli, J. R., & Greenwood, M. R. C. Development of obesity in Zucker obese (fa/fa) rat in the absence of hyperphagia. *American Journal of Physiology*, 1980, *238*, E284-E292.

Cohn, C., & Joseph, D. Influence of body weight and body fat on appetite of "normal" lean and obese rats. *Yale Journal of Biology and Medicine*, 1962, *34*, 598-607.

Fabry, P., & Tepperman, J. Meal frequency: A possible factor in human pathology. *American Journal of Clinical Nutrition*, 1970, *23*, 1059-1068.

Faust, I. M., Johnson, P. R., & Hirsch, J. Surgical removal of adipose tissue alters feeding behavior and the development of obesity in rats. *Science*, 1977, *197*, 393-396.

Faust, I. M., Johnson, P. R., & Hirsch, J. Long-term effects of early nutritional experience on the development of obesity in the rat. *Journal of Nutrition*, 1980, *110*, 2027-2034.

Faust, I. M., Johnson, P. R., Stern, J. S., & Hirsch, J. Diet-induced adipocyte number increase in adult rats: A new model of obesity. *American Journal of Physiology*, 1978, *235*, E279-E286.

Forbes, G. B., & Reina, J. C. Adult lean body mass declines with age: Some longitudinal observations. *Metabolism*, 1970, *19*, 653-663.

Garrow, J. S. *Energy balance and obesity in man* (2nd ed.). Amsterdam: Elsevier, 1978, pp. 70-91.

Heald, F. P. The natural history of obesity. *Advances in Psychosomatic Medicine*, 1972, *7*, 102-115.

Hirsch, J. Regulation of food intake: Discussion. In F. Reichsman (Ed.), *Advances in psychosomatic medicine* (Vol. 7, *Hunger and satiety in health and disease*). Basel: Karger, 1972, pp. 229-242.

Hirsch, J., & Knittle, J. L. Cellularity of obese and nonobese human adipose tissue. *Federation Proceedings*, 1970, *29*, 1516-1521.

Jordan, H. A., Stellar, E., & Duggan, S. Z. Voluntary intragastric feeding in man. *Behavioral Biology*, 1968, *1*, 65-67.

Kanarek, R. B., & Hirsch, E. Dietary-induced overeating in experimental animals. *Federation Proceedings*, 1977, *36* (2), 154-158.

Kaufmann, N. A., Poznanski, R., & Guggenheim, K. Eating habits and opinions of teen-agers on nutrition and obesity. *Journal of the American Dietetic Association*, 1975, *66*, 264-268.

Keen, H., Thomas, B. J., Jarret, R. J., & Fuller, J. H. Nutrient intake, adiposity and diabetes. *British Medical Journal*, 1979, *1*, 655-658.

Keene, H. J., Sklair, I. L., & Hoerman, K. C. Caries immunity in naval recruits and ancient Hawaiians. In S. E. Mergenhagen & H. W. Sherp (Eds.), *Comparative immunology of the oral cavity* (DHEW Publ. No. 73-438). Washington, D.C.: U.S. Government Printing Office, 1973, pp. 71-117.

Keesey, R. E. A set-point analysis of the regulation of body weight. In A. J. Stunkard (Ed.), *Obesity*. Philadelphia: W. B. Saunders, 1980, pp. 144-165.

Keesey, R. E., Boyle, P. C., & Storlien, L. H. Food intake and utilization in lateral hypothalamically lesioned rats. *Physiology and Behavior*, 1978, *21*, 265-268.

Kennedy, G. C. The role of depot fat in the hypothalamic control of food intake in the rat. *Proceedings of the Royal Society of London (Biology)*, 1953, *140*, 578-582.

Knittle, J. L. In *Proceedings of Serono Symposium No. 17 on Obesity in Childhood*, Bologna, Italy, 1977.

Knittle, J. L., & Hirsch, J. Effect of early nutrition on the development of rat epididymal fat pads: Cellularity and metabolism. *Journal of Clinical Investigation*, 1968, *47*, 2091-2098.

Krotkiewski, M., Sjostrom, L., Bjorntorp, P., Calgren, C., Garrelik, G., & Smith, U. Adipose tissue cellularity in relation to prognosis for weight reduction. *International Journal of Obesity*, 1977, *1*, 395.

Krotkiewski, M., Sjostrom, L., Bjorntorp, P., & Smith, U. Regional adipose tissue cellularity in relation to metabolism in young and middle-aged women. *Metabolism*, 1976, *24*, 703-710.

LeMagnen, J. Sur le mécanisme d'établissement des appétits caloriques. *Comptes Rendus de l'Académie des Sciences*, 1955, *240*, 2436-2438.

McCance, R. A., & Widdowson, E. M. Nutrition and growth. *Proceedings of the Royal Society of London*, Ser. B., 1962, *156*, 326.

McKenna, R. J. Some effects of anxiety level and food cues on the eating behavior of obese and normal subjects. *Journal of Personality and Social Psychology*, 1972, *22*, 311-319.

Mrosovsky, N., & Powley, T. Set points for body weight and fat. *Behavioral Biology*, 1977, *20*, 205-223.

Nisbett, R. E. Taste, deprivation and weight behavior. *Journal of Personality and Social Psychology*, 1968, *10*, 107-116.

Nisbett, R. E., & Storms, M. D. Cognitive, social physiological determinants of food intake. In H. London & R. E. Nisbett (Eds.), *Cognitive modification of emotional behavior.* Chicago: Aldine, 1975.

Pliner, P. L. Effect of liquid and solid preloads on eating behavior of obese and normal persons. *Physiology and Behavior*, 1973, *11* (3), 285-290.

Price, J. M., & Grinker, J. Effects of degree of obesity, food deprivation, and palatability on eating behavior of humans. *Journal of Comparative and Physiological Psychology*, 1973, *85*, 265.

Rodin, J. The role of perception of internal and external signals on regulation of feeding in overweight and nonobese individuals. In T. Silverstone (Ed.), *Appetite and food intake.* Braunschweig: Pergamon Press/Viewing, 1976.

Rodin, J. Has the distinction between internal versus external control of feeding outlived its usefulness? In G. Bray (Ed.), *Recent advances in obesity research* (Vol. 2). London: Newman, 1978, pp. 75-110.

Rodin, J. The externality theory today. In A. J. Stunkard (Ed.), *Obesity.* Philadelphia: W. B. Saunders, 1980, pp. 226-240.

Rolls, B. J., Rowe, E. A., & Turner, R. C. Persistent obesity in rats following a period of consumption of a mixed high energy diet. *Journal of Physiology*, in press.

Ross, L. Effects of manipulating the salience of food upon consumption by obese and normal eaters. In S. Schachter & J. Rodin (Eds.), *Obese humans and rats.* Washington, D. C.: Erlbaum/Halsted, 1974.

Rothwell, N. J., & Stock, M. J. Mechanisms of weight gain and loss in reversible obesity in the rat (Proceedings). *Journal of Physiology*, 1978, *276*, 66.

Scala, J. Weight control and the food industry. In G. Bray (Ed.), *Recent advances in obesity research* (Vol. 2, *Proceedings of the Second International Congress on Obesity*). London: Newman, 1978, pp. 494-503.

Schachter, S. Obesity and eating. *Science*, 1968, *161*, 751-756.

Schachter, S., Goldman, R., & Gordon, A. The effects of fear, food deprivation and obesity on eating. *Journal of Personality and Social Psychology*, 1968, *10*, 91.

Schachter, S., & Gross, L. Manipulated time and eating behavior. *Journal of Personality and Social Psychology*, 1968, *10*, 98–106.

Schachter, S., & Rodin, J. *Obese humans and rats.* New York: Wiley, 1974.

Schemmel, R., Mickelsen, O., & Gill, J. L. Dietary obesity in rats: Body weight and body fat accretion in seven strains of rats. *Journal of Nutrition*, 1970, *100*, 1041–1048.

Sclafani, A., & Springer, D. Dietary obesity in adult rats: Similarities to hypothalamic and human obesity syndromes. *Physiology and Behavior*, 1976, *17*, 461–471.

Silverstone, J. T., Gordon, R. P., & Stunkard, A. J. Social factors in obesity in London. *Practitioner*, 1969, *202*, 682–688.

Sims, E. A. H., Danforth, E., Jr., Horton, E. S., et al. Endocrine and metabolic effects of experimental obesity in man. *Recent Progress in Hormone Research*, 1973, *29*, 457–496.

Sims, E. A. H., & Horton, E. S. Endocrine and metabolic adaption to obesity and starvation. *American Journal of Clinical Nutrition*, 1968, *21*, 1455–1470.

Stunkard, A. J. Obesity and the social environment. In A. Howard (Ed.), *Recent advances in obesity research* (Vol. 1, *Proceedings of the First International Congress on Obesity*). London: Newman, 1975, pp. 178–190. (a)

Stunkard, A. Satiety is a conditioned reflex. *Psychosomatic Medicine*, 1975, *37*, 383–387. (b)

Stunkard, A. J., & McLaren-Hume, M. The results of treatment for obesity: A review of the literature and report of a series. *AMA Archives of Internal Medicine*, 1959, *103*, 79.

Trayhurn, P., & James, W. P. T. Thermoregulation and non-shivering thermogenesis in the genetically obese (ob/ob) mouse. *Pflügers Archiv*, 1978, *373*, 189.

Trayhurn, P., Thurlby, P. L., Woods, C. J. H., et al. Thermoregulation in genetically obese rodents: The relationship to metabolic efficiency. In M. F. W. Festing (Ed.), *Genetic models of obesity in laboratory animals.* In press.

U.S. Department of Agriculture, Consumer Nutrition Center. *National food review.* Washington, D.C.: U.S. Government Printing Office, 1980.

U.S. Department of Health, Education and Welfare. Ten State Nutrition Survey, 1968–1970. Publication No. HSM 72-8131, 1972.

Wooley, S. C. Physiologic versus cognitive factors in short term food regulation in the obese and non-obese. *Psychosomatic Medicine*, 1972, *34*, 62–68.

Wooley, O. W., Wooley, S. C., & Dunham, R. B. Can calories be perceived and do they affect hunger in obese and non-obese humans? *Journal of Comparative and Physiological Psychology*, 1972, *80*, 250–258.

Wooley, S. C., & Wooley, O. W. Salivation to the sight and thought of food: A new measure of appetite. *Psychosomatic Medicine*, 1973, *35*, 136–142.

Chapter 7

The Physiology of Thirst

ALAN N. EPSTEIN

Animals seek water when the state of thirst arises in their brains and the tonic activity of that state governs their behavior as they select water and ingest it. The problem of the physiology of drinking behavior is therefore essentially that of the brain mechanisms that are the state of thirst. That is, drinking behavior would be understood if we had intimate knowledge of the complex and specific state of brain activity that currently (1) leads the animal to search out water and *expect* that it will be consumed, (2) arouses appetitive behaviors, often highly *individuated*, that bring the animal into contact with water, (3) is accompanied by an *affect* that, in the case of thirst, is usually pleasurable but can, when water intake is deficient, be agonizing, and lastly (4) controls ingestion in harmony with needs for water. As is argued in the preceding review (Chapter 2, this volume), the cognitive and affective aspects of thirst are essential for its full understanding just as they are for our understanding of motivated behavior in general. But we know so little about their physiology or their neurological bases that nothing more can be added here. We do know something about the mechanisms for the control of water ingestion itself because these are closely linked to water losses. We have some understanding of the physiology of the events that lead to the initiation of drinking and to the satiation of water intake. These matters will be the subject of this review.

Fitzsimons' monograph (1979) should be read for a more comprehensive discussion of thirst. It treats aspects not reviewed here, such as the history of the research enterprise, the comparative physiology of thirst, sodium appetite, and thirst as a symptom of disease.

Introduction

Our present understanding of the physiology of thirst began with Andersson's report (1953) of the elicitation of drinking by hyperosmotic treatment of the brain of the goat. Conscious animals showing no interest in water drank avidly, sometimes massively, when stimulated briefly in the anterior hypothalamus with small volumes of hypertonic saline or, in later experiments, with weak electric currents. In addition, simple tasks that the animals had previously learned in order to gain access to water after deprivation were performed in the absence of normal thirst while stimulation was applied to the same sites in the goats' brains from which drinking had been obtained (Andersson & Wyrwicka, 1957). These reports, vividly demonstrating the arousal of thirst by stimulation of the brain, had two important conceptual consequences. First, they ended preoccupation with thirst as a mere sensation, and with drinking behavior as a reflexive response to the reduced salivary flow produced by dehydration (Cannon, 1918); and second, they made a reality of predictions of a central neural basis for thirst as a form of instinctive (Lashley, 1938) and motivated (Stellar, 1954) behavior.

Lesion studies confirmed the existence of a "thirst center" (or more properly, a major focus of the neurological systems for thirst) in the hypothalamus when dogs (Andersson & McCann, 1956) and rats (Montemurro & Stevenson, 1957) were rendered adipsic by ablations of tissues within the medial forebrain bundle of the lateral hypothalamus. The failure to drink was prolonged and in the Andersson and McCann experiments was quite specific. Their dogs refused water for the rest of their postoperative lives but would eat palatable diets and drink nutritive fluids such as beef broth and thereby maintained themselves alive and well.

In this work of the mid 1950s and early 1960s emphasis was given almost exclusively to the thirst of cellular dehydration, first proposed by Wettendorff (1901) and then established as a mechanism of thirst by Gilman's well-known experiments (1937) showing that solutes that are excluded from cells and therefore dehydrate them are the most effective dipsogens.

But the more complex context of current research on the neural mechanisms of thirst was not achieved until Fitzsimons established hypovolemia (reduced blood volume) as an independent stimulus for thirst (1961). He did so by eliciting water intake in rats with a variety of experimental manipulations (hemorrhage, ligation of the inferior vena cava, hyperoncotic colloid dialysis). All these reduce the circulating blood volume without increasing the osmolarity of the remaining plasma, and therefore without withdrawing water from cells. This essential point has been confirmed most clearly by Tang (1976), whose work shows (1) that these treatments reduce the plasma volume of rats without altering serum electrolytes or osmolarity; and (2) that if the reduction in intravascular volume is prevented by intravenous infusion of an isotonic plasma substitute, drinking is suppressed.

Earlier work had suggested that the causes of thirst were complex (Adolph, Barker, & Hoy, 1954) and that changes in extracellular volume, among others, must be considered. But this did not express the idea of hypovolemia as a second and potent cause of thirst capable of operating under normal conditions of dehydration and having an independent sensory system utilizing detectors of reduced blood volume. This concept we owe to Fitzsimons (see Fitzsimons, 1979, for a full summary). Hypovolemia has since been shown to have a low threshold for the initiation of drinking (Stricker, 1968), to generate water intake as a function of the magnitude of the reduction in blood volume (Stricker, 1968), and to yield thirst with the expected properties of motivation (Rolls, Jones, & Fallows, 1972). In addition, the hormone system renin–angiotensin has been shown to be an important participant in its arousal (Fitzsimons, 1969).

The demonstration that both cellular dehydration and extracellular volume loss are each separately competent for the arousal of thirst has suggested the *double depletion hypothesis of thirst* (Epstein, Kissileff, & Stellar, 1973). Evidence for the hypothesis comes from several sources. First, water losses that occur normally, such as deprivation (Hatton & Almli, 1969; Hall & Blass, 1975) and defense against hyperthermia (Hainsworth, Stricker, & Epstein, 1968), deplete *both* cellular water and plasma volume. Second, as described below, water loss arouses thirst by two qualitatively different mechanisms with afferent systems that are separately tuned to either the cellular or the extracellular compartments for body water. Third, cellular dehydration and hypovolemia add quantitatively to produce drinking in rats (Blass & Fitzsimons, 1970; Fitzsimons & Oatley, 1968) and in dogs (Wood, Rolls, & Ramsay, 1977). That is, when applied concurrently, two different thirst challenges produce a total water intake that is the simple sum of the intakes that each produces when it is acting alone. In the Blass and Fitzsimons experiment, for example, cellular dehydration (hypertonic saline administered subcutaneously) produced 20 ml of intake, hypovolemia (hyperoncotic colloid in saline administered intraperitoneally) produced 7 ml, and the combination resulted in 28 ml of water intake. In these experiments excretion of the administered solutes was prevented by ureteric ligation. And, fourth, the hypothesis is supported by the fact that the separate restoration of each deficit produces a partial reduction of drinking. This is also a simple summative effect, and is true in the rat (Ramsay, Rolls, & Wood, 1977a), dog (Ramsay, Rolls, & Wood, 1977b), and monkey (Rolls, Wood, & Rolls, 1981). The dog experiments are summarized in Figure 7-1. The animals were deprived of water for 24 hours and then allowed to drink

168 A. N. Epstein

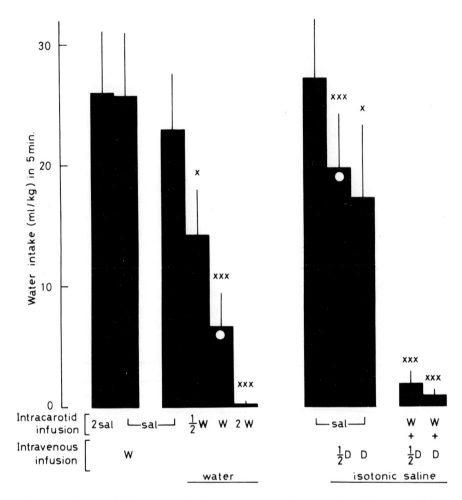

Figure 7-1. Water intake of eight 24-hour water-deprived dogs during depletion restoration experiments. Left to right: Control treatments, intracarotid water infusions, intravenous saline infusions, and combined water and saline infusions. Intracarotid water infusions attenuate the central cellular thirst stimulus and intravenous saline infusions attenuate the extracellular thirst stimulus. White circles indicate treatments that restore central plasma tonicity and systemic plasma volume to predeprivation values. *Intracarotid infusions* (bilateral, 10 minutes): water infusions at a total rate of .6 ml/kg per minute (W) or at half (½W) or twice (2W) this rate. Intracarotid isotonic (.15 M NaCl) saline infusions (sal) were a control procedure to replicate any discomfort of the water infusions, and they accompanied all intravenous infusions. *Intravenous infusions* (40 minutes): isotonic (.15 M NaCl) saline given in volumes equivalent to half (½D) or all (D) of the total fluid loss, by weight, during deprivation. Water (W) given intravenously at .6 ml/kg per minute was to control for peripheral effects of equivalent intracarotid water infusions. Significant differences: x, $p < .05$; xxx, $p < .001$, compared to control. (Modified from Ramsay et al., 1977.)

just after restoration of their cellular or plasma water losses or after the combined restoration of both. Depletions of cellular water were reversed in the forebrain by infusion of water into both carotid arteries (indicated by W in the "Intracarotid infusion" row at the bottom of Figure 7-1). Plasma depletions of the whole body were reversed by intravenous infusion of isotonic saline (as shown by D in the "Intravenous infusions" row). Restoration of the cellular deficit in the forebrain reduced intake by 72% (fifth bar from the left; white dot signifies that the treatment restored central hydration to predeprivation levels as determined by return of jugular venous plasma to normal osmotic pressure), restoration of the systemic volume deficit reduced drinking by 27% (eighth bar from the left; again white dot signifies that treatment succeeded, in this case by restoring blood volume to predeprivation levels as measured by return of plasma protein and hematocrit to normal), and the concurrent restoration of both deficits resulted in a 93% reduction, or virtual elimination, of water intake (last bar on the right). The other bars show that intracarotid isotonic saline by itself (first, second, third, and seventh bars) had no effect, even when combined with intravenous water (given at the same slow rate as that for intracarotid infusion) and that the effects of the treatments were graded when their volume was halved or doubled.

These experiments show that for thirst provoked by deprivation, the double depletion hypothesis gives a very satisfactory account of the causes of drinking behavior. Cellular dehydration of the brain and systemic hypovolemia add to produce the urge to drink, and the concurrent restoration of each deficit results in a summative suppression of drinking. The nature of the receptors for the two depletions, the portions of the brain devoted to their appreciation, and the manner of their joint function in the control of spontaneous drinking behavior are major concerns of current research on the physiology of thirst.

Cellular Dehydration and Brain Osmosensors for Thirst

Lateral Preoptic Osmosensors for Thirst

The operation of the cellular dehydration mechanism of thirst requires that the brain somehow detect water loss from cells. The experiments of Peck and Novin (1971) using the rabbit and of Blass and Epstein (1971) using the rat show that, as is the case for release of ADH, the antidiuretic hormone (Verney, 1947), the principal sensors that arouse thirst during cellular water loss are within the brain itself. The two sets of experiments, performed independently and published in the same year, converge with remarkable agreement on the identification of the lateral preoptic area (LPO) as the site of maximum concentration of the osmosensors for thirst.

Both the Peck and Novin and the Blass and Epstein studies used lesions and both found that brain damage limited to the lateral preoptic area selectively impairs drinking stimulated by a sudden increase in the osmolarity of the blood reaching the brain. Figure 7-2 shows these results. Peck and Novin's reconstructions are shown on the left. They show one of the three (of 28 attempted) lesions that severely impaired cellular dehydration drinking induced by hypertonic sodium chloride given intravenously. It destroyed the tissue within the area of vertical striping. Diagonal and horizontal striping describe lesions that did not produce the deficit. The smallest effective lesion ablated the bed nucleus of the stria terminalis and the lateral preoptic area as well as the intervening anterior commissure. Although deficient in drinking to cellular dehydration, the animals with effective lesions drank normally to water deprivation. Blass and Epstein's lesion results are strikingly similar and more convincing. Larger groups of animals were studied and selectivity of deficit was shown specifically for cellular dehydration versus hypovolemia. Animals whose lesions ablated the LPO bilaterally (at the bottom of Figure 7-2) did not drink or drank less than 20% of normal to cellular dehydration induced by intraperitoneal injection of hypertonic saline, but they drank normally to hypovolemia induced by subcutaneous dialysis with polyethylene glycol. The lesion therefore produced a selective deficit in drinking induced by cellular dehydration. Again, as in the Peck and Novin study, only a minority of the attempted lesions were successful in reducing or eliminating drinking in response only to cellular dehydration. More

Figure 2-2. *Top:* The schematic frontal section of Peck and Novin (1971) drawn ▶ through the anterior commissure (AC) to show the extent of lesions abolishing and sparing drinking induced in the rabbit by cellular dehydration. Vertical striping represents the tissue destroyed bilaterally by the smallest lesion producing the deficit; horizontal striping, the tissue destroyed bilaterally by the largest lesions centered in the LPO that produced no deficit; diagonal striping, the tissue destroyed bilaterally centered in the BST that produced no deficit.

Bottom: The reconstruction from Blass and Epstein (1971) of the minimal neural damage in the rat brain that resulted in selective loss of drinking in response to cellular dehydration. The lesions are drawn in outline on a section through the anterior commissure. The area of bilateral destruction common to all lesions is shown in shading. (Abbreviations: AA, amygdala; AC or CA, anterior commissure; BST, bed nucleus of stria terminalis; C or cp, caudate; CO, optic chiasm; FX, fornix; FMP, medial forebrain bundle; GP, globus pallidus; IC, internal capsule; LPO or pol, lateral preoptic area; MPO or pom, medial preoptic area; OT, optic tract; poma, magnocellular preoptic nucleus; SO, supraoptic nucleus. SP or sl, septum; st, nucleus of the stria terminalis; TCC, corpus callosum; TD, diagonal band; V_{III} or IIIV, third ventricle; VEN, lateral ventricle.)

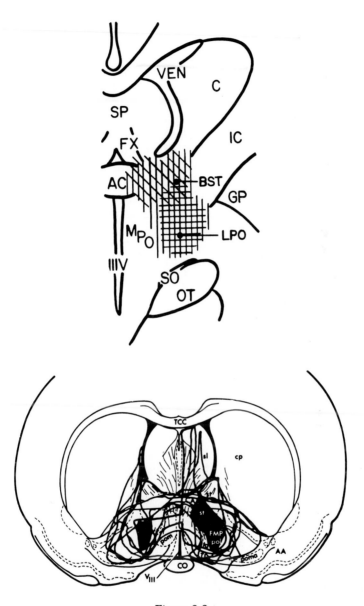

Figure 2.2

frequently, lesions in the preoptic–anterior hypothalamic zone impair thirst nonselectively or not at all.

Both the Peck and Novin and the Blass and Epstein studies relied heavily on elicitation of thirst by direct intracranial injection. The Peck and Novin study, in particular, made meticulous and extensive use of the technique. They chose their solutes carefully, selecting (1) urea, which enters cells freely when inside the blood–brain barrier and therefore does not exert an osmotic pressure; (2) sodium chloride, which was used by Andersson because it is an effective osmotic solute but which, like electrical stimulation, is also a nonspecific excitant of neural tissue; and (3) sucrose, which is the ideal osmotic solute because it is excluded from cells and is therefore capable of establishing an osmotic gradient between the cells and their ambient fluid, but is otherwise inert.

Peck and Novin recognized that the more conservative and most compelling criterion for identification of an osmosensitive zone in the brain for thirst was that it yield drinking behavior when perfused with equiosmotic sodium chloride *and* sucrose, but *not* with equiosmotic urea. Applying this criterion, they injected hypertonic but equiosmotic urea, sodium chloride, and sucrose (1.15 Osmols) into more than 600 sites within the hypothalamus, amygdala, and septum. The majority of them were insensitive to injection of all three solutes. The experimenters found a band of tissue caudal to the LPO running along the medial forebrain bundle from the dorsal–anterior hypothalamus to the posterior-lateral hypothalamus from which drinking could be induced with hyperosmotic saline, but not with sucrose. This reproduced Andersson's original phenomenon but forced a reinterpretation of it as the result of nonspecific activation of neurons within tracts mediating drinking behavior. Feeding and gnawing were also elicited by hyperosmotic saline either singly or with drinking in the same region (three sites within it were sensitive to all three solutes), as would be expected if the behavior were the result of nonspecific activation.

As is shown in Figure 7-3, six sites that clustered tightly within the LPO under the anterior commissure yielded drinking to both sodium chloride *and* sucrose, but not to urea. Sucrose alone was not effective in eliciting behavior of any kind outside this small zone. The crucial criterion of selective activation of thirst by an extracellular solute that is not a general neural excitant was met only by tissue within the lateral preoptic area. Note the obvious congruence of this osmosensitive zone with that shown in Figure 7-2 from which the identical function is inferred from lesions.

The same conclusions about the anatomy of the system emerged from the injection studies of Blass and Epstein. Injections of hyperosmotic sodium chloride and sucrose (but not urea) elicited drinking in the satiated rat, but only when they were made into the lateral preoptic area. Moreover, Blass and Epstein showed that the thirst induced

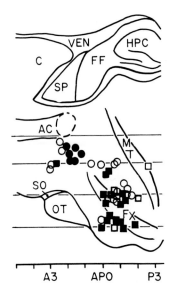

Figure 7-3. The schematic sagittal section from Peck and Novin (1971) of the rabbit diencephalon taken through the vertical plane joining the fornix and the mammillothalamic tracts to indicate the distribution of loci sensitive to cellular dehydration per se, or to hypertonic saline. (Symbols: Drinking induced by cellular dehydration, filled circles; drinking induced by hypertonic saline, open circles; eating induced by hypertonic saline, filled squares; gnawing, scratching, or licking induced by hypertonic saline, open squares.) Note the tight cluster of loci (just under the anterior commissure) from which drinking was elicited by cellular dehydration. (Abbreviations as in Figure 7-2, and HPC, hippocampus; FF, column of the fornix; MT, mammillothalamic tract.)

by cellular dehydration was temporarily suppressed by injection of several microliters of water into the LPO. This demonstrated that, as would be required of a brain sensor, rehydration of the crucial osmosensitive zone satiates cellular dehydration thirst. Second, they demonstrated that the effects of osmotic manipulation of the LPO are behaviorally specific. They found that neither thirst induced by systemic renin nor hunger for a liquid diet was suppressed by watering the LPO.

   Other work has shown the cellular dehydration treatment to have a low threshold, and the same characteristic must be expected of the LPO osmosensors. Increases of only 1–2% in systemic osmotic pressure (.30 OsM) are sufficient to arouse drinking when solute is given intravenously (Wolf, 1950) or subcutaneously (Hatton & Almli, 1969). Sensitivity as low has not been reported for elicitation of thirst by injection of solute directly into the osmosensitive zone of the brain. But Blass has succeeded (1974) in arousing drinking with 2-μl injections of

.33–.34 OsM NaCl or sucrose provided the injections are made bilaterally into the tissue of the LPO and immediately adjacent tissue. A strong case is therefore made for the existence within the LPO of cells that are sensitive to their own water content and have afferent inputs into the brain mechanisms of thirst and drinking behavior.

Electrophysiological Studies of Osmosensitive Sites in the Brain

Since the publication of the Peck and Novin and the Blass and Epstein studies, the lateral preoptic area has been shown to be activated by intracarotid injections of hyperosmotic solutions. Malmo and Mundl (1975) compared the multiple-unit activity of the medial and lateral preoptic areas of the rat while the animals received intracarotid injections of saline over a wide range of concentrations (.1 ml over 5 sec of .15–.75 M NaCl). Sites of activation were found in the lateral preoptic area and in tissue immediately lateral and ventral to it at all injection concentrations above isotonic, and the strength of activation increased with increasing concentration. Medial preoptic area sites were only weakly activated and then only by concentrations above .45 M.

Malmo and Malmo (1979) have also shown that the LPO is activated by osmotically active solutes whether they increase the sodium content of the brain or not. Sucrose and sodium chloride solutions were found to be equally effective when infused directly into the carotid circulation. This important result is shown in Figure 7-4 from their work, which shows the multiunit recordings from a site just dorsal to the LPO. Note the striking similarity of the activation produced by both solutes. They studied 11 sites in or adjacent to the LPO in as many animals (one site per animal) and could find no differences between sucrose and sodium chloride in the latency of the onset of activation, and in the mean percentage change from baseline.

Other studies have found a broader distribution and more variety in the responsiveness to saline stimulation of cells in the brain (Nicolaïdis, 1968; Weiss & Almli, 1975; Blank & Wayner, 1975). These have been unit studies which rely on the preselection of spontaneously active cells. They do not have the virtue of multiple-unit recordings which measure the changes in the summed activity of a population of neurons that may have been active or silent before stimulation, and as a group, these studies do not reveal the relationship of these units to cellular dehydration thirst because they are not supported by behavioral studies.

A complex neurological mechanism can be expected for the cellular dehydration control of thirst. Both zona incerta (Walsh & Grossman, 1973; Evered & Mogenson, 1976) and globus pallidus (Neill & Linn, 1975) lesions have been reported to abolish drinking selectively to systemic hypertonic saline, and midline damage to the brain adjacent

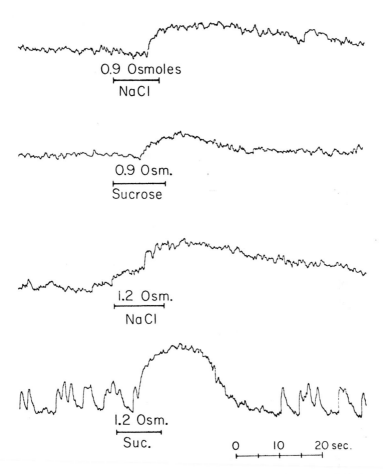

Figure 7-4. Integrated multiple-unit recording of Malmo and Malmo (1979) from a site within the lateral preoptic area of the rat showing the identity of response to intracarotid injection of hypertonic NaCl and sucrose.

to the lamina terminalis produces a complex of deficits that includes failure to drink in response to cellular dehydration (Andersson, Leksell, & Lishajko, 1975; Johnson, Buggy, & Housh, 1976).

In species other than the rat, osmosensors for thirst may be concentrated in brain regions other than the LPO. In dogs (Thrasher, Simpson, & Ramsay, 1980) and sheep (McKinley, Denton, Graham, Leksell, Mouw, Scoggins, Smith, Weisinger, & Wright, 1980) lesions of the anterior wall of the third ventricle which include the lamina terminalis and its organum vasculosum (one of the circumventricular organs of the ependyma) have recently been reported to abolish drinking induced by cellular dehydration.

Alternative Mechanisms for Cellular Dehydration Thirst

Objection has been raised to the thesis of Peck and Novin/Blass and Epstein in lesion studies that have failed to confirm the selective loss of the dipsogenic response to cellular dehydration after lateral preoptic damage (Almli & Weiss, 1974). Instead, a variety of more subtle deficits (elevated thresholds and prolonged latencies to drink to cell dehydration), or combined deficits to both cellular dehydration and hypovolemia, have been reported after lesions in the preoptic area, or in the anterior and lateral hypothalamus. Almli and his colleagues propose that parallel osmosensor systems for thirst may exist in the lateral preoptic area and the lateral hypothalamus (Tondat & Almli, 1976). However, when lesions of the lateral preoptic area and surrounding tissue were made in the 10-day-old suckling a most interesting confirmation was obtained (Almli, Golden, & McMullen, 1976). When tested as juveniles (30–42 days of age) and as adults (43–160 days) animals with such lesions gave attenuated responses to cellular dehydration and exaggerated responses to water deprivation and to the hypovolemia of polyethylene glycol. In addition, they were spontaneously hyperdipsic after weaning and drank enormous excesses of water when allowed to eat and drink after food deprivation. This suggests that the suppression of the LPO by hydration may function in ontogeny to limit water intake.

Others have succeeded in reproducing the Blass and Epstein preparation in the adult rat (Colburn & Stricker, 1976). That is, they have produced animals with only very mild deficits in ingestive behavior immediately after surgery that drink normally to the hypovolemia of hyperoncotic colloid but are behaviorally unresponsive to cellular dehydration. Coburn and Stricker have suggested that such animals may retain a delayed responsiveness to cellular dehydration. This suggestion should be tested in nephrectomized rats, which cannot be drinking in response to the hypovolemia that may result from the excretion of the administered solute load.

Ironically, a more fundamental objection was raised by Andersson, who, having initiated the work leading to the discovery of the LPO osmosensors, has entirely abandoned the idea of sensors for cellular water loss within the brain (Andersson, 1971). He and his colleagues (Andersson, Dallman, & Olsson, 1969) find, in experiments on the goat that rely heavily on intraventricular injection, that thirst (and ADH release) is stimulated by infusions of sodium solutions but not by equiosmolar infusions of other electrolytes (K, NH_4) and not by infusions of sucrose or monosaccharides. In fact, they find that intraventricular infusion of fructose *depresses* the thirst induced by intracarotid infusion of hyperosmotic sodium chloride (Olsson, 1973). Andersson proposes that there are sodium receptors in the walls of the third ventricle that are aroused by the increase in cerebrospinal fluid (CSF) sodium that would accompany a loss of water from the blood.

Andersson's sodium receptor hypothesis is not helpful in understanding how thirst is aroused by cellular dehydration. Sucrose (Peck & Novin, 1971; Blass & Epstein, 1971; Buggy, Hoffman, Phillips, Fisher, & Johnson, 1979) and monosaccharides such as glucose (McKinley, Blaine, & Denton, 1974) or 2-deoxy-D-glucose (Miselis, personal communication) are effective dipsogens when injected into the brain of the rat or sheep, and sucrose is more effective when injected directly into the tissues of the LPO than when injected into adjacent ventricles (Blass, 1974), all of which demonstrates that increases in CSF or brain ECF sodium are not necessary for the arousal of thirst. And recently it has been shown (McKinley, Denton, & Weisinger, 1978; Thrasher, Ramsay, Keil, & Brown, 1978) that such increases are also not sufficient for the arousal of thirst. When equiosmolal solutes are infused intravenously they produce equivalent changes in CSF sodium (and potassium) whether or not they are dipsogenic. That is, 2 M urea or glucose, which are weakly dipsogenic or nondipsogenic, respectively, raise CSF sodium when they are given intravenously to rats, and they do so with latencies, magnitudes, and durations that are indistinguishable from the changes produced by sodium chloride or sucrose (Epstein, 1978).

But sodium is a more effective stimulant of thirst than is sucrose when injected into the CSF and it must be present in the saccharide solutions in order for them to be maximally dipsogenic in the sheep (McKinley et al., 1974). These effects may be understood as the result of the potent nonspecific excitatory effects of strong salt solutions with which Andersson began this line of investigation (1953). In addition, the failure of glucose and fructose to arouse thirst when injected into the ventricles of the goat may be related to their demonstrated soporific effects when injected into the brain of other species (Booth, 1968a).

Lastly, Andersson's idea of sodium receptors within the brain as the principal mediators of thirst is not addressed to the thirst of hypovolemia, which occurs, of necessity, when the sodium content and osmolarity of the body fluids is unchanged.

Hypovolemia and the Neuroendocrine Mechanism of Thirst

As noted in the introduction, hypovolemia is now established as a separate cause of thirst. The demonstration of its independence from cellular dehydration comes from experiments in which rats drink water in response to an isotonic reduction of blood volume (Fitzsimons, 1961;

Stricker, 1969, Tang, 1976). The osmolarity of the plasma is not increased and their thirst cannot be caused by the dehydration of cells.

The Dipsogenic Role of Angiotensin

The discovery of a hormonal control of drinking came from Fitzsimon's demonstration that the kidneys must be in the circulation in order for hypovolemic treatments to have their full dipsogenic effects (1964, 1969). This was shown most clearly in his studies of the thirst that follows caval ligation. By this treatment the principal means by which blood returns to the heart from the abdomen and hind limbs in occluded, thereby reducing cardiac output by some 40%. The result is an acute and severe hypovolemia without change in the chemical composition or water content of the blood that remains in the circulation. The surgery was performed under ether so that the animals were behaviorally competent within a short time after the ligation. Drinking began in the first hour, continued throughout most of the 6-hour observation period, and was considerable (15–20 ml per rat). Sham litigation produced very little drinking, and the impressive water intake produced by the ligation occurred only if the kidneys remained in the circulation. Nephrectomized animals drank, but much less than those whose kidneys were intact, and abolishing the kidney's excretory function by ureteric ligation did not reduce the drinking. Fitzsimons concluded from these and similar data that the kidneys played a major role in the thirst of hypovolemia, but as an endocrine rather than an excretory organ.

Kidney extracts prepared in his laboratory and shown to contain renin by pressor assay were dipsogenic when given to rats by intraperitoneal injection. The dipsogenic action was destroyed by boiling and enhanced by prior nephrectomy, as would be expected of renin. Renin was then shown to be dipsogenic in a dose-dependent manner, and angiotensin II (A II) infused intravenously stimulated thirst in the satiated rat (Fitzsimons & Simons, 1969). The relationship between renin and angiotensin II is given in Figure 7-5, which shows the enzyme cascade that generates the octapeptide. The several target organs and actions of angiotensin are shown at the right. The synthetic cascade is initiated whenever renin is released by hypovolemia, hyponatremia, hypotension, or sympathetic activation of the kidney (Page & Bumpus, 1974). The actions of the hormone reverse the circulatory changes that cause the release of renin. Note, in particular, that the participation by angiotensin in the conservation of water and sodium and in their ingestion will reverse the hypovolemia and hyponatremia, and are essential for the long-term defense of blood volume. In addition to its presence in the kidneys, renin is found in other organs such as the uterus, rodent salivary glands, and, of particular interest, in the brain itself (Ganten, Hutchinson, Schelling, Ganten, & Fischer, 1975). This renin, referred

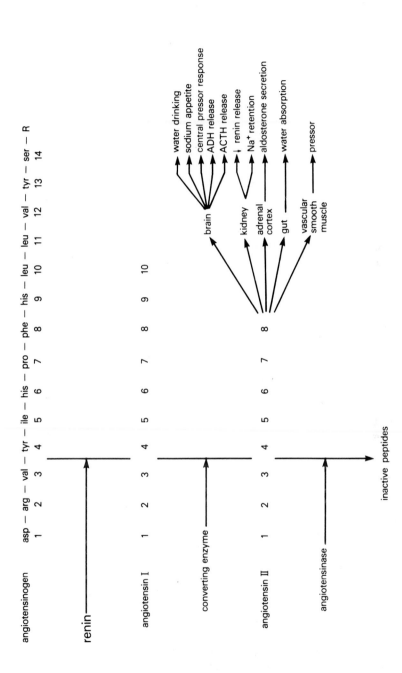

Figure 7-5. From top to bottom: The synthetic cascade for production and degradation of angiotensin II, with the principal target organs and actions of the hormone shown at the right. (Courtesy of James T. Fitzsimons, and modified.)

to as cerebral isorenin, can generate angiotensin intracerebrally. Suggestions have been offered of a role for it in drinking behavior. They are discussed below.

A series of experiments has now shown that angiotensin stimulates thirst at reasonable physiological doses when testing is done under conditions that mimic those that must prevail when the hormone participates in spontaneous drinking (Hsiao, Epstein, & Camarado, 1977). That is, as shown in Figure 7-6, when the hormone is given intravenously after full recovery from the artifacts of surgery, with the animal in its home cage and without the disturbance of restraint and manipulation, rats drink reliably to doses of the hormone (10 ng per rat or 25 ng/kg per minute) that are the same as those that provoke a mild to moderate pressor response (Gross, Bock, & Turrian, 1961), release physiological amounts of aldosterone (Campbell, Brooks, & Pettinger, 1974), and are similar to or less than those employed to produce the other effects of the hormone in animals that have not been nephrectomized (Page & Bumpus, 1974).

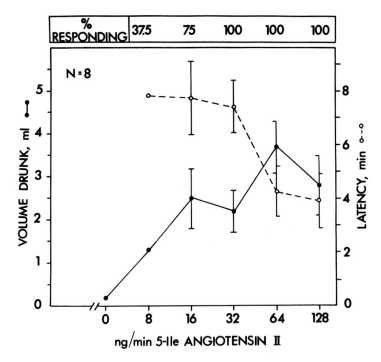

Figure 7-6. Dose–response curve of drinking (left ordinate) and latency to the onset of drinking (right ordinate) as a function of intravenous dose of angiotensin II. Percentage of animals responding at each dose is given in the box at the top. (From Hsiao, Epstein, & Camardo, 1977.)

Direct measurements have now been made by radioimmunassay of the plasma levels of A II that are reached during intravenous infusions of the hormone that produce drinking in the rat, and these have been compared with the levels of A II that are generated endogenously by several normal dipsogenic treatments (12, 24, and 48 hours of water deprivation; ingestion of a dry meal), as well as with those that result from ether anesthesia and from experimental hypertension (unilateral and renal artery constriction) (Johnson, Mann, Housh, & Ganten, 1978; Mann, Johnson, & Ganten, 1979). Before infusion, resting levels of A II were found to be between 50 and 90 pg/ml of plasma. After 1 hour of infusion with the Hsiao and Epstein method and with their lowest effective dipsogenic dose (25 ng/minute), levels of A II were 204 pg/ml. This was designated the "dipsogenic threshold" for the hormone. The animals were water replete and were tested at times when they normally do not drink. The threshold is, therefore, the level to which plasma angiotensin must be raised by intravenous infusion in order to produce drinking when the hormone is the sole dipsogen operating, and when it must act against a neural background of satiation for water and a predisposition to sleep. It could be thought of more as a "ceiling" than a threshold. That is, it is the range of plasma angiotensin levels within which angiotensin is dipsogenic when conditions are unfavorable for drinking. The normal dipsogenic treatments resulted in plasma levels of the hormone that were well above the resting level (12- and 24-hour deprivation, 173% and 134% increase, respectively; dry meal, 151% increase) and somewhat below the conservative threshold for intravenous infusion. The more prolonged dehydration raised plasma levels to twice the dipsogenic threshold and the pathological states raised them as much as 15-fold. The authors conclude, first, that relatively mild dehydrations elevate blood-borne endogenous angiotensin to levels that are dipsogenically effective; and second, that more vigorous challenges to the endogenous renin–angiotensin system result in hormone levels that are far in excess of those that produce drinking.

Drinking to physiological doses of angiotensin has also been shown for the dog (Trippodo, McCaa, & Guyton, 1976; Fitzsimons, Kuchanczyk, & Richards, 1978). And elevations of plasma renin produced in man by several pathological conditions (Conn, Cohen, Lucas, McDonald, Mayor, Blough, Eveland, Bookstein, & Lapides, 1972) are associated with excessive water intake (Brown, Curtis, Lever, Robertson, DeWardener, & Wing, 1969) and complaints of thirst. Rogers and Kurtzman (1973) have used the excess intake, which complicates the management of patients with chronic kidney disease, as an indication for bilateral nephrectomy. They have reported that plasma renin levels fell postoperatively and the excess thirst disappeared. The failure of sheep to drink intravenous angiotensin (Abraham, Baker, Blaine, Denton, & McKinley, 1975) is the result either of differences between species or of experimental design. And lastly, we have known for some time that water deprivation provokes renin release (Maebashi & Yoshinaga, 1967), as does the ingestion of a meal (Blair-West & Brook, 1969). Both, of course, are reliable predictors of drinking behavior.

Central Receptors for the Dipsogenic Action of Angiotensin

The hormone elicits thirst by direct action on the brain (Booth, 1968b; Epstein, Fitzsimons, & Rolls, 1970; Severs, Summy-Long, Taylor, & Connor, 1970). In these experiments, rats drank copiously and repeatedly within tens of seconds or minutes after injection of angiotensin II into their brains. The response was quite specific, both behaviorially, because only drinking behavior was elicited, and chemically, because among the many agents tested (ADH, aldosterone, bradykinin, adrenaline), only angiotensin was dipsogenic (Epstein et al., 1970). Subsequent experiments showed that (1) the precursors of angiotensin II (renin, renin substrate, and angiotensin I) were all highly dipsogenic in the brain (Fitzsimons, 1971). (2) The receptors within the brain for the dipsogenic action of angiotensin are best accommodated by the octapeptide A-II (Fitzsimons, Epstein, & Johnson, 1978). (3) The drinking is blocked or attenuated by prior treatment of the brain with antibodies against angiotensin II (Epstein, Fitzsimons, & Johnson, 1972). (4) The phenomenon is biologically ubiquitous. All species that have been tested drink to intracranial angiotensin. This includes a variety of rodents, several ungulates (sheep and goat), carnivores (dog and cat), the monkey, birds (ringdove and chicken), and the iguana (Fitzsimons, 1979). (5) The thirst elicited by angiotensin has normal motivational characteristics (Rolls & Jones, 1972; Rolls et al., 1972; Kirkstone & Levitt, 1974; Graeff, Gentil, Perex, & Covian, 1973). Intracranial administration suppresses feeding, produces drinking despite quinine adulteration of the water, and generates level pressing for water in animals that have been trained to do so after water deprivation.

As it became increasingly likely that the renin–angiotensin system could function as a hormone of thirst, progress in understanding how it interacts with the brain was obstructed by the demonstrated impenetrability of the blood–brain barrier to circulating angiotensin II. Tritium-labeled angiotensin II with high biological activity, even when used in intravenous doses as high as 2 μg, did not concentrate in any portion of the parenchyma of the brain (Osborne, Pooters, Angles d'Auriac, Epstein, Worcel, & Meyer, 1971; Shrager, Osborne, Johnson, & Epstein, 1975). If angiotensin could not reach cerebral tissue, how did it affect the brain to produce thirst? Where were the receptors for its dipsogenic action? The solution to this vexing problem was provided by the important work of Simpson and his colleagues, who showed, beginning in

1973 (Simpson & Routtenberg), that the subfornical organ, which is on
the surface of the third ventricle, contains the required receptors.

They were led to their precedent-making work by an interest in the
thirst induced by intracranial carbachol (Grossman, 1960). Believing
that it exerts its dipsogenic effect by acting on tissue lining the ventricles, they focused their attention on the subfornical organ of the
third ventricle because of the richness of its cholineacetylase and acetyl-
cholinesterase content. They found that its ablation reduced or abolished the rat's drinking response to carbachol (Simpson & Routtenberg,
1972), and that injection of cholinergic agents, including both acetylcholine and physostigmine, directly into the organ elicited drinking at
low doses and with short latencies (Simpson & Routtenberg, 1974).

The position of the subfornical organ on the anterior–dorsal surface
of the third ventricle is shown in Figure 7-7, a photomicrograph of a
midsagittal section through the rat forebrain. The organ lies between
the foramina of Monro (not shown). It is composed of a highly vascular-

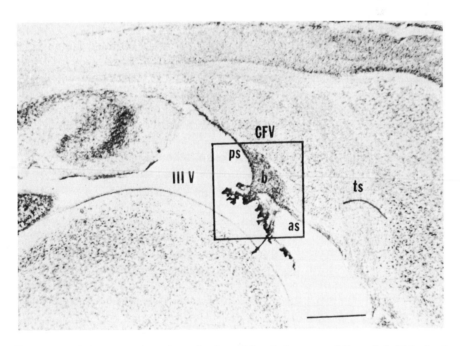

Figure 7-7. Sagittal section through the subfornical organ of the rat (within box)
and surrounding ventricle and parenchyma. The structures adherent to the body of
the organ are portions of the choroid plexus. (Abbreviations: as, anterior stalk of
the subfornical organ; ps, posterior stalk of the organ; b, body of the organ; ts,
triangular nucleus of the septum; CFV, ventral commissure of the fornix; IIIV, third
ventricle. Bar at lower right = 1 mm.) (Photomicrograph courtesy of John B.
Simpson.)

ized body which elongates anteriorly and posteriorly into structures called stalks. It contains neurosecretory cells, tanicytes, and neurons that receive synapses. It is one of the family of circumventricular structures (Akert, 1969; Weindl, 1973) which are midline specializations of ependyma, richly vascularized, in contact over one surface with the cerebrospinal fluid, and outside the blood–brain barrier (Wislocki & Leduc, 1952). This last characteristic made it an attractive candidate for the brain's sensor of angiotensin in its dipsogenic role, particularly when the area postrema, the circumventricular organ of the fourth ventricle, had already been shown to be a receptor organ for the central pressor response of angiotensin II (see Dickenson & Ferrario, 1974, for a review) in the dog.

In addition, the location of the subfornical organ at the dorsal-anterior extremity of the third ventricle between the foramina of Monro placed it in the ideal position for exposure to angiotensin that was injected into the lateral ventricle, which at the time of Simpson and Routtenberg's work was either deliberately or inadvertently the most frequent route of administration of the hormone. They therefore ablated the organ in rats that were drinking an average of 14 ml in response to 100 or 500 ng of angiotensin II injected into the anterior forebrain. Despite the high dose of hormone employed, six of seven animals did not drink in response to the hormone postoperatively (Simpson & Routtenberg, 1973). Lesions in adjacent tissue had no effect. Moreover, drinking (spontaneous or induced by deprivation) was not disturbed by the subfornical organ ablations, except for a brief postoperative hypodipsia.

Lesions studies by themselves, even when they produce specific deficits, cannot demonstrate hormore receptor structures in the brain. They must be complemented by a demonstration that the presumed receptor organ has uniquely high sensitivity to direct application of the active agent. The effect produced should be a faithful mimic of that which occurs when the hormone reaches the brain from the blood. In addition, direct application of specific inhibitors of the hormone to the presumed receptor organ should suppress its action. The suppression should be limited to the effects of the blood–borne hormone, and it should be reversible. The subfornical organ has satisfied all of these criteria.

Figure 7-8, from Simpson, Epstein, and Camardo (1978), is the dose-response curve for drinking elicited by angiotensin II injected directly into the subfornical organ of the rat. The hormone was injected (in a volume of 1.0 μl) from a remote syringe while the animal rested quietly in its home cage. Experiments were conducted during the daylight hours when spontaneous drinking is rare and were completed in 15–20 minutes. Data from nine animals compose the dose–response curve. In all, the tip of the injector lay in the body of the subfornical organ

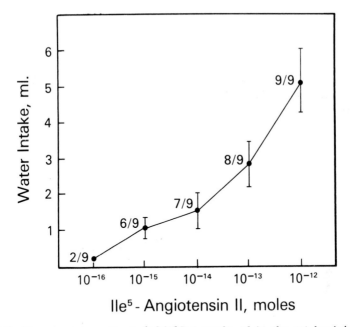

Figure 7-8. Dose–response curve of drinking produced in the rat by injection of angiotensin II directly into the subfornical organ. Doses in moles of hormone. Fractions at each dose give the number of animals responding (numerator) and the number tested (denominator). (From Simpson, Epstein, & Camardo, 1977.)

without rupture of the limiting ependyma of the third ventricle. The fractions adjacent to the curve are response fractions that give the number of animals tested at each dose (denominator) and the number drinking to that dose (numerator). The dose range explored extended from 10^{-16} to 10^{-12} moles of hormone and shows that the threshold dose is between .1 and 1.0 pg of angiotensin II or 10^{-16} and 10^{-15} moles. Intake grows as the dose increases to 1 ng. At that dose all of the animals drink, and the average intake is considerably greater than the average draft size for the rat when it is drinking spontaneously (Kissileff, 1969). The behavior elicited appears quite normal in all respects. It is indistinguishable from that which is elicited by low intravenous doses of the hormone (Hsiao et al., 1977). In animals in which the cannulas had penetrated the ependyma and opened into the ventricular space, or had missed the body of the organ and lay in adjacent tissue such as the ventral commissure of the fornix, the threshold for drinking rose 2 or 3 orders of magnitude.

The requirement of specific and reversible blockade was met in the Simpson, Epstein, and Camardo experiments with the use of a competitive inhibitor of angiotensin II with low intrinsic activity, Saralasin (or P-113), the sarcosine-1, alanine-8 analogue of angiotensin. This analogue has been shown to block the pressor response of intravenous angiotensin II (Pals, Masucci, Denning, Sipos, & Fessler, 1971), and the dipsogenic actions of both intravenous (Tang & Falk, 1974) and intraventricular angiotensin (Fitzsimons et al., 1978a). It was infused into the subfornical organ for a 30-minute period during the last 20 minutes of which the animal received an intravenous infusion of angiotensin II at a high and reliable dose (50 ng/minute). When isotonic saline was infused, drinking occurred, and was quite comparable to that which is produced by the same dose of intravenous angiotensin when the subfornical organ is not irrigated by exogenous solutions. But when the specific competitive inhibitor of angiotensin II perfused the organ, drinking induced by intravenous angiotensin was suppressed. The animals drank no more than when the organ was treated with Saralasin alone, which was shown, in other experiments, to be weakly dipsogenic at the very high doses that were used here in the subfornical organ. As required, the suppression was reversible. Termination of the Saralasin treatment of the subfornical organ restored the dipsogenic action of the blood-borne angiotensin. As is the case for surgical ablation of the organ, the effect of the inhibitor was specific for angiotensin-induced thirst. Thirst induced by systemic cellular dehydration was not suppressed.

Lastly, the Simpson, Epstein, and Camardo experiments showed that ablation of the organ abolishes the drinking produced by intravenous infusion of angiotensin. Animals that suffer a loss of 90% or more of the organ do not drink to intravenous angiotensin even when it is given in doses that are frankly hypertensive (128 ng/minute per rat). Drinking to cellular dehydration or deprivation is not reduced, nor do there appear to be abnormalities of spontaneous drinking once the animals have recovered from the brief hypodipsia that follows SFO damage. The failure to drink seems specific to antiotensin-induced thirst. Complete unresponsiveness to intravenous A II is found as long as 80–84 days after subfornical ablation. The organ is therefore essential for the dipsogenic action of the hormone.

This body of evidence is strengthened by the following additional demonstrations: (1) as shown by radioimmune assay, blood levels of renin (Miselis, Nicolaïdis, Menard, & Siatitsas, 1976) and of angiotensin II (Russell, Abdelaal, & Mogenson, 1975; Abdelaal, Mercer, & Mogenson, 1976) rise impressively after hypovolemic treatments; (2) as shown by radioautography, when doses of hormone as low as 400 ng are used, tritiated angiotensin II can reach the circumventricular organs from the blood (Shrager et al., 1975); (3) the essentiality of the subfornical organ for the drinking induced by blood-borne angiotensin has now been confirmed in the American opossum (Findlay, Elfont, & Epstein, 1980) and in the dog (Thrasher et al., 1980); and (4) as shown by electrophysiology, there are cells within the subfornical organ that respond selectively to angiotensin II.

In this work (Felix & Akert, 1974; Phillips & Felix, 1976) the sub-fornical organ of the cat was exposed in situ and studied by micro-iontophoretic application of angiotensin II, Saralasin (the sar-1, ala-8 competitive analogue of angiotensin II, also known as P-113) and acetyl-choline. Twenty-two units responded to A II. Of these, 19 increased their rate of discharge as the injection current increased, confirming Felix and Akert's earlier demonstration of a dose–response relationship between ejected A II and unit discharge rate (see the top of Figure 7-9). Eighteen of these units ceased their response to A II during concurrent ejection of the specific peptide antagonist (P-113). A unit of this kind is shown in Figure 7-9 at the bottom. It is responsive to both A II and acetylcholine (7 of the 22 units showed such dual responsiveness). Note that the ejection of the blocker produces an immediate slowing of the rate of spontaneous firing followed by a blockade of the excitation pro-duced by exogenous A II. The acetylcholine response is unaffected. Ten units that responded exclusively to A II were all completely suppressed by P-113, whereas the same dose of P-113 did not completely inhibit the seven units with dual responsiveness. Units with similar selective responsiveness to angiotensin have also been found in the rat SFO (Buranarugsa & Hubbard, 1979).

Recent anatomical work of Miselis, Shapiro, and Hand (1979) dem-onstrates that the rat SFO has direct efferent connections that are quite appropriate for a diverse role in the control of body water content. Using autographic transport techniques, both anterograde and retro-grade, they have discovered a set of large SFO neurons that send axons out the anterior stalk of the organ to the organum vasculosum lamina terminalis, or OVLT, the other circumventricular organ of the anterior third ventricle; to the supraoptic nucleus; and to the nucleus medianus of the preoptic area, which may be an important integrative zone for defense of body water by drinking and ADH release (Shrager & Johnson, 1980). Transection of these axons has the same effect as ablation of the SFO, drinking induced by blood-borne angiotensin is abolished (Eng et al., 1980; Lind & Johnson, 1980). Other efferent connections to the posterior forebrain and to the brain stem, as well as the afferent inputs to the SFO, remain to be described with modern neuroanatomical methods.

It seems very clear therefore that the subfornical organ contains receptors for angiotensin, that they can be reached by blood–borne hormone, and that they can provide the means by which the hormone participates in the arousal of thirst.

Nonhormonal Afferents of Hypovolemic Thirst

The thirst of hypovolemia is not explained simply by the operation of angiotensin on the brain. Drinking to hypovolemia has a low threshold and is proportional to the decrease in circulating blood volume over a

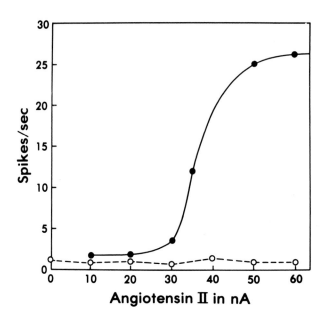

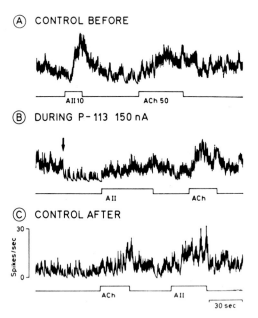

Figure 7-9. *Top:* Dose–response curve of a subfornical unit excited by microionto-phoretically applied angiotensin II (approximate amount of hormone in nanoam-peres, nA, of injection current). Dotted line is absence of response to isotonic saline. (From Felix & Akert, 1974.) *Bottom:* Specific blockade of angiotensin II-sensitive unit by concurrent application of angiotensin II and Saralasin (P-113); ACh is acetylcholine. (From Phillips & Felix, 1976.)

wide range when produced by treatments such as hyperoncotic colloid dialysis, which can be varied quantitatively. But this thirst is not attenuated by nephrectomy (Fitzsimons & Stricker, 1971). Low-pressure baroreceptors in the walls of the great vessels are known to send vagal afferents to the brain that disinhibit ADH secretion when blood volume decreases by only 10% (Share, 1969). Unfortunately, we have no information about their neurology, but their role in hypovolemic thirst is now clearly demonstrated. Fitzsimons and Moore-Gillon (1980) have simulated hypovolemia by inflating an obstructive balloon in the upper abdominal vena cava of dogs thereby reducing their venous return acutely and reversibly. The animals drank repeatedly to this hypovolemic challenge, and they did so promptly, drinking an amount of water that correlated with the severity of the reduction in their central venous pressure. Blockade of the left cervical vagosympathetic nerve (by infiltration of the skin loop containing the nerve with xylocaine), by which much of the low-pressure baroreceptive discharge reaches the brain, enhanced the drinking, demonstrating that, as is the case for ADH release, these afferents exert a tonic inhibitory control over drinking. As expected from this idea, blockade of the nerve in the otherwise normal dog provoked drinking. Similar increases in drinking in response to hypovolemia have been demonstrated in the rat after left cervical vagotomy (Zimmer, Meliza, & Hsiao, 1976; Moore-Gillon, 1980).

Vagal afferents from below the diaphragm may play a more important role in the arousal of thirst than has been previously suspected. Smith and his colleagues (Kraly, Gibbs, & Smith, 1975) have recently reported surprisingly severe deficits in responses to thirst challenges (cellular dehydration, beta-adrenergic activation, hypovolemia, and water deprivation) by rats after recovery from abdominal vagotomy. The animals drank to some of the challenges (hypovolemia and water deprivation) but they did so sluggishly and in diminished volume. Their inertia in drinking is due, in part, to sluggish gastric emptying of water (Kraly, 1978).

Hypovolemia causes renin release and, as noted earlier, a blockade of angiotensin's actions (Abdelaal, Mercer, & Mogenson, 1974) or ablation of the subfornical organ (Simpson et al., 1977) reduce hypovolemic drinking by half in the rat. In their recent experiments Fitzsimons and Moore-Gillon demonstrated that acute obstruction of the venous return raised the plasma renin levels of their dogs, and that competitive inhibition of angiotensin action with infusions of Saralasin prolonged the latency of the onset of their drinking and reduced its amount. As in the rat, the reduction was approximately 50%.

It therefore seems well established that hypovolemic thirst is provoked by a synergy of reduced baroreceptive inputs from the thorax (decreased filling of the great vessels reduces the tonic inhibitory input) and the direct action of angiotensin on the brain. Either is capable of producing thirst when acting alone, but the full behavioral effect is not produced unless they act together. This idea was suggested by earlier work showing that the reduction in the thirst threshold for cellular-dehydration drinking that is produced by blood withdrawal or systemic infusion of angiotensin is lost in dogs that have had left vagosympathetic blockade or transection (Koslowski, Drzewieki, & Sobocinska, 1968; Koslowski & Szczepanska-Sadowska, 1975). This synergy does not appear to operate in the sheep, which is peculiarly insensitive to the dipsogenic action of circulating angiotensin (Abraham et al., 1975). In this animal hypovolemic drinking appears to be mediated almost entirely by the baroreceptors (Zimmerman, Blaine, & Stricker, 1980).

Controversial Issues in Research on Angiotensin-Induced Thirst

Alternatives to Subfornical Organ Receptors

Objections have been raised to the claim of exclusivity for the subfornical organ as the receptor site for the dipsogenic action of angiotensin. First, Mogenson and his colleagues have proposed additional receptor sites in the preoptic area (Mogenson & Kucharczyk, 1975). They have recorded excitation of single units in the lateral hypothalamic area and the ventral tegmentum of the midbrain after injection of angiotensin into the ipsilateral preoptic area, and have reported (Black, Kucharczyk, & Mogenson, 1974), first, that lesions of the lateral hypothalamus ipsilateral to the preoptic cannula through which angiotensin is injected into the rat brain produce more severe impairment of drinking than symmetrical contralateral lesions, and second, that bilateral injection into the preoptic area is more dipsogenic than unilateral injection of the same amount of hormone (Richardson & Mogenson, 1981). All of these data suggest that the preoptic area contains receptors for the dipsogenic action of angiotensin. Fitzsimons et al. (1978b) have drawn similar conclusions from intracranial injection studies in the dog. However, the idea of a preoptic receptive zone is contradicted by the failure of injection into the preoptic area of the rat to elicit thirst, even at high doses of angiotensin, unless the cannula traverses the anterior ventricles (Johnson & Epstein, 1978).

Secondly, recovery of the dipsogenic action of angiotensin has been reported (Buggy, Fisher, Hoffman, Johnson, & Phillips, 1975) within 10–14 days after what have been described as complete lesions of the subfornical organ. In this work the hormone was injected into the lateral ventricle, and the temporary reduction of its dipsogenic action was attributed to blockade of the foramen of Monro by lesion debris and edema. A very similar result has come from recent work with the opossum (Findlay & Epstein, 1980), which recovers responsiveness to angiotensin some weeks after ablation of the subfornical organ, but only to hormone injected directly into the anterior cerebral ventricles. That is, these possums did not respond to intravenous angiotensin, but did drink when the hormone was given into the third ventricle. Alternate receptors that are somehow responsive to angiotensin generated within the brain (recall that there is a renin–angiotensin system within the brain itself) but that are insensitive to blood-borne angiotensin are implicated by this work. Buggy and his colleagues may have been activating just such receptors in their earlier work.

Thirdly, deliberate obstruction of the ventricular lumen with injected cold cream (Buggy & Fisher, 1976; Hoffman & Phillips, 1976) has produced two results that can be explained only with recourse to hypothetical receptors for the dipsogenic action of angiotensin at some site in the brain other than the subfornical organ. In these experiments commercial cold cream is injected into the ventricular space of unanesthetized rats in order to fill portions of its lumen. Angiotensin is then injected into the ventricles elsewhere and is apparently excluded from the cream-filled areas. The procedure is benign. It does not compromise the animals' behavioral competence. High doses of the hormone are used, but in this instance they support the argument of the work. On the one hand, drinking occurred when the cold cream occluded access to the subfornical organ. On the other hand, drinking did not occur when the cold cream covered the anterior–ventral third ventricle, in the region of the lamina terminalis and organum vasculosum lamina terminalis (OLVT), leaving the dorsal third ventricle and the subfornical organ uncovered and exposed to hormone reaching it through the foramen of Monro.

Angiotensin employs receptors in the area postrema (Ueda, Katayama, & Kato, 1972; Dickenson & Ferrario, 1974) and in the central grey of the midbrain (Deuben & Buckley, 1970) for its central pressor action, and it is a potent releaser of ADH (Severs & Daniels-Severs, 1973; Mouw, Bonjour, Malvin, & Vander, 1971; Peck, 1973). It may act in both these roles and others on receptors that have been identified pharmacologically (Bennett & Snyder, 1976) and microiontophoretically (Wayner, Ono, & Nolley, 1973; Gronan & York, 1976) in many parts of the forebrain. Research in hand supports the possibility that alternative receptors for dipsogenic action of the hormone exist within the parenchyma of the brain. But we do not yet know where they are, and they cannot mediate thirst induced by blood-borne angiotensin because subfornical organ ablation completely abolishes that effect even when high intravenous doses are employed (Simpson et al., 1977). In addition, they cannot be sensitive to blood-borne angiotensin that may reach the CSF from the blood because this has now been excluded by careful radioimmune assay of CSF during intravenous infusion of

high doses of angiotensin II (Shelling et al., 1976). The alternative receptors, if they exist, may appreciate changes in the levels within the
brain of angiotensin that may be generated by the cerebral isorenin
system (Ganten, Hutchinson, Schelling, Ganten, & Fischer, 1975),
but it must be noted that the proposals of such receptors (Phillips
& Hoffman, 1974) rest heavily on lesion studies (Andersson et al.,
1975; Johnson et al., 1976).

Satiety Systems for Thirst

Septal Inhibitory System

Massive septal lesions enhance the drinking induced by dipsogenic treatments that are mediated in whole or in part by angiotensin. Rats with
such lesions are spontaneously hyperdipsic postoperatively (Harvey &
Hunt, 1965), but their excessive drinking is selective. They do not drink
more to cellular dehydration and in most cases do not drink prandially
as a consequence of salivary deficits (Blass & Hanson, 1970). They
drink more than normal rats to ligation of the vena cava, release of
endogenous renin by beta-adrenergic agonists, injection of exogenous
renin, and intravenous infusion of angiotensin. Electrical stimulation of
the septum has been reported to specifically suppress thirst in which
the renin–angiotensin system participates (Blass & Moran, 1975). This
has led to the suggestion that the septum contains a neural system that
is specifically inhibitory for the thirst mediated by angiotensin (Blass &
Hanson, 1970; Blass, Nussbaum, & Hanson, 1974). Although this idea
remains an attractive one, recent studies of this problem have left the
neurological basis of the phenomenon unclear. Cells have been found in
the septum (Bridge & Hatton, 1973) that respond to thirst challenges,
but they respond to both cellular dehydration and hypovolemia, imply-
ing a more general role in thirst. The full meaning of this interesting
phenomenon is therefore still unclear.

Prostaglandins of Cerebral Origin

The prostaglandin E's (PGEs) synthesized within the brain provide another interesting possibility for an inhibitory control of thirst, and
particularly of those forms of thirst in which angiotensin plays a role.
Kenney and Epstein (1978) reported that when injected into the lateral
cerebral ventricle, prostaglandin E_1 and E_2 (but not prostaglandin A
or $F_{2\alpha}$) suppress drinking induced by angiotensin. The suppression is effective at doses as low as 10 ng per rat, is not an artifact of the anorexia
associated with the intracranial injection of the PGEs, and appears to

increase with increasing dependence of the thirst challenge upon angiotensin. Moreover, Fluharty (1981) has shown that the suppression is produced by intracranial injection of arachidonic acid, the precursor of the prostaglandins. Kenny and Epstein have proposed that as angiotensin activates thirst, it concurrently stimulates the synthesis of the prostaglandin E's, which then participate in the suppression of drinking by their vasodilator action. The effective prostaglandin may be produced on the periphery. Kenny and Moe (1981) have shown, in recent work, that the drinking produced by intravenous angiotensin is enhanced in the rat by prior treatment of the animals with a blocker of prostaglandin synthesis. It was administered to the animals in their food and would therefore have suppressed PG synthesis in peripheral tissues.

This idea has the interesting conceptual corollary that the activation of thirst by angiotensin is itself vasoactive. That is, the hormone may act on specialized vascular beds in the brain just as it does in the peripheral blood vessels. It may produce vasoconstriction which is then transduced into a neural signal contributing to the arousal of thirst (Kenney & Epstein, 1978; Nicolaïdis & Fitzsimons, 1975). This idea is encouraged by the fact that the suppressive effect can be produced by vasodilator drugs such as nitroprusside and papavarine as well as by the PGEs, and by the fact that vasoconstrictors (norepinephrine, serotonin) are dipsogenic when delivered at high dose into the brain ventricles.

Several of the neuropeptides are also antidipsogenic. These include substance P (DeCaro, Massi, & Micossi, 1978), enkephalin (DeCaro, Micossi, & Venturi, 1979), and bradykinin (Kenney, 1980). Others such as elidoisin and physalamine are also antidipsogens in the rat, but are dispogenic in the pigeon (Evered, Fitzsimons & DeCaro, 1977).

The Satiety of Rehydration

We have no account of the neurological system that mediates satiety for thirst. The septal and prostaglandin contributions to satiety that are mentioned above are both only poorly understood and both appear to be closely linked to thirst aroused by angiotensin. The more powerful and ubiquitous satiator of thirst is cellular rehydration (Adolph, 1969). Providing water, either intragastrically or parenterally, so that it enters cells and restores their diminished water content, reduces or eliminates the thirst of both cellular dehydration (Holmes & Montgomery, 1960) and hypovolemia (Stricker, 1969).

We do not know how the brain appreciates the rehydration of its cells. It may do so in some circumstances by restoration of the volume of the lateral preoptic osmosensors. Blass and Epstein (1979) suppressed the thirst of cellular dehydration by watering that part of the brain, but the LPO osmosensors do not appear to be necessary for satiety, since animals with LPO ablations sufficient to abolish cell dehydration thirst do not overdrink to other thirst challenges such as water deprivation. Moreover, Blass and Hall (1974) have shown that it is not simply restoration of cellular water that yields full satiety. For optimal effect the cellular rehydration must take place while the animal is drinking water, that is, there must be contiguity between the restoration of the internal state of the cells and the sensory feedback from the acts of drinking and from gastric distension.

This analysis places a burden of complexity on the neurological mechanism for the mediation of thirst satiety. It cannot be simply a population of cells that are sensitive to their own rehydration and that deliver inhibition to thirst mechanisms elsewhere in the brain. At the very least, satiety must be mediated by a neurological system that utilizes converging outputs from rehydrated cells and from receptors in the oropharynx and upper gastrointestinal tract. Projections from afferents into the hypothalamus have been reported recently (Norgren, 1976) and suggest that convergences of the required kind may exist in the forebrain.

Cells have been found in the diencephalon and forebrain of the rat (Edinger, 1971), the rabbit (Ranck, 1976), and the monkey (Vincent, Arnauld, & Bioulac, 1972) that decrease their electrical discharge when drinking begins. They could certainly contribute to satiety, but the abruptness with which they reduce their activity at the very onset of drinking does not match the temporal course of satiety.

The Neuropharmacology of Thirst

Neurochemical Mediation of Thirst

At this writing there is no neuropharmacology of thirst, although one or several can be expected from the fragmentary evidence in hand. The strong case that has been made for mediation by dopamine of the thirst induced by angiotensin (Setler, 1973) is of particular interest. The dipsogenic action of angiotensin is blocked by prior application to the brain of haloperidol, but not by either an alpha- or beta-adrenergic blocker. Selective depletion of dopamine, but not norepinephrine, reduces the dipsogenic effectiveness of intracranial angiotensin without affecting the thirst induced by carbachol. Furthermore, deprivation-induced drinking (but not feeding) is reduced by haloperidol, is unaffected by alpha- or beta-adrenergic blockers, and is increased, relative to food intake, after overnight starvation, by a combination of drugs within the brain that increases the amount of available dopamine (a beta-hydroxylase inhibitor plus L-DOPA). Dopamine itself is dipsogenic when given into the lateral ventricle, but the very high doses that must be used (about 200 μg) produce weakness and ataxia. It is most remarkable that animals drink during such treatments despite the disabling artifacts of the amine.

These experiments relate directly to Ungerstedt's (1971) important observations of severe deficits in thirst and hunger that follow destruction of the biogenic pathways of the midbrain. With local injections of 6-hydroxydopamine and subsequent histochemical verification, he showed that rats with combined loss of both dopamine and norepinephrine ascending pathways suffered a syndrome of aphagia and adipsia that mimicked the early stages of the lateral hypothalamic syndrome (Teitelbaum & Epstein, 1962). Depletion of norepinephrine alone did not impair ingestive behavior. Similar animals prepared by others (Smith, Strohmeyer, & Reis, 1972; Marshall, Richardson, & Teitelbaum, 1974) have many of the residual deficits that characterize the lateral hypothalamic syndrome (failure to drink to all thirst challenges and failure to eat to glucoprivation). The thirst deficits, in particular, have been associated with damage to the nigrostriatal bundle and subsequent depletion of forebrain dopamine (Oltmans & Harvey, 1972).

It has been proposed (Stricker & Zigmond, 1976) that the failure of animals with lateral hypothalamic damage to drink and eat to acutely imposed metabolic imbalances is caused by depletions of forebrain monoamines (dopamine, in particular), rather than by disruption of specific systems for the response to physiological imbalances. By this interesting argument, the loss of the monoamines deprives the brain of a background of neurochemical activation that is essential for rapid mobilization of homeostatic behaviors. Marshall and Ungerstedt (1976) recently supported this idea by comparing the restoration of responsiveness to thirst challenges that is produced by apomorphine when it was given, on the one hand, to rats made adipsic and aphagic by intraventricular injection of 6-OH-dopamine, and on the other hand, to those made adipsic and aphagic by lateral hypothalamic lesions. They report a transient recovery of function with apomorphine treatment in the former group but not in the latter. That is, animals whose forebrains had been depleted of dopamine by injection of 6-OH-DA into the ventral tegmental area and were not drinking to cellular dehydration and isoproterenol, responded to both thirst challenges while under the influence of a powerful dopamine agonist (systemic apomorphine). But the failure of animals with electrocoagulation of the lateral hypothalamic area to respond to thirst challenges was not reversed by apomorphine. The lateral hypothalamic syndrome (Teitelbaum & Epstein, 1962; Epstein, 1971) therefore appears to be a complex result of neurochemical depletion of the forebrain and destruction of additional neural systems essential for homeostatic behavior in response to specific physiological challenges.

Norepinephrine has a well-established role in feeding behavior

(Grossman, 1960), and manipulations of brain norepinephrine also affect drinking. Large amounts (1–20 µg) injected into the tissue of the medial preoptic area attenuate but do not abolish drinking induced by water deprivation and by cellular dehydration, but not that induced by hypovolemia or angiotensin (Setler, 1973). This effect is most effectively prevented by alpha-adrenergic blockers. In food- and water-satiated animals, injection of similar amounts into the paraventricular nucleus and its immediate vicinity provoke a brief bout of drinking that precedes eating but nevertheless will occur in the absence of food (Liebowitz, 1976).

There is some evidence of a role for serotonin in thirst (Lehr & Goldman, 1973). The amine is dipsogenic when injected into the anterior ventricles, and destruction of the raphe nuclei of the midbrain produces a transient increase in water intake (Lorens & Yunger, 1974). Histamine has also been reported to produce thirst when injected into the brain (Liebowitz, 1973) and has been implicated in the thirst of cellular dehydration (Goldstein & Halperin, 1977) and in food-associated drinking in the rat (Kraly, 1981).

Although intracranial carbachol is a potent and reliable dipsogen in the rat (Grossman, 1960), it is not dipsogenic in most other animals. And atropinization of the brain, although it blocks the drinking produced by carbachol (Levitt & Fisher, 1966), does not affect the thirst of cellular dehydration or water deprivation (Blass & Chapman, 1971), nor does it suppress drinking induced by angiotensin. This is true in the cat (Cooling & Day, 1973) as well as the rat (Fitzsimons & Setler, 1971; Covian, Gentil, & Antunes-Rodrigues, 1972). Nevertheless, there may be a cholinergic component in the neuropharmacology of thirst, because lesions of the septum that result in hyperdipsia are correlated with decreased brain acetylcholine (Sorenson & Harvey, 1971). Myers and his colleagues have reported an intriguing overlap of nicotinic and angiotensin sites for thirst in the monkey brain (Myers, Hall, & Rudy, 1973). These are the only current fragments of evidence for a cholinergic system. They invite further investigation.

Convergence of Systems Arousing Thirst

The Role of the Lateral Hypothalamic Area

Water losses from the lungs, skin, gut, and kidneys deplete both the cellular and extracellular compartments, and concurrent experimental depletion of each compartment yields drinking that is the sum of that which would have occurred if each had acted alone (Fitzsimons & Oatley, 1968; Blass & Fitzsimons, 1970). Although each depletion alone is competent to generate thirst, their cooperation in the arousal of spontaneous drinking behavior is fundamental to the double depletion hypothesis of thirst (Epstein et al., 1973). They must converge within the brain to produce a single motivational state. More than two decades ago it was shown that small lesions within the posterior–lateral lateral hypothalamic area produce prolonged adipsia in the rat (Montemurro & Stevenson, 1957). Animals with these lesions, sometimes produced by mere insertion of the electrodes, ate palatable foods but did not drink water for as long as 55 days. Larger lesions of the lateral hypothalamic area and adjacent tissues (Epstein & Teitelbaum, 1964) including the nigrostriatal bundle (Oltmans & Harvey, 1972), produce severe and permanent adipsia for all acutely administered thirst challenges. These tissues remain the favored candidates for the zone of convergence of thirst afferents and for their transformation into the urge to drink. This appears to require the joint action of neural systems mediating specific depletion signals (Epstein, 1971) and neurochemical systems for arousal and vigilance (Stricker & Zigmond, 1976).

The double depletion hypothesis assumes that prior to convergence the several determinants of thirst and drinking behavior are mediated by separate neurological systems. Support for this idea is provided by the work, discussed earlier in this review, on the medial preoptic osmosensitive zone (Peck & Novin, 1971; Blass & Epstein, 1971; Malmo & Malmo, 1979) and the subfornical organ (Simpson et al., 1977). The idea is further strengthened by the work of Grossman and his students (see Grossman, 1979, for a review) which shows, first, that knife cuts which interrupt fibers passing between the globus pallidus and the caudate nucleus do not interfere with spontaneous drinking which occurs largely at mealtime, but reduce or abolish drinking induced by specific thirst challenges (cellular dehydration, hypovolemia); and second, these studies show that ablation of the anterior zona incerta (Walsh & Grossman, 1978) essentially eliminates drinking in response to cellular dehydration and to isoproterenol and intracranial angiotensin, but does not impair hypovolemic or spontaneous drinking. Lesions of the more posterior zona incerta, on the other hand, increase the animals' sensitivity to quinine adulteration but do not result in deficits in drinking to specific depletions (Evered & Mogenson, 1976), suggesting interference with a system concerned with the hedonic evaluation of fluids rather than with homeostatic drinking. The selectivity of these effects and the facts that they occur in animals without sensorimotor or arousal deficits and that they are not accompanied by catecholamine depletions of the forebrain make it likely that specific and anatomically separate neural systems have been disrupted by the surgical interventions.

Issues That Await Neurological Explanation

Thermal Control of Drinking Behavior

It was proposed some time ago from work on the goat (Andersson &
Larsson, 1961) that brain temperature exerted a direct control over
water intake. Specifically, it was found that heating of the anterior
hypothalamus and preoptic area induced water intake and other de-
fenses against hyperthemia (vasodilation, panting). This finding has now
been confirmed and extended in sheep (Baldwin & Cooper, 1980), in
which it is found that heating the hypothalamus aguments drinking,
and cooling it decreases drinking. Neither treatment affects feeding
behavior. But there are species differences here. Rats drink less, not
more, when the same portions of the brain are heated to temperatures
that are within the upper limit of the physiological range (Hamilton &
Ciaccia, 1971), and they do not drink at all in the heat despite life-
threatening hyperthermia unless they are dehydrated (Hainsworth
et al., 1968). Rats and most small mammals cool themselves by spreading saliva on their body surfaces. In doing so they lose blood volume,
their cells become dehydrated, and they drink as a consequence of
these water losses. The desalivate rat does not dehydrate in the heat
and does not drink despite rapid and potentially lethal hyperthermia.
A role for peripheral heat sensation has been suggested. Small water
intakes are associated with exposure to high ambient temperatures and
this may represent drinking that is under direct thermal control (Grace
& Stevenson, 1971), but it will have to be distinguished from the drinking that is learned by rats in anticipation of heat exposure. Ollove (personal communication) has recently shown that rats that do not drink
when first brought to an unheated antechamber just prior to heat stress
in an adjacent compartment drink increasing amounts of water in the
antechamber as the experience is repeated.

The Role of Mouth Dryness

Having rejected the exaggerated role that ideas about dryness of the
mouth once played in our thinking about thirst, we should be prepared
to reconsider its proper place among the several determinants of drinking behavior. The evidence against a primary and exclusive role for the
sensation is strong. Drinking behavior continues spontaneously when
the water consumed does not pass through the oropharynx. That is,
rats that are not given access to water for ingestion by mouth will
operate levers for intragastric (Epstein, 1960) or intravenous (Rowland
& Nicolaïdis, 1974) water and in doing so maintain constant daily intakes. Their total intake is constant, albeit reduced, and sufficient for

long-term maintenance, and the water is consumed in discrete "drafts" taken mostly at night. Moreover, we know now that the chronic dryness of the mouth that is produced by desalivation does *not* exaggerate water intake except under the special circumstances of a dry diet. When compelled to swallow dry food from a dry mouth the rat acquires the habit of drinking a very small draft of water immediately after each morsel of food is taken into the mouth. The result is what Kissileff and Epstein (1969) called prandial drinking. The accumulation of a very large number of such drafts results in daily hyperdipsia. Prandial drinking does not occur in normal animals. In fact it was first observed in rats that had recovered from the immediate postoperative aphagia and adipsia of lateral hypothalamic lesions (Teitelbaum & Epstein, 1962) and which were found to have severely deficient salivary flow (Hainsworth & Epstein, 1966). Analysis of the phenomenon in the brain-damaged animal led to an understanding of its mechanism. It is due entirely, both in the recovered lateral-lesioned and in the neurologically normal rat without salivary glands, to the solution that prandial drinking provides for the difficulty of swallowing dry food in the absence of saliva (see Kissileff, 1973). The extraordinary fact for this discussion is that the desalivate rat drinks *less* than normal under several thirst-provoking circumstances and does not drink excessively except when prandial drinking is required. It drinks less to water deprivation (Epstein, Spector, Samman, & Goldblum, 1964), hypovolemia (Stricker & Wolf, 1969; Gutman et al., 1967), constant access to water in the absence of food (Vance, 1965), and in the heat (Hainsworth et al., 1968). The only exception is the desalivate's normal response to cellular dehydration (Epstein et al., 1964). The desalivate human also does not drink excessively, and distinguishes between water drunk simply to wet the mouth and that which is drunk to satisfy thirst (Austin & Steggerda, 1936). Clearly dryness of the mouth is not thirst, and the emphasis on it that we owe to Cannon's authority (1918) was a caricature of the problem of drinking behavior.

But it is an undeniably prominent sensation in the human experience of dehydration, and its relief affords much of the pleasure of fluid intake. What is its proper role in the physiology of thirst? How can we account for the paradoxical fact that the desalivate appears to be less thirsty than normal? Mouth and throat dryness may, in fact, serve as a salient cue of water loss, and wetting of the mouth appears to be an effective reinforcer of drinking, but the desalivate, having a chronically dry oropharynx, or at least one in which decreases in surface hydration are greatly attenuated, may no longer experience the increase in dryness that accompanies dehydration and may be less motivated to drink water. It may therefore drink only minimally, relying on renal conservation to defend body water constancy, except when it must swallow dry food. The sluggishness with which the desalivate drinks may, therefore, conceal something of importance for our understanding of the sensory events within the oropharynx that arouse and maintain the state of thirst. They merit further investigation.

Drinking Without Deficits

Although providing a productive framework for the promotion of research on the brain mechanisms of thirst, the double depletion hypothesis is an incomplete description of the controls of drinking behavior. Its major premise is that drinking is initiated by the additive effects of deficits in cellular and plasma water, and this implies that drinking will not occur in the absence of such deficits. As discussed earlier, this concept accounts for drinking when depletions have been produced by water deprivation, but it does not appear to be broad enough to explain the drinking done spontaneously by animals such as the rat. First, the selective abolition of one control of thirst does not reduce the total daily intake of the rat when it is allowed to drink as part of its spontaneous behavior. This is true both of the animal with effective LPO lesions (Blass & Epstein, 1971) and of the animals with ablation of the SFO (Simpson et al., 1977). It appears that the several controls of thirst are compensatory. That is, drinking behavior can still be emitted in a normal fashion despite the absence of one control because the others are sufficient to arouse and terminate drinking and to meter intake in accordance with water needs.

Secondly, the double depletion hypothesis does not account for the drinking that occurs in apparent absence of deficits. Animals such as the rat can satisfy their water needs in a small number of large drafts, but when allowed to drink spontaneously they do so frequently, taking small drafts periodically when they are unlikely to be in water deficit, and when they could rely on urine concentration to defer drinking for many hours. Kissileff (1969) recorded drinking continuously in rats that were allowed to drink freely in their home cages, and showed that they drank 15-18 drafts, mostly at night, and all were small in volume (78% between .5 and 2.5 ml, median = 1.2 ml). The question then for an animal like the rat is why does it drink so often and so little in each draft when, in a homeostatic sense, it does not have to do so. Even in animals like the carnivores that drink infrequently and in large drafts these questions cannot be evaded. Although it has been easier in the dog than in the rat to demonstrate body water deficits just prior to spontaneous drinking (Rolls et al., 1981), the question remains, why do they drink before they are compelled to do so by exhaustion of their several means of water conservation?

The question is answered by acknowledging that there are controls of drinking that appear to operate in the absence of significant water loss.

In the typical adult mammal, they may be the dominant controls of spontaneous drinking behavior. We are only beginning to characterize them and have just begun the study of their neurological mechanisms. Cognitive and hedonic controls appear to be prominent among them. In animals like ourselves ingestive behavior is preceded by expectations and is accompanied by feelings. It is the anticipation of water intake that begins an episode of drinking behavior. Most often, in fact, an animal becomes thirsty in the absence of water and the brain mobilizes the search for the missing commodity in anticipation of it.

This is well illustrated by several studies of drinking behavior. In the first, Fitzsimons and LeMagnen (1969) examined the adjustments in water intake that are imposed upon rats by the substitution of high-protein for high-carbohydrate diets. The former requires more water for excretion, and animals that have been eating high-protein diets for some time drink more and do so at meal time. Fitzsimons and LeMagnen found that water intake did indeed increase when they introduced the high-protein diet, but for the first few days the extra drinking was not done in association with meals. The synchronization of the extra water intake with meal taking was delayed for several days. They pointed out that such synchronization of the drinking with meals cannot be a mere consequence of the increased water losses because they occur long after both the food and water have been ingested. Fitzsimons and LeMagnen suggest that the sensory qualities of the food themselves become an immediate stimulus for excess drinking by which the animal meets needs for water before they actually arise.

A second example comes from the work of Kriekhaus and Wolf (1968). They showed that rats that had prior experience operating levers that delivered plain or salty water will, when made salt deficient for the first time, approach the "salty" bar from a distance in preference to the "water" bar, and will work at it vigorously even when both bars are disengaged and deliver no fluids. That is, having learned where salt was and how to get it, the rats expected to find it there and worked for it when made salt deficient.

Thirdly, Nicolaïdis (1968) found cells in the lateral hypothalamus that were activated or suppressed with equal effectiveness by water or hypertonic saline given into the carotid circulation or directly onto the tongue. They may be serving an anticipatory function, as he suggests in a subsequent review (Nicolaïdis, 1974), and it would be most interesting to reinvestigate them in the unanesthetized animal. Units that appear to anticipate the availability of food or water that has not yet been taken into the mouth have been found in the hippocampus of rats that have been trained to expect them, and they are differentially activated by signals that have been associated with the presentation of either food or water (Olds & Hirano, 1969).

The hedonic aspects of ingestion must also be considered in completing the picture of the physiology of thirst. Once it has been initiated, drinking behavior is charged with feeling. The animal seeks the water and drinks it with an avidity that is somehow generated by the sensory qualities of the fluid it finds and ingests. The palatability of the fluid therefore contributes to the amount of water drunk, either reducing it when the fluid is aversive or increasing it, sometimes to the limits of overhydration, when its flavor is enhanced. Supersweet fluids have been devised from combinations of glucose and saccharin. These are drunk in daily volumes that often exceed the animal's body weight (Valenstein, Cox, & Kakolewski, 1967). There is precious little that can be said about the neural mechanisms of these effects of palatability except to recall the intriguing fact that projections from the brain-stem nuclei of the chemical senses have now been traced into the hypothalamus (Norgren, 1976).

The photoperiod is also an important control of ingestion. The spontaneous drinking (and feeding) behavior of virtually all animals is obedient to the light/dark cycle (Richter, 1965), with good evidence of an endogenous or circadian periodicity (Gutman, Benzakein, & Chaimovitz, 1969) that, in the rat, appears to be acquired during weaning (Levin & Stern, 1975). Again, neurological investigation has only begun. Lesions of the suprachiasmatic nucleus of the basal hypothalamus abolish the circadian cyclicity of ingestive behavior as well as that of locomotion (Stephan & Zucker, 1972). The nucleus appears to receive photoperiodic information via a direct retinohypothalamic pathway (Moore, 1974).

The Ontogeny of Drinking Behavior

The depletional controls of drinking are operative in the neonatal rat, long before they are employed in adult behavior. Their competence so early in ontogeny suggests a means by which the double depletion mechanisms may provide a basis on which the more complex physiology of thirst is built in the adult. The facts are these. When behavioral testing is limited to consumatory responding by allowing rat pups to ingest or reject water that is infused into their mouths, it is found that they drink to cellular dehydration as early as 2 days after birth (Wirth & Epstein, 1976). Other deficits control drinking shortly thereafter, hypovolemia at 4 days and renin release (provoked by treatment with isoproterenol) at 6. Intracranial angiotensin is an effective dipsogen at the transition of 4 to 5 days of age (Misantone, Ellis, & Epstein, 1980). The infant rat is therefore equipped by its ontogeny with an impressive set of controls of drinking behavior by the end of its first week of postnatal life, one week at least before it will ingest water (Krecek & Krecekova, 1957) and more than two weeks before it is weaned. A similar precocity has been shown for the controls of feeding (Houpt & Epstein, 1973). These depletional controls may be the earliest elements with which the cognitive, hedonic, and circadian controls are combined in later development to produce the ultimate and complex drinking behavior of the mature animal (Epstein, 1976).

It is tempting to suggest that in ontogeny, and especially during weaning, ingestive behaviors are frequently and episodically aroused by depletions that are made more salient to the animal by their accompanying peripheral sensations such as dryness of the oropharynx. As maturation proceeds, the depletions and their accompanying sensations may be used to organize ingestion into short bouts of feeding and drinking that occur frequently as punctuations in the animal's daily round of spontaneous behaviors. The close contiguity of feeding and drinking is a well-established fact. In Kissileff's studies (1969), 84% of all drafts occurred either 20 minutes before or 20 minutes after meals. In other words, as the animal develops, drinking and feeding may occur as natural complements of each other, and they may occur frequently and in modest amounts, not because the animal is compelled to restore accumulated deficits, but because it anticipates the pleasures of ingestion and thereby avoids the deficits entirely.

References

Abdelaal, A. E., Mercer, P. F., & Mogenson, G. J. Drinking elicited by polyethylene glycol and isoproterenol reduced by antiserum to angiotensin II. *Canadian Journal of Physiology and Pharmacology*, 1974, *52*, 362–363.

Abdelaal, A. E., Mercer, P. F., & Mogenson, G. J. Plasma angiotensin II levels and water intake following α-adrenergic stimulation, hypovolemia, cellular dehydration and water deprivation. *Pharmacology, Biochemistry and Behavior*, 1976, *4*, 317–321.

Abraham, S. F., Baker, R. M., Blaine, E. H., Denton, D. A., & McKinley, M. J. Water drinking induced in sheep by angiotensin—a physiological or pharmacological effect? *Journal of Comparative and Physiological Psychology*, 1975, *8*, 503–518.

Adolph, E. F. Regulation of water intake in relation to body water content. In *Handbook of physiology*, Section 6: *Alimentary canal* (Vol. 1). Washington, D.C.: American Physiological Society, 1969, pp. 163–171.

Adolph, E. F., Barker, J. P., & Hoy, P. A. Multiple factors in thirst. *American Journal of Physiology*, 1954, *178*, 538–562.

Akert, K. The mammalian sub-fornical organ. *Journal of Neuro-Visceral Relationships*, 1969, Suppl. 9, 78–93.

Almli, C. R., & Weiss, C. R. Drinking behaviors: Effects of lateral preoptic and lateral hypothalamic destruction. *Physiology and Behavior*, 1974, *13*, 527–538.

Almli, C. R., Golden, G. T., & McMullen, N. T. Ontogeny of drinking behavior of preweaning rats with lateral preoptic damage. *Brain Research Bulletin*, 1976, *1*, 437–442.

Andersson, B. The effect of injections of hypertonic NaCl-solutions in different parts of the hypothalamus of goats. *Acta Physiologica Scandinavica*, 1953, *28*, 188-201.

Andersson, B. Thirst and brain control of water balance. *American Scientist*, 1971, *59*, 408-415.

Andersson, B., Dallman, M. F., & Olsson, K. Observations on central control of drinking and release of antidiuretic hormone (ADH). *Life Sciences*, 1969, *8* p. 1, 425-432.

Andersson, B., & Larsson, B. Influence of local temperature changes in the preoptic area and rostral hypothalamus on the regulation of food and water intake. *Acta Physiologica Scandinavica*, 1961, *52*, 75-89.

Andersson, B., Leskell, G., & Lishajko, F. Perturbations in fluid balance induced by medially placed forebrain lesions. *Brain Research*, 1975, *99*, 261-275.

Andersson, B., & McCann, S. M. The effect of hypothalamic lesions on the water intake of the dog. *Acta Physiologica Scandinavica*, 1956, *35*, 312-320.

Andersson, B., & Wyrwicka, W. The elicitation of a drinking motor conditioned reaction by electrical stimulation of the hypothalamic "drinking area." *Acta Physiologica Scandinavica*, 1957, *41*, 194-198.

Austin, V. T., & Steggerda, F. R. Congenital dysfunction of the salivary glands with observations on the physiology of thirst. *Illinois Medical Journal*, 1936, *69*, 127-138.

Baldwin, B. A., & Cooper, T. R. Effects of warming and cooling the hypothalamus on food and water intake in sheep. Paper presented to the *7th International Conference on the Physiology of Food and Fluid Intake*, Warsaw, July 1980.

Bennett, J. P., Jr., & Snyder, S. Angiotensin II binding to mammalian brain membranes. *Journal of Biological Chemistry*, 1976, *251*, 7423-7430.

Black, S. L., Kucharczyk, J., & Mogenson, C. J. Disruption of drinking to intracranial angiotensin by a lateral hypothalamic lesion. *Pharmacology, Biochemistry and Behavior*, 1974, *2*, 515-522.

Blair-West, J. R., & Brook, A. H. Circulatory changes and renin secretion in sheep in response to feeding. *Journal of Physiology (London)*, 1969, *204*, 15-30.

Blank, D. L., & Wayner, M. J. Lateral preoptic single unit activity: Effects of various solutions. *Physiology and Behavior*, 1975, *15*, 723-730.

Blass, E. M. Evidence for basal forebrain thirst osmoreceptors in rats. *Brain Research*, 1974, *82*, 69-76.

Blass, E. M., & Chapman, H. W. An evaluation of the contribution of cholinergic mechanisms to thirst. *Physiology and Behavior*, 1971, *7*, 679-686.

Blass, E. M., & Epstein, A. N. A lateral preoptic osmosensitive zone for thirst in the rat. *Journal of Comparative and Physiological Psychology*, 1971, *76*, 378-394.

Blass, E. M., & Fitzsimons, J. T. Additivity of effect and interaction of a cellular and an extracellular stimulus of drinking. *Journal of Comparative and Physiological Psychology*, 1970, *70*, 200-205.

Blass, E. M., & Hall, W. G. Behavioral and physiological bases of drinking inhibition in water deprived rats. *Nature*, 1974, *249*, 485-486.

Blass, E. M., & Hanson, D. G. Primary hyperdipsia in the rat following septal lesions. *Journal of Comparative and Physiological Psychology*, 1970, *70*, 87-93.

Blass, E. M., & Moran, J. S. Specific inhibition of angiotensin mediated drinking in rats by stimulation of the septum. *Neuroscience Abstracts*, 1975, *1*, 470.

Blass, E. M., Nussbaum, A. E., & Hanson, D. G. Septal hyperdipsia: Specific enhancement of drinking to angiotensin in rats. *Journal of Comparative and Physiological Psychology*, 1974, *81*, 422-439.

Booth, D. A. Effects of intrahypothalamic glucose injection on eating and drinking elicited by insulin. *Journal of Comparative and Physiological Psychology*, 1968, *65*, 13-16. (a)

Booth, D. A. Mechanism of action of norepinephrine in eliciting an eating response on injection into the rat hypothalamus. *Journal of Pharmacology and Experimental Therapeutics*, 1968, *160*, 336-348. (b)

Bridge, J. G., & Hatton, G. I. Septal unit activity in response to alterations in blood volume and osmotic pressure. *Physiology and Behavior*, 1973, *10*, 769-774.

Brown, J. J., Curtis, J. R., Lever, A. F., Robertson, J. I. S., DeWardener, H. E., & Wing, A. J. Plasma renin concentration and the control of blood pressure in patients on maintenance haemodialysis. *Nephron*, 1969, *6*, 329-349.

Buggy, J., & Fisher, A. E. Anteroventral third ventricle site of action for angiotensin induced thirst. *Pharmacology, Biochemistry and Behavior*, 1976, *4*, 651-660.

Buggy, J., Fisher, A. E., Hoffman, W. E., Johnson, A. K., & Phillips, M. I. Ventricular obstruction: Effect of drinking induced by intracranial angiotensin. *Science*, 1975, *190*, 72-74.

Buggy, J., Hoffman, W. E., Phillips, M. I., Fisher, A. E., & Johnson, A. K. Osmosensitivity of the rat third ventricle and interactions with angiotensin. *American Journal of Physiology*, 1979, *236*, R75-R82.

Buranarugsa, P., & Hubbard, J. I. The neuronal organization of the rat subfornical organ *in vitro* and a test of the osmo- and morphine receptor hypotheses. *Journal of Physiology (London)*, 1979, *291*, 101-116.

Campbell, W. B., Brooks, S. N., & Pettinger, W. A. Angiotensin II- and angiotensin III-induced aldosterone release in vivo in the rat. *Science*, 1974, *184*, 994-996.

Cannon, W. B. The physiological basis of thirst. *Proceedings of the Royal Society (London)*, 1918, Ser. B, *90*, 283-301.

Coburn, P. C., & Stricker, E. M. Osmoregulatory thirst in rats following lateral preoptic lesions. *Neuroscience Abstracts*, 1976, *2*, 298.

Cooling, M. J., & Day, M. D. Antagonism of central dipsogenic and peripheral vasoconstrictor responses to angiotensin II with Sar^1-Ala^8-angiotensin in the conscious rat. *Journal of Pharmacy and Pharmacology*, 1973, *25*, 1005-1006.

Conn, J. W., Cohen, E. L., Lucas, C. P., McDonald, W. J., Mayor, G. H., Blough, W. M., Jr., Eveland, W. C., Bookstein, J. J., & Lapides, J. Primary reninism. *Archives of Internal Medicine*, 1972, *130*, 682-686.

Covian, M. J., Gentil, C. G., & Antunes-Rodrigues, J. Water and sodium chloride intake following microinjections of angiotensin II into the septal area of the rat. *Physiology and Behavior*, 1972, *9*, 373-377.

DeCaro, G., Massi, M., & Micossi, L. G. Antidipsogenic effect of intracranial injections of substance P in rats. *Journal of Physiology (London)*, 1978, *279*, 133-140.

DeCaro, G., Micossi, L. G., & Venturi, L. Drinking behavior induced by intracerebroventricular administration of enkephalins to rat. *Nature*, 1979, *277*, 51.

Deuben, R. R., & Buckley, J. P. Identification of a central site of action of angiotensin II. *Journal of Pharmacology and Experimental Therapeutics*, 1970, *175*, 139-146.

Dickenson, C. J., & Ferrario, C. M. Central neurogenic effects of angiotensin. In

I. H. Page & F. M. Bumpus (Eds.), *Angiotensin.* Heidelberg: Springer-Verlag, 1974, pp. 408-414.

Edinger, H. M. Single unit firing patterns during drinking. *Proceedings of the 4th International Conference of Regulation of Food and Water Intake.* Cambridge, England, 1971.

Eng, R., Miselis, R. R., & Salanga, G. Knife cuts of the anterior stalk of the subfornical organ produce drinking deficits to angiotensin II but not to other dipsogenic challenges. *Neuroscience Abstracts,* 1980, *6,* 33.

Epstein, A. N. Water intake without the act of drinking. *Science,* 1960, *131,* 497-498.

Epstein, A. N. The lateral hypothalamic syndrome. In E. Stellar & J. M. Sprague (Eds.), *Progress in physiological psychology.* New York: Academic Press, 1971, pp. 263-317.

Epstein, A. N. Feeding and drinking in suckling rats. In D. Novin, W. Wyrwicka, & G. Bray (Eds.), *Hunger: Basic mechanisms and clinical implications.* New York: Raven Press, 1976, pp. 193-202.

Epstein, A. N. Consensus, controversies, and curiosities. (In M. J. Fregly (Ed.), Angiotensin-Induced Thirst: Peripheral and Contral Mechanisms.) *Federation Proceedings,* 1978, *37,* 2711-2715.

Epstein, A. N., Fitzsimons, J. T., & Johnson, A. K. Prevention by angiotensin II antiserum of drinking induced by intracranial angiotensin. *Journal of Physiology (London),* 1972, *230,* 42-43P.

Epstein, A. N., Fitzsimons, J. T., & Rolls, B. J. Drinking induced by injection of angiotensin into the brain of the rat. *Journal of Physiology (London),* 1970, *210,* 474.

Epstein, A. N., Kissileff, H. R., & Stellar, E. (Eds.). *The neuropsychology of thirst.* Washington, D.C.: V. H. Winston & Sons, 1973.

Epstein, A. N., Spector, D., Samman, A., & Goldblum, C. Exaggerated prandial drinking in the rat without salivary glands. *Nature,* 1964, *201,* 1342-1343.

Epstein, A. N., & Teitelbaum, P. Severe and persistent deficits in thirst produced by lateral hypothalamic damage. In M. J. Wayner (Ed.), *Thirst: Proceedings of the 1st International Symposium on Thirst in the Regulation of Body Water.* Oxford: Pergamon Press, 1964, pp. 395-406.

Evered, M. D., Fitzsimons, J. T., & DeCaro, G. Drinking behaviour induced by intracranial injections of eledoisin and substance P in the pigeon. *Nature (London),* 1977, *268,* 332-333.

Evered, M. D., & Mogenson, G. J. Regulatory and secondary water intake in rats with lesions of the zona incerta. *American Journal of Physiology,* 1976, *230,* 1049-1057.

Felix, D., & Akert, K. The effect of angiotensin II on neurons of the cat subfornical organ. *Brain Research,* 1974, *76,* 350-353.

Findlay, A. L. R., Elfont, R. M., & Epstein, A. N. The site of the dipsogenic action of angiotensin II in the American opossum. *Brain Research,* 1980, *198,* 85-94.

Fitzsimons, J. T. Drinking by rats depleted of body fluid without increase in osmotic pressure. *Journal of Physiology (London),* 1961, *159,* 297-309.

Fitzsimons, J. T. Drinking caused by constriction of the inferior vena cava in the rat. *Nature,* 1964, *204,* 479-480.

Fitzsimons, J. T. The role of renal thirst factor in drinking induced by extracellular stimuli. *Journal of Physiology (London),* 1969, *201,* 349-369.

Fitzsimons, J. T. The effect on drinking of peptide precursors and of shorter chain peptide fragments of angiotensin II injected into the rat's diencephalon. *Journal of Physiology (London)*, 1971, *214*, 295–303.

Fitzsimons, J. T. *The physiology of thirst and sodium appetite.* Cambridge, England: Cambridge University Press, 1979.

Fitzsimons, J. T., Epstein, A. N., & Johnson, A. K. Peptide antagonists of the renin-angiotensin system in the characterization of the receptors for angiotensin-induced thirst. *Brain Research*, 1978, *153*, 319–331. (a)

Fitzsimons, J. T., Kucharczyk, J., & Richards, G. Systemic angiotensin-induced drinking in the dog: A physiological phenomenon. *Journal of Physiology (London)*, 1978, *276*, 435–448. (b)

Fitzsimons, J. T., & LeMagnen, J. Eating as a regulatory control of drinking in the rat. *Journal of Comparative and Physiological Psychology*, 1969, *67*, 273–283.

Fitzsimons, J. T., & Moore-Gillon, M. J. Drinking and antidiuresis in response to reductions in venous return in the dog: Neural and endocrine mechanisms. *Journal of Physiology (London)*, 1980, *308*, 403–416.

Fitzsimons, J. T., & Oatley, K. Additivity of stimuli for drinking in rats. *Journal of Comparative and Physiological Psychology*, 1968, *66*, 450–455.

Fitzsimons, J. T., & Setler, P. E. Catecholaminergic mechanisms in angiotensin-induced drinking. *Journal of Physiology (London)*, 1971, *218*, 43–44P.

Fitzsimons, J. T., & Simons, B. J. The effect on drinking in the rat of intravenous infusion of angiotensin, given alone or in combination with other stimuli of thirst. *Journal of Physiology (London)*, 1969, *203*, 45–57.

Fitzsimons, J. T., & Stricker, E. M. Sodium appetite and the renin–angiotensin system. *Nature, New Biology*, 1971, *231*, 58–60.

Fluharty, S. J. Cerebral prostaglandin biosynthesis and angiotensin-induced drinking in rats. *Journal of Comparative and Physiological Psychology*, 1981, in press.

Ganten, D., Hutchinson, J. S., Schelling, P., Ganten, U., & Fischer, H. The iso-renin angiotensin systems in extrarenal tissue. *Clinical Experimental Pharmacology and Physiology*, 1975, *2*, 127–151.

Gilman, A. The relation between blood osmotic pressure, fluid distribution and voluntary water intake. *American Journal of Physiology*, 1937, *120*, 323–328.

Goldstein, D. J., & Halperin, J. A. Mast cell histamine and cell dehydration thirst. *Nature*, 1977, *267*, 250–252.

Grace, J. E., & Stevenson, J. A. F. Thermogenic drinking in the rat. *American Journal of Physiology*, 1971, *220*, 1009–1015.

Graeff, F. G., Gentil, C. G., Perex, V. L., & Covian, M. R. Lever-pressing behavior caused by intraseptal angiotensin II in water satiated rats. *Pharmacology, Biochemistry and Behavior*, 1973, *1*, 357–359.

Gronan, R. J., & York, D. H. Effects of angiotensin on cells in the preoptic area of rats. *Neuroscience Abstracts*, 1976, *2*, 300.

Gross, F., Bock, K. D., & Turrian, H. Untersuchen über die Blutdruckwinkung von Angiotensin. *Helvetica Physiologica et Pharmocologica Acta*, 1961, *19*, 42–47.

Grossman, S. P. Eating or drinking elicited by direct adrenergic or cholinergic stimulation of hypothalamus. *Science*, 1960, *132*, 301–302.

Grossman, S. P. The biology of motivation. *Annual Review of Psychology*, 1979, *30*, 209–242.

Gutman, Y., Benzakein, F., & Chaimovitz, M. Kidney factors affecting water consumption in the rat. *Israel Journal of Medicine and Science*, 1967, *3*, 910–911.

Gutman, Y., Benzakein, F., & Chaimovitz, M. Effect of illumination on water intake, thirst, and urine output in the rat. *American Journal of Physiology*, 1969, *217*, 471-474.

Hainsworth, F. R., & Epstein, A. N. Severe impairment of heat-induced saliva-spreading in rats recovered from lateral hypothalamic lesions. *Science*, 1966, *153*, 1255-1257.

Hainsworth, F. R., Stricker, E. M., & Epstein, A. N. Water metabolism of rats in the heat: Dehydration and drinking. *American Journal of Physiology*, 1968, *214*, 983-989.

Hall, G. H., & Blass, E. M. Orogastric, hydrational, and behavioral controls of drinking following water deprivation in rats. *Journal of Comparative and Physiological Psychology*, 1975, *89*, 939-954.

Hamilton, C. L., & Ciaccia, P. J. Hypothalamus, temperature regulation, and feeding in the rat. *American Journal of Physiology*, 1971, *221*, 800-807.

Harvey, J. A., & Hunt, H. F. Effect of septal lesions on thirst in the rat as indicated by water consumption and operant responding for water reward. *Journal of Comparative and Physiological Psychology*, 1965, *59*, 49-56.

Hatton, G. I., & Almli, C. R. Plasma osmotic pressure and volume changes as determinants of drinking thresholds. *Physiology and Behavior*, 1969, *4*, 207-214.

Hoffman, W. E., & Phillips, M. I. Regional study of cerebral ventricle sensitive sites to angiotensin II. *Brain Research*, 1976, *110*, 313-330.

Holmes, J. H., & Montgomery, A. V. Relation of route of administration and types of fluid to satisfaction of thirst in dog. *American Journal of Physiology*, 1960, *199*, 907-911.

Houpt, K. A., & Epstein, A. N. The ontogeny of the controls of food intake in the rat: GI fill and glucoprivation. *American Journal of Physiology*, 1973, *225*, 58-66.

Hsiao, S., Epstein, A. N., & Camardo, J. S. The dipsogenic potency of intravenous angiotensin. *Hormones and Behavior*, 1977, *8*, 129-140.

Johnson, A. K., Buggy, J., & Housh, M. W. Effects of lesions surrounding the anteroventral third ventricle (AC3V) on fluid homeostasis. *Neuroscience Abstracts*, 1976, *2*, 301.

Johnson, A. K., & Epstein, A. N. The cerebral ventricles as the avenue for the dipsogenic action of intra-cranial angiotensin. *Brain Research*, 1975, *86*, 399-418.

Johnson, A. K., Mann, J. F. E., Housh, M. W., & Ganten, D. Plasma Angiotensin II (A II) levels and thirst. *Neuroscience Abstracts*, 1978, *4*, 175.

Kenney, N. J. A case study in the neuroendocrine control of goal-directed behavior: The interactions between angiotensin II and prostaglandin E_1 in the control of water intake. In R. F. Thompson, L. H. Hicks, & V. B. Shvyrkov (Eds.), *Neural mechanisms of goal-directed behavior and learning.* New York: Academic Press, 1980, pp. 437-446.

Kenney, N. J., & Epstein, A. N. The antidipsogenic role of the E-prostaglandins. *Journal of Comparative and Physiological Psychology*, 1978, *92*, 204-219.

Kenney, N. J., & Moe, K. E. The role of endogenous prostaglandin E in angiotensin-II-induced drinking. *Journal of Comparative and Physiological Psychology*, 1981, in press.

Kirkstone, B. J., & Levitt, R. A. Comparisons between drinking induced by water deprivation or chemical stimulation. *Behavioral Biology*, 1974, *11*, 547-559.

Kissileff, H. R. Food associated drinking in the rat. *Journal of Comparative and Physiological Psychology*, 1969, *67*, 284-300.

Kissileff, H. R. Nonhomeostatic controls of drinking. In A. N. Epstein, H. R. Kissileff, & E. Stellar (Eds.), *The neuropsychology of thirst*. Washington, D. C.: V. H. Winston & Sons, 1973, pp. 163-194.

Kissileff, H. R., & Epstein, A. N. Exaggerated prandial drinking in the recovered lateral rat without saliva. *Journal of Comparative and Physiological Psychology*, 1969, *67*, 301-308.

Koslowski, S., Drzewieki, K., & Sobocinska, J. The influence of expansion of extracellular fluid volume on the thirst threshold. *Bulletin Academy Pol. Sci.*, 1968, *16*, 47-51.

Koslowski, S., & Szczepanska-Sadowska, E. Mechanisms of hypovolemic thirst and interactions between hypovolemia, hyperosmolarity and the antidiuretic system. In G. Peters, J. T. Fitzsimons, & L. Peters-Haefeli (Eds.), *Control mechanisms of drinking*. New York: Springer-Verlag, 1975, pp. 25-35.

Kraly, F. S. Abdominal vagotomy inhibits osmotically induced drinking in the rat. *Journal of Comparative and Physiological Psychology*, 1978, *92*, 999-1013.

Kraly, F. S. The role of histamine in food-associated drinking. *Journal of Comparative and Physiological Psychology*, 1981, in press.

Kraly, F. S., Gibbs, J., & Smith, G. P. Disordered drinking after abdominal vagotomy in rats. *Nature*, 1975, *258*, 226-228.

Krecek, J., & Krecekova, J. The development of the regulation of water metabolism, III: The relation between water and milk intake in infant rats. *Physiologica Bohemoslovenica*, 1957, *6*, 26-34.

Kriekhaus, E. E., & Wolf, G. Acquisition of sodium by rats: Interaction of innate mechanisms and latent learning. *Journal of Comparative and Physiological Psychology*, 1968, *65*, 197-201.

Lashley, K. S. The experimental analysis of instinctive behavior. *Psychological Review*, 1938, *45*, 445-471.

Lehr, D., & Goldman, W. Continued pharmacologic analysis of consummatory behavior in the albino rat. *European Journal of Pharmacology*, 1973, *23*, 197-210.

Leibowitz, S. F. Histamine: A stimulatory effect on drinking behavior in the rat. *Brain Research*, 1973, *63*, 440-444.

Leibowitz, S. F. Brain catecholaminergic mechanisms for control of hunger. In D. Novin, W. Wyrwicka, & G. Wray (Eds.), *Hunger: Basic mechanisms and clinical implications*. New York: Raven Press, 1976, pp. 1-18.

Levin, R., & Stern, J. M. Maternal influences on ontogeny of suckling and feeding rhythms in the rat. *Journal of Comparative and Physiological Psychology*, 1975, *89*, 711-721.

Levitt, R. A., & Fisher, A. E. Anticholinergic blockade of centrally induced thirst. *Science*, 1966, *154*, 520-522.

Lind, R. W., & Johnson, A. K. Knift cuts between the subfornical organ (SFO) and antero-ventral third ventricle (AV3V) block drinking to peripheral angiotensin II. *Neuroscience Abstracts*, 1980, *6*, 33.

Lorens, S. A., & Yunger, L. M. Morphine analgesia, two-way avoidance and consummatory behavior following lesions in the midbrain raphe nuclei of the rat. *Pharmacology, Biochemistry and Behavior*, 1974, *2*, 215-221.

Maebashi, M., & Yoshinaga, K. Effect of dehydration on plasma renin activity. *Japanese Circulation Journal*, 1967, *31*, 609-613.

Malmo, R. B., & Malmo, H. P. Responses of lateral preoptic neurons in the rat to hypertonic sucrose and NaCl. *Electroencephalography and Clinical Neurophysiology*, 1979, *46*, 401-408.

Malmo, R. B., & Mundl, W. J. Osmosensitive neurons in the rat's preoptic area: Medial–lateral comparison. *Journal of Comparative and Physiological Psychology*, 1975, *88*, 161–175.

Mann, J. F. E., Johnson, A. K., & Ganten, D. Plasma angiotensin II: Dipsogenic levels and the angiotensin-generating capacity of the renin–angiotensin system. *American Journal of Physiology*, 1980, *238*, R372–R377.

Marshall, J. F., Richardson, J. S., & Teitelbaum, P. Nigrostriatal bundle damage and the lateral hypothalamic syndrome. *Journal of Comparative and Physiological Psychology*, 1974, *87*, 808–830.

Marshall, J. F., & Ungerstedt, U. Apomorphine-induced restoration of drinking to thirst challenges in 6-hydroxydopamine-treated rats. *Physiology and Behavior*, 1976, *17*, 817–822.

McKinley, M. J., Blaine, E. H., & Denton, D. A. Brain osmoreceptors, cerebrospinal fluid electrolyte composition and thirst. *Brain Research*, 1974, *70*, 532–537.

McKinley, M. J., Denton, D. A., Graham, W. F., Leksell, L. G., Mouw, D. R., Scoggins, B. A., Smith, M. H., Weisinger, R. S., & Wright, R. D. Lesions of the organum vasculosum of the lamina terminalis inhibit water drinking to hypertonicity in sheep. Paper presented to the *7th International Conference on the Physiology of Food and Fluid Intake*, Warsaw, July 1980.

McKinley, M. J., Denton, D. A., & Weisinger, R. S. Sensors for antidiuresis and thirst-osmoreceptors or CSF sodium detectors? *Brain Research*, 1978, *141*, 89–103.

Misantone, L. J., Ellis, S., & Epstein, A. N. Development of angiotensin-induced drinking in the rat. *Brain Research*, 1980, *186*, 195–202.

Miselis, R., Nicolaïdis, S., Menard, M., & Siatitsas, Y. Concurrent measures of renin and drinking in response to hypovolemia. *Neuroscience Abstracts*, 1976, *2*, 305.

Miselis, R. R., Shapiro, B., & Hand, P. J. Subfornical organ efferents to neural systems for control of body water. *Science*, 1979, *205*, 1022–1025.

Mogenson, G. J., & Kucharczyk, J. Evidence that the lateral hypothalamus and midbrain participate in the drinking response elicited by intracranial angiotensin. In G. Peters, J. T. Fitzsimons, & L. Peters-Haefeli (Eds.), *Control mechanisms of drinking.* New York: Springer-Verlag, 1975, pp. 127–131.

Montemurro, D. G., & Stevenson, J. A. F. Adipsia produced by hypothalamic lesions in the rat. *Canadian Journal of Biochemistry and Physiology*, 1957, *35*, 31–37.

Moore-Gillon, M. J. Effects of vagotomy on drinking in the rat. *Journal of Physiology (London)*, 1980, *308*, 417–426.

Mouw, D., Bonjour, J. P., Malvin, R. L., & Vander, A. Central action of angiotensin in stimulating ADH release. *American Journal of Physiology*, 1971, *220*, 239–242.

Myers, R. D., Hall, G. H., & Rudy, T. A. Drinking in the monkey evoked by nicotine or angiotensin II microinjected in hypothalamic and mesencephalic sites. *Pharmacology, Biochemistry and Behavior*, 1973, *1*, 15–22.

Neill, D. B., & Linn, C. L. Deficits in consummatory responses to regulatory challenges following basal ganglia lesions in rats. *Physiology and Behavior*, 1975, *14*, 617–624.

Nicolaïdis, S. Réponses des unités osmosensibles hypothalamiques aux stimulations salines et aqueuses de la langue. *Comptes Rendus de l'Académie des Sciences*, 1968, *267*, 2352–2355.

Nicolaïdis, S. Role des récepteurs internes et externes dan la prise d'eau régulatrice et non régulatrice. *Journées Internationales de Néphrologie*, 1974, *16B*, 159–174.

Nicolaïdis, S., & Fitzsimons, J. T. La dépendance de la prise d'eau induite par l'angiotensine II envers la fonction vasomotrice cérébrale locale chez le rat. *Comptes Rendus de l'Académie des Sciences*, Séries D, 1975, *281*, 1417-1420.

Norgren, R. Taste pathways to hypothalamus and amygdala. *Journal of Comparative Neurology*, 1976, *166*, 17-30.

Olds, J., & Hirano. Conditioned responses of hippocompal and other neurons. *Journal of Electroencephalography and Clinical Neurophysiology*, 1969, *26*, 159-166.

Olsson, K. Further evidence for the importance of CSF Na^+ concentration in central control of fluid balance. *Acta Physiologica Scandinavica*, 1973, *88*, 183-188.

Oltmans, G. A., & Harvey, J. A. The LH Syndrome and brain catecholamine levels after lesions of the nigrostriatal bundle. *Physiology and Behavior*, 1972, *8*, 69-78.

Osborne, M. J., Pooters, N. Angles d'Auriac, G., Epstein, A. N., Worcel, M., & Meyer, P. Metabolism of tritiated angiotensin II in anaesthetized rats. *Pflügers Archiv*, 1971, *326*, 101-114.

Page, I. H., & Bumpus, F. M. *Angiotensin.* New York: Springer-Verlag, 1974.

Pals, D. T., Masucci, F. D., Denning, G. S., Jr., Sipos, F., & Fessler, D. C. Role of the pressor action of angiotensin II in experimental hypertension. *Circulation Research*, 1971, *29*, 673-681.

Peck, J. W. Discussion: Thirst(s) resulting from bodily water imbalances. In A. N. Epstein, H. R. Kissileff, & E. Stellar (Eds.), *The neurophyschology of thirst.* Washington, D. C.: V. H. Winston & Sons, 1973, pp. 99-110.

Peck, J. W., & Novin, D. Evidence that osmoreceptors mediating drinking in rabbits are in the lateral preoptic area. *Journal of Comparative and Physiological Psychology*, 1971, *74*, 134-147.

Phillips, M. I., & Felix, D. Specific angiotensin II receptive neurons in the cat subfornical organ. *Brain Research*, 1976, *109*, 531-540.

Phillips, M. I., & Hoffman, W. E. Sensitive sites in the brain for the blood pressure and drinking responses to angiotensin II. In J. P. Buckley, C. Ferrario, & M. F. Lokhandwala (Eds.), *Central actions of angiotensin and related hormones.* New York: Pergamon Press, 1974, pp. 325-356.

Ramsay, D. J., Rolls, B. J., & Wood, R. J. Body fluid changes which influence drinking in the water deprived rat. *Journal of Physiology (London)*, 1977, *266*, 453-469. (a)

Ramsay, D. J., Rolls, B. J., & Wood, R. J. Thirst following water deprivation in dogs. *American Journal of Physiology*, 1977, *232*, R93-R100. (b)

Ranck, J. Behavioral correlates and firing repertoires of neurons in septal nuclei in unrestrained rats. In J. DeFrance (Ed.), *The septal nuclei.* New York: Plenum Press, 1976, pp. 423-461.

Richter, C. P. *Biological clocks in medicine and psychiatry.* Springfield: C. C. Thomas, 1965.

Rogers, P. W., & Kurtzman, N. A. Renal failure, uncontrollable thirst and hyperreninemia. *Journal of the American Medical Association*, 1973, *225*, 1236-1238.

Rolls, B. J., & Jones, B. P. Cessation of drinking following intracranial injections of angiotensin in the rat. *Journal of Comparative and Physiological Psychology*, 1972, *80*, 26-29.

Rolls, B. J., Jones, B. P., & Fallows, D. J. A comparison of the motivational properties of thirst induced by intracranial angiotensin and water deprivation. *Physiology and Behavior*, 1972, *9*, 777-782.

Rolls, B. J., Wood, R. J., & Rolls, E. T. Thirst: The initiation, maintenance, and termination of drinking. In J. M. Sprague and A. N. Epstein (Eds.), *Progress in psychobiology and physiological psychology* (Vol. 9). New York: Academic Press, 1981.

Rowland, N., & Nicolaïdis, S. Periprandial self-intravenous drinking in the rat. *Journal of Comparative and Physiological Psychology*, 1974, *87*, 16-25.

Russell, P. J. D., Abdelaal, A. E., & Mogenson, G. J. Graded levels of hemorrhage, thirst and angiotensin II in the rat. *Physiology and Behavior*, 1975, *15*, 117-119.

Setler, P. E. The role of catecholamines in thirst. In A. N. Epstein, H. R. Kissileff, & E. Stellar (Eds.), *The neuropsychology of thirst*. Washington, D.C.: V. H. Winston & Sons, 1973, pp. 279-291.

Severs, W. B., & Daniels-Severs, A. E. Effects of angiotensin on the central nervous system. *Pharmacological Review*, 1973, *25*, 415-449.

Severs, W. B., Summy-Long, J., Taylor, J. S., & Connor, J. D. A central effect of angiotensin: Release of pituitary pressor material. *Journal of Pharmacology and Experimental Therapeutics*, 1970, *174*, 27-34.

Share, L. Extracellular fluid volume and vasopressin secretion. In W. F. Ganong and L. Martini (Eds.), *Frontiers in neuroendocrinology 1969*. New York: Oxford Press, 1969, pp. 183-210.

Shelling, P., Ganten, D., Heckl, R., Hayduk, K., Hutchinson, J. S., Sponer, G., & Ganten, U. On the origin of angiotensin-like peptides in cerebrospinal fluid. In J. P. Buckley, C. Ferrario, & M. F. Lokhandwala (Eds.), *Central actions of angiotensin and related hormones*. New York: Pergamon Press, 1974, pp. 325-356.

Shrager, E. E., Osborne, M. J., Johnson, A. K., & Epstein, A. N. Entry of angiotensin into cerebral ventricles and circumventricular structures. In D. S. Davies and J. L. Reid (Eds.), *Central action of drugs in blood pressure regulation*. Baltimore: University Park Press, 1975, pp. 65-67.

Shrager, E. E., & Johnson, A. K. Contributions of periventricular structures of the rostral third ventricle to the maintenance of drinking responses to humoral dipsogens and body fluid homeostasis. *Neuroscience Abstracts*, 1980, *6*, 128.

Simpson, J. B., Epstein, A. N., & Camardo, J. S. The localization of receptors for the dipsogenic action of angiotensin II in the subfornical organ. *Journal of Comparative and Physiological Psychology*, 1977, *92*, 581-608.

Simpson, J. B., & Routtenberg, A. The subfornical organ and carbachol-induced drinking. *Brain Research*, 1972, *45*, 135-142.

Simpson, J. B., & Routtenberg, A. Subfornical organ: Site of drinking elicitation by angiotensin II. *Science*, 1973, *181*, 1172-1174.

Simpson, J. B., & Routtenberg, A. Subfornical organ: Acetylcholine application elicits drinking. *Brain Research*, 1974, *79*, 157-164.

Smith, G. P., Strohmeyer, A. J., & Reis, D. J. Effect of lateral hypothalamic injections of 6-hydroxydopamine on food and water intake in rats. *Nature*, 1972, *235*, 27-29.

Sorenson, J. D., Jr., & Harvey, J. A. Decreased brain acetylcholine after septal lesions in rats: Correlation with thirst. *Physiology and Behavior*, 1971, *6*, 723-725.

Stellar, E. The physiology of motivation. *Psychological Review*, 1954, *61*, 5-22.

Stephan, F. K., & Zucker, I. Circadian rhythms in drinking behavior and locomotor activity of rats are eliminated by hypothalamic lesions. *Proceedings of the National Academy of Sciences*, 1972, *69*, 1583-1586.

Stricker, E. M. Some physiological and motivational properties of the hypovolemic stimulus for thirst. *Physiology and Behavior*, 1968, *3*, 379-385.

Stricker, E. M. Osmoregulation and volume regulation in rats: Inhibition of hypovolemic thirst by water. *American Journal of Physiology*, 1969, *217*, 98-105.

Stricker, E. M., & Wolf, G. Behavioral control of intravascular fluid volume: Thirst and sodium appetite. In P. J. Morgane (Ed.), *Neural Regulation of Food and Water Intake. Annals of the New York Academy of Sciences*, 1969, *157*, 533-567.

Stricker, E. M., & Zigmond, M. J. Recovery of function after damage to central catecholamine-containing neurons: A neurochemical model for the lateral hypothalamic syndrome. In J. M. Sprague & A. N. Epstein (Eds.), *Progress in psychobiology and physiological psychology* (Vol. 6). New York: Academic Press, 1976.

Tang, M. Dependence of polyethylene glycol-induced dipsogenesis on intravascular fluid volume depletion. *Physiology and Behavior*, 1976, *17*, 811-816.

Tang, M., & Falk, J. L. Sar[1]-Ala[8] angiotensin II blocks renin-angiotensin but not beta-adrenergic dipsogenesis. *Pharmacology, Biochemistry and Behavior*, 1974, *2*, 401-408.

Teitelbaum, P., & Epstein, A. N. The lateral hypothalamic syndrome: Recovery of feeding and drinking after lateral hypothalamic lesions. *Psychological Review*, 1962, *69*, 74-90.

Thrasher, T. N., Ramsay, D. J., Keil, L. C., & Brown, C. J. Thirst and vasopressin release: An osmoreceptor or sodium receptor mechanism? *Federation Proceedings*, 1978, *37*, 815.

Thrasher, T. N., Simpson, J. B., & Ramsay, D. J. Drinking responsiveness following ablation of the subfornical organ (SFO) or organum vasculosum of the lamina terminalis (OVLT) in dogs. Paper presented to the *7th International Conference on the Physiology of Food and Fluid Intake*, Warsaw, July 1980.

Tondat, L. M., & Almli, C. R. Hyperdipsia produced by severing ventral septal fiber systems. *Physiology and Behavior*, 1975, *15*, 701-706.

Trippodo, N. C., McCaa, R. E., & Guyton, A. C. Effect of prolonged angiotensin II infusion on thirst. *American Journal of Physiology*, 1976, *230*, 1063-1066.

Ueda, H., Katayama, S., & Kato, R. Area postrema-angiotensin-sensitive site in brain. *Advances in Experimental Biology and Medicine*, 1972, *17*, 109-116.

Ungerstedt, U. Adipsia and aphagia after 6-hydroxydopamine induced degeneration of the nigrostriatal dopamine systems. *Acta Physiologica Scandinavica Supplement*, 1971, *367*, 95-122.

Valenstein, E. S., Cox, V. C., & Kakolewski, J. W. Polydipsia elicited by the synergistic action of a saccharin and glucose solution. *Science*, 1967, *157*, 552-554.

Vance, W. B. Observations on the role of the salivary secretions in the regulation of food and fluid intake in the white rat. *Psychological Monographs*, 1965, *79*, No. 598.

Verney, E. B. The antidiuretic hormone and the factors which determine its release. *Proceedings of the Royal Society (London)*, 1947, Ser. B., *135*, 25-106.

Vincent, J. D., Arnauld, E., & Bioulac, B. Activity of osmosensitive cells in the hypothalamus of the behaving monkey during drinking. *Brain Research*, 1972, *44*, 371-384.

Walsh, L. L., & Grossman, S. P. Zona incerta lesions: Disruption of regulatory water intake. *Physiology and Behavior*, 1973, *11*, 885-887.

Walsh, L. L., & Grossman, S. P. Dissociation of responses to extracellular thirst stimuli following zona incerta lesions. *Pharmacology, Biochemistry and Behavior*, 1978, *8*, 409–415.

Wayner, M. J., Ono, T., & Nolley, D. Effects of angiotensin II on central neurons. *Pharmacology, Biochemistry and Behavior*, 1973, *1*, 679–691.

Weindl, A. Neuroendocrine aspects of circumventricular organs. In W. F. Ganong and L. Martini (Eds.), *Frontiers in neuroendocrinology, 1973*. New York: Oxford University Press, 1973, pp. 3–32.

Weiss, C. S., & Almli, C. R. Lateral preoptic and lateral hypothalamic units: In search of the osmoreceptors for thirst. *Physiology and Behavior*, 1975, *15*, 713–722.

Wettendorff, H. Modifications de sang sous l'influence de la privation d'eau: Contribution à l'étude de la soif. *Travaux du Laboratoire de Physiologie, Institut de Physiologie, Instituts Solvay*, 1901, *4*, 353–384.

Wirth, J. R., & Epstein, A. N. The ontogeny of thirst in the infant rat. *American Journal of Physiology*, 1976, *230*, 188–198.

Wislocki, G. B., & Leduc, E. H. Vital staining of the hematoencephalic barrier by silver nitrate and trypan blue and cytological comparisons of the neurohypophysis, pineal body, area postrema, intercolumnar tubercle and supraoptic crest. *Journal of Comparative Neurology*, 1952, *96*, 371–413.

Wood, R. J., Rolls, B. J., & Ramsay, D. J. Drinking following intracarotid infusions of hypertonic solutions in dogs. *American Journal of Physiology*, 1977, *232*, R88–92.

Zimmer, L. J., Meliza, L., & Hsaio, S. Effects of cervical and subdiaphragmatic vagotomy on osmotic and volemic thirst. *Physiology and Behavior*, 1976, *16*, 665–670.

Zimmerman, M. B., Blaine, E. H., & Stricker, E. M. Water intake in hypovolemic sheep: Effects of crushing in the left atrial appendage. *Science*, 1980, *211*, 489–491.

Part Three

Thermal, Maternal, and Sexual Motivation

Chapter 8

Are There Similarities Between Thermoregulation and Sexual Behavior?

EVELYN SATINOFF

In several previous reviews I have described a model for the neural control of thermoregulation (Satinoff, 1978, 1982). This model, which is outlined below, derived from data that were not comfortably explained by existing models. A consideration of *why* the brain should be organized in this way to regulate body temperature led to speculations on how it might have evolved to be so arranged. Those speculations, in turn, led to the idea that the brain is similarly organized for many forms of motivated behaviors. If this is the case, then even in systems that appear unrelated to each other, there should be similarities that are not obvious. In this chapter I have chosen to compare thermoregulation with sexual behavior because they are so apparently unlike each other.

The chapter is divided into four sections. The first reviews the model for the neural control of thermoregulation. The second considers possible evolutionary constraints on the brain that make such an organization likely. This is really the heart of the argument, since the constraints must have been the same on all behaviors evolving at the same time. In the third section the possible heuristic value of this approach will be presented. Finally, parallels between thermoregulation and sexual behavior will be discussed.

Neural Organization of Thermoregulation

The major premises of the model for the neural control of thermoregulation are as follows:

1. There are separate channels from thermal detector to motor effector for every thermoregulatory response in an animal's repertoire.

2. These "miniature thermoregulatory systems" are located at several levels of the neuraxis from spinal cord to cortex.

3. They are not independent of each other; rather, the activity of lower structures is facilitated and inhibited by those above.

This way of looking at the brain, which may seem absurdly complicated for so apparently simple a function as maintaining a normal body temperature, adequately accounts for many puzzling facts that cannot be handled by the traditional model, in which the hypothalamus is considered to be *the* thermostat.

There are two main categories of results that cannot be explained by a model that locates a single thermostat in the preoptic/anterior hypothalamic area (Figure 8-1) or by an even older model in which the preoptic/anterior hypothalamus is a "heat-loss" center and the posterior hypothalamus a "heat-production" center (Ranson, 1940). First, there is abundant evidence that animals whose brains have been transected below the level of the hypothalamus are still capable of making appropriate thermoregulatory responses. Keller and co-workers (Keller, 1938; Keller & McClaskey, 1964) did a series of studies showing that cats and dogs whose brains were transected through the rostral midbrain or upper pons were able to maintain near-normal body temperatures in the heat. Thauer (1935) reported that rabbits with a high cervical spinal section slowly regained the ability to maintain normal body temperature in the cold. Results such as these were never incorporated into either of the prevalent models because they did not fit.

The second category of results concerns lesions of the preoptic/

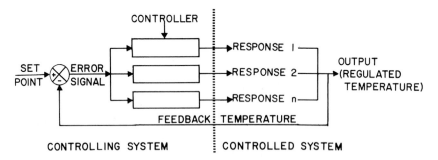

Figure 8-1. Control diagram of the relation between set point (or reference input), actual body temperature, and a reflexive response. The comparators (circles) are mixing points. Whenever the pluses and minuses do not cancel one another, an error signal is generated. When this occurs (i.e., whenever there is a disturbance such that heat-gain and heat-loss mechanisms are not at minimum levels), a response is activated that alters the regulated body temperature. Information from temperature receptors is then fed back to the comparator and the error signal is adjusted. (From Satinoff & Hendersen, 1977.)

anterior hypothalamus itself. If there were a single integrative center located under the electrode tip, then one would expect that a lesion would impair all responses designed to maintain a normal body temperature in the face of heat or cold stress. But this is not what happens. Large preoptic lesions impair thermoregulatory reflex responses so completely that an animal will die if left in a hot or cold environment. Yet the same animal under the same thermal stress can maintain its body temperature quite adequately by using an operant response. Thus, one form of behavioral regulation remains intact even though important reflexive regulations are virtually abolished. When one looks more closely at several thermoregulatory responses, one sees large variability in the effects of the lesions. For instance, as mentioned, after preoptic/anterior hypothalamic lesions, operant responding for heat in the cold is left almost intact (Carlisle, 1969; Satinoff & Rutstein, 1970), as is vasoconstriction (Satinoff, Valentino, & Teitelbaum, 1976), but such lesioned rats do not build good nests (Van Zoeren & Stricker, 1977), increase their food intake or activity as much as normals do (Hamilton & Brobeck, 1964, 1966), or shiver adequately (Satinoff et al., 1976). In the heat they will press a bar for cool air (Lipton, 1968) and will groom and show increased locomotion (two common responses to heat stress) (Roberts & Martin, 1977), but they do not sprawl (Roberts & Martin, 1977) or reduce their food intake appropriately (Hamilton & Brobeck, 1964).

These experiments so clearly point to multiple thermostats that one may reasonably wonder how anyone could have overlooked them. The answer is very simple. The results just cited were not published until 1964 and later, by which time the single-thermostat model was well established. Furthermore, they are mostly experiments involving behavioral thermoregulatory responses, performed by psychologists; most of the work on the neural control of thermoregulation was done on decerebrate or spinal preparations by physiologists who did not study behavior or who did not think that behavior would lead to any new insights into body temperature control (e.g., Hardy, Stolwijk, & Gagge, 1971).

The results discussed so far establish two points. First, after preoptic/anterior hypothalamic lesions, some thermoregulatory responses remain whereas others do not. Second, animals without a hypothalamus can respond appropriately to thermal stresses (see Simon, 1974, and Satinoff, 1974, for reviews). The latter point implies that subhypothalamic tissue is capable of organizing thermoregulatory responses. Given the assumption of separate integrating systems located at several levels of the brain and spinal cord, a reasonable question to ask is, why do all thermoregulatory responses appear in the same sequence when a normal animal is in a thermally extreme environment? One of the major reasons for this is that the separate thermoregulatory systems are not independent of each other; rather, they are under hierarchical control. This concept is illustrated beautifully in an experiment by Chambers, Siegel, Liu, and Liu (1974). Cats with high-level decerebrations did not shiver, vaso-constrict, or piloerect in response to cooling of the skin or core or both; lowering the level of decerebration to the caudal pons or medulla rein-stated these responses. Thus, in the mesencephalon and upper pons, there appears to be a tonic inhibition of responses to cold stress. When medullary and spinal centers are released from this inhibition, they can and do initiate such responses. These results have been replicated in monkeys (Liu, 1979). The tonic inhibitory area in cats has been further localized by Amini-Sereshki (1977). When a local anesthetic, procaine, was microinjected into the ventromedial pontine tegmentum in high-level decerebrates (which do not shiver), heat-gain responses were released.

The organization of the brain for controlling thermoregulation that is proposed here follows the Jacksonian concept of levels of integra-tion, each level adjusting and regulating the activities of lower levels (Jackson, 1958). It is an alternative to the classical concept of the hypothalamus as the controller for all thermoregulatory responses, with other parts of the brain merely supplying it with thermal information. In a Jacksonian framework, the hypothalamus is near the top of a hier-archy, directing the activities of thermoregulatory systems lower down. These other systems are capable of independent action, but without the hypothalamus they are much less effective. With diencephalic direc-tion, appropriate reflexes and behaviors are activated promptly and inappropriate ones are suppressed. [The hypothalamus is near, not at, the top of the hierarchy, because more encephalized mesocortical and neocortical systems influence the activity of the hypothalamus in tem-perature regulation. For truly normal reflexive thermoregulation, all levels of the nervous system, from spinal cord to cortex, are necessary (Satinoff, 1974)].

This scheme, with the hypothalamus (and in particular the preoptic/ anterior hypothalamus) near the top, applies only to thermoregulatory reflexes. Although the same Jacksonian framework can also be applied to the many varieties of thermoregulatory behaviors, the neuroanatomi-cal site of the top of the behavioral hierarchy remains to be described. Since one judges the top of a hierarchy by whether the behavior either disappears or becomes largely unintegrated when it is damaged, the lat-eral hypothalamic area would certainly qualify as being at or near the top. When this area of the brain is damaged, thermoregulatory reflexes are sufficient to allow animals to maintain normal body temperatures in the cold. However, rats with such lesions do not press a bar to turn on a heat lamp until many weeks postoperatively, nor do they build ade-quate nests (Satinoff & Shan, 1971; Van Zoeren & Stricker, 1977).

Evolution of Thermoregulation

Models similar to the foregoing one, applied here to thermoregulation, have previously been used to explain the neural control of micturition (Ruch, 1960), the galvanic skin reflex (Ingram, 1960), and autonomic responses in general (Koizumi & Brooks, 1972). The model is extremely complicated because not only are there separate integrating systems for each individual thermoregulatory response, but each system is represented at several different levels of the neuraxis. Furthermore, these responses are influenced by other functional systems of which they are a part. Vasoconstriction, for instance, is a heat-conservation response, but it is also part of a general sympathetic arousal mechanism that is activated when an animal is emotionally stressed, and it is also critical in the control of blood pressure. However, the neural organization of temperature regulation is so complicated because of the evolutionary constraints on its design.

The major points of the evolutionary argument are the following:

1. Many changes are needed to evolve from an ectotherm like a lizard into a well-regulating endotherm like a bird or a mammal. These include the development of fur, feathers, and fat; vasoconstriction; shivering; an internal means of heat production (chemical thermogenesis); panting; sweating; and vasodilation. Some of these changes are merely changes in degree and efficiency, like panting: lizards and dogs both pant. Some, like chemical thermogenesis, are unique in the mammalian line.
2. Evolution takes a long time. Each response took millions of years to become efficient for thermoregulatory purposes, and while it was evolving it was constrained by other responses evolving for other purposes.
3. These responses did not evolve concurrently. Most if not all of them were originally used for other purposes and only over eons came to be integrated with temperature detectors. Whenever a response came under the control of thermal stimuli, it became one complete thermal integrating system, from receptor to effector. Eventually there came to be many such systems, each having evolved at separate times and each independent of the others but not destined to remain independent.
4. Given the tremendous variety of thermoregulatory mechanisms, given that no species has all of them, and given that many if not all of them are also used for nonthermal purposes, there is no reason to suppose that there should be a single site of thermal integration in the central nervous system.

The key point for present purposes is the third—most thermoregulatory responses were originally used for other purposes. This point is discussed more fully in Satinoff (1982); here I shall give only one example.

All animals breathe, and panting in mammals, which is an excellent heat-losing response, is simply a sophisticated overlay on basic respiratory mechanisms. Thus, a rudiment of one pattern can be a refinement of another. Several different levels of this single thermal response can be identified from reptiles to birds and mammals. For our purposes, the simplest refinement is breathing with the mouth open, or gaping. Gaping is a characteristic activity in crocodilians when they are ashore, and experiments in the laboratory show that it is a moderately effective heat-loss mechanism. The heads of anesthetized alligators with their mouths propped open at an angle that simulated normal gaping become hot at a lower rate than the heads of alligators whose mouths are taped shut (Spotila, Terpin, & Dodson, 1977).

The next step up from simple mouth opening is to alter the rate and depth of respiration. Rapid shallow breathing, or panting, is found in many species of desert lizards and it is also effective in regulating body temperature. Panting in chuckwallas, for instance, is a complicated function of brain and peripheral temperatures and when it is initiated it can keep the lizard's brain temperature about 3°C cooler than the environment for many hours (Crawford & Barber, 1974; Crawford, 1972). The panting response is very little changed in mammals like dogs, but because it is initiated at a much lower core temperature and because the dog's highly vascularized tongue protrudes very far out of the mouth, it is much more effective than in lizards.

Gaping, panting, and gular fluttering (a response seen in some birds that augments panting for respiratory evaporation) are all well under the control of central and/or peripheral thermosensitive units. In other cases, however, thermal sensations may have no control over a response that would be thermally useful. Sweating on paws and palms is such a response. Humans sweat on their palms and the soles of their feet when they are emotionally stressed or when they are exercising, but not in response to heat. Adelman, Taylor, and Heglund (1975) studied several species of animals that sweat on their footpads when running. Blocking the sweating with atropine sulfate greatly decreased the coefficient of static friction between the paw and the tread of an inclined treadmill. A similar dose of atropine had no effect on the coefficient of static friction in a rabbit, an animal that does not have sweat glands on its paws. The authors concluded that a major function of footpad sweating is to prevent slippage between the foot and the substrate when running or climbing, and they speculated that the sweating seen in response to stress may play a role in preparing an animal for fleeing the situation. If sweating on paws or palms were thermally useful, and if such heat-induced sweating were not detrimental to the animal, then in the future thermal systems may gain control over this response.

Thermoregulatory responses were not only *once* used for other purposes; most if not all are *still* components of other integrative systems. Furred animals piloerect in response to cold or to unpleasant emotional stimuli. Rodents build nests in the cold and, if they have newborn pups, at neutral temperatures also. Reptiles change skin color both as camouflage and as thermoregulatory devices (Templeton, 1970). The vasomotor system is involved in blood pressure regulation and regional blood flow as well as in thermoregulation. This third function may have been added over the course of evolution. Cowles (1958) has argued that the vasomotor system is used as a supplementary respiratory organ in amphibia, which have moist skin. It was inherited by dry-skinned reptiles, where its function changed to control the influx of radiant heat and to transfer the heat to the deep tissues of the body via the blood. In mammals, peripheral vasomotor changes control the rate of heat flow in the opposite direction, from the organism to the environment.

So, in a highly speculative and of course unprovable chain of events, we start with an organism that senses temperature and has some form of behavior (locomotion) that turns out to be useful in allowing the animal to be somewhat independent of its thermally changing environment (it can shuttle between sun and shade). If temperature sensors gain all or partial control over this behavior, we have one primitive (in the sense of evolutionarily early), yet efficient (it enables the animal to maintain its body temperature within narrow limits), thermoregulatory integrative system. Eons later the animal's posture evolves from the sprawling stance of a reptile to the limb-supported posture of a therapsid, a mammal-like reptile. As a side effect of this postural change, the animal's internal heat production is increased (Heath, 1968). Eventually temperature sensors gain control over this new form of heat production, and that is another integrating system. Too high a rate of internal heat production may be deleterious, and it would be advantageous to lose some of the heat more quickly. The animal already breathes and has a good vasomotor system, and when changes in respiratory rate and peripheral blood flow come under the influence of thermal detectors, we have two more integrating systems; and so on. The same principle of new controls over an already existing mechanism for a new function can be used to understand the nervous organization of many forms of motivated behavior.

In summary, the neural control of thermoregulation, when viewed from an evolutionary perspective, does not require a single center or coordinator for behaviors that to our eyes look coordinated, any more than Darwin required the existence of an "adaptor" to explain adaptations. Rather, Darwin detailed the sorts of complex conditions that brought about adaptation. This chapter makes a similar argument for complex behaviors and their neural organization. Fractions of control systems evolved as integrated entities to start with. The individual components in a pattern such as breathing must be useful for making respiration more efficient at the same time that these components are being modified by a different regulatory system, such as thermoregulation, for its own end—more effective heat loss. The accommodation that is worked out between competing systems is called integration. Most patterns are represented at many levels of the nervous system because if a particular response accidentally turns out to be useful for several different patterns, higher level controls must be added to handle the new arrangement, in particular to establish which control system has dominance over a shared component when priorities change. During heat stress, for example, an animal may be lying sprawled on its side, panting, with flattened fur. In the presence of an emotionally upsetting stimulus the animal will get up, crouch, and piloerect, and its breathing pattern will change. Both heat and emotion control posture, respiration, and fur position, but in opposite directions. One function of higher level centers is to activate the appropriate switching circuits—in other words, to organize dominance hierarchies.

Applications of the Model

The value of any approach ultimately lies in its ability to generate new, unexpected findings, and so it is with the one outlined here. The position advanced so far has four correlates:

1. All complex behavior patterns are built up out of simple components, or elements.
2. The components, evolved for use by a particular system, were opportunistically taken over by other systems if the need arose and the conditions allowed.
3. Any component, at any level, can be broken down into smaller subcomponents.
4. Any stimulus that affects a (sub)component of one system will affect that (sub)component in any other system of which it is a part.

The characterization of a set of responses as a system or subsystem and of the response itself as a component or subcomponent depends on the level of discourse at the time. If, for instance, the class of motivated behaviors is taken as the system, then thermoregulation is a subsystem. The crouched, immobile stance of a rat in the cold is one of its components and postural support is a subcomponent. If the class of thermoregulatory responses is considered to be the system, then crouched immobility is a subsystem and postural support is a component. Bullock (1970) has stated it succinctly.

There are many subsystems. They embrace larger and smaller sets of elements; they overlap and are delimited arbitrarily, in some cases by function, in others by structure. Examples are the visual, olfactory, somesthetic, limbic, reticular activating, extrapyramidal, temperature-regulating, startle response, and hypophyseal control systems—any fractions we wish to define.... (Classically, many of these are "systems," which is quite appropriate when considered by themselves; in the context of the whole nervous system, they are subsystems.)

These propositions are presumed to hold both for complex behavior and for its neural organization. The most important point is the fourth —that a stimulus that affects an element of a system will affect that element wherever it is embedded. In this section I will take one stimulus, environmental temperature, and show how it affects one arbitrarily isolatable subcomponent of many behavior patterns—postural support. I will also show how it affects rapid eye movement (REM) sleep, of which postural support, or rather its inhibition, is a subcomponent.

Postural support is an obvious unit to choose for someone working in thermoregulation, because the postures of animals are strikingly different depending upon the ambient temperature. Normal rats in the cold sit in a hunched-up position that is efficient for conserving heat because less of the animal's surface area is exposed to the cold. If the air is warmed, support disappears and the animals lie prone on the ground with bodies sprawled and limbs extended. The sprawled posture is efficient for losing heat, since as much of the body surface as possible is exposed and more heat is removed (assuming, of course, that ambient temperature is lower than body temperature).

The point here is that if a treatment (warming) affects one subcomponent (postural support) of a complex behavior (thermoregulation), then it is likely that the same treatment will affect that subcomponent wherever it is found, even as part of what look like completely unrelated behaviors where temperature would not be thought to play any role.

Schallert, Whishaw, DeRyck, and Teitelbaum (1978) view catalepsy as a state in which postural and motor subsystems are organized to maintain static stable equilibrium. Early after large lateral hypothalamic lesions or intraventricular injection of the neurotoxin 6-hydroxydopamine (6-ODHA) rats are akinetic and rigid at normal laboratory temperatures of 22–24°C (below thermoneutrality). They also sit in the hunched-up position. In fact, they will sit this way for hours without moving. However, if the skin of such rats is warmed slightly, the rigid posture is replaced by a sprawled prone position and by a torpor so profound that the animals do not right themselves if they are rolled over on their backs (Figure 8-2). Deep hypothermia can produce the same cataleptic-like state in normal rats. The only movement subsystem they have left is postural support and this is the one that permits them

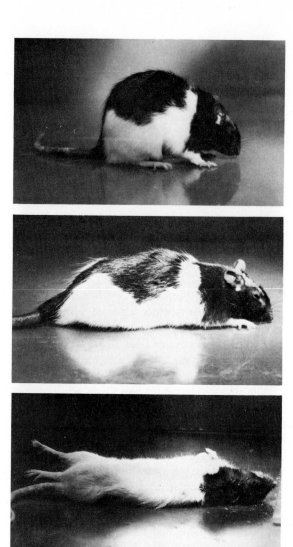

Figure 8-2. *Top:* The crouched, immobile posture of catalepsy/akinesia, produced in this rat by electrolytic lateral hypothalamic damage. *Middle:* Slight warming by a heat lamp causes the rat to lose support and subside into a prone posture. *Bottom:* So profound is the torpor induced by such warmth that if the animal is slowly rolled over onto its back, it no longer rights itself. (From Schallert, Whishaw, DeRyck, & Teitelbaum, 1978.)

to shiver. Thus, the postures of cataleptic rats not only maintain static equilibrium but are also adaptive for thermoregulation.

Postural support is also a prominent feature of sexual behavior in female rodents. It is manifested particularly in the raised hind legs that, together with a deflected tail, concave, dorsiflexed back, and flattened ears, make up the lordosis posture (Figure 8-3). Lordosis in hamsters is a fixed, stereotyped pattern that may be maintained unchanged for 10 minutes or longer (Carter, 1973). When Carter-Porges, Schallert, and I placed an estrual female in a hot environment, she sprawled; when her flanks were stimulated, lordosis was induced, but the hind-limb support subcomponent was absent (Figure 8-4). The hamster became lordotic for several minutes, with ears flattened and tail deflected, but postural support was inhibited by the heat. Thus, the seemingly unitary lordosis response can be further fragmented by applying a stimulus that affects only one of its several subcomponents.

Ambient temperature also affects more complicated behaviors of which postural support is a part. Rats sleep more and have concomitantly more REM sleep when they are housed at an environmental temperature that is within their thermoneutral zone—that range of ambient temperatures at which metabolic rate is minimal and constant. Szymusiak, Satinoff, Schallert, and Whishaw (1980) found that when rats were in slow wave sleep (SWS) at ambient temperatures above or below their thermoneutral zones a few minutes of brief convective cooling or warming, respectively, which returned skin temperature to more neutral ranges, triggered REM sleep on 70–80% of the trials

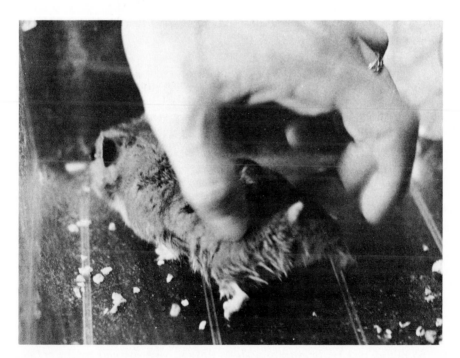

Figure 8-3. Lordosis posture in an estrogen/progesterone-primed ovariectomized hamster. Ambient temperature 23°C.

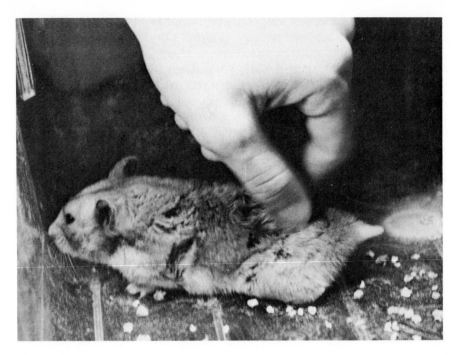

Figure 8-4. Lordosis posture in the same hamster at an ambient temperature of 34°C. Note that the posture is normal except that the hind limbs are no longer elevated.

(Figure 8-5). When no thermal stimuli were applied the SWS bouts ended in REM on only 21–23% of the trials (the rest of the time the rats woke up). The same warming or cooling stimuli applied when the rats were in SWS at an ambient temperature within their thermoneutral zone reduced the transition into REM sleep from 46% to 9–22%. Thus, REM sleep mechanisms are very sensitive to relatively mild thermal stress and its alleviation.

REM sleep is even more sensitive to ambient temperature than is minimal metabolic rate, the most commonly used indicator of thermo-neutrality in rats. Szymusiak and Satinoff (1981) found that metabolic rate was minimal and constant between 25 and 31°C, whereas REM sleep time varied significantly over this range (Figure 8-6). At 29°C REM sleep time was more than double the amount seen at 23°C, a common laboratory temperature. Because the REM sleep of normal rats is so sensitive to ambient temperature, Szymusiak and I recently conjectured that the reduced sleep of rats (Nauta, 1946) and cats with basal forebrain lesions (McGinty & Sterman, 1968; Lucas & Sterman, 1975) might not be primarily a sleep deficit, but instead might reflect the exaggerated sensitivity of these rats to changes in the ambient tem-

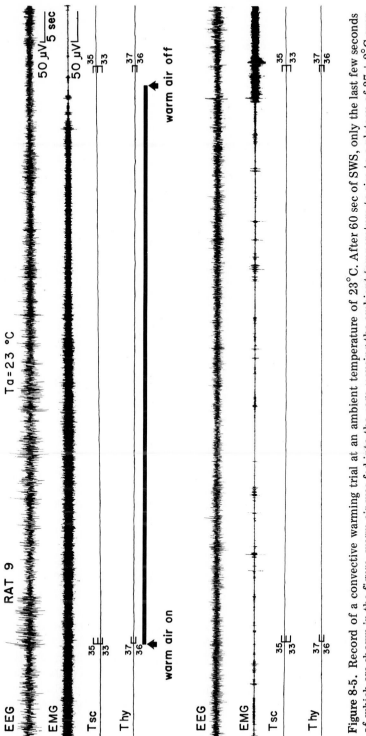

Figure 8-5. Record of a convective warming trial at an ambient temperature of 23°C. After 60 sec of SWS, only the last few seconds of which are shown in the figure, warm air was fed into the cage, causing the ambient temperature to rise to a plateau of 37 ± 2°C over 3 minutes. After 91 sec of warming the rat enters REM sleep, and warming is discontinued by switching back to air at 23 ± 2°C. The REM sleep continues for 117 sec. (Abbreviations: EEG, cortical electroencephalogram; EMG, dorsal neck electromyograph; Tsc, subcutaneous temperature; Thy, hypothalamic temperature; Ta, ambient temperature.) (From Szymusiak, Satinoff, Schallert & Whishaw, 1981.)

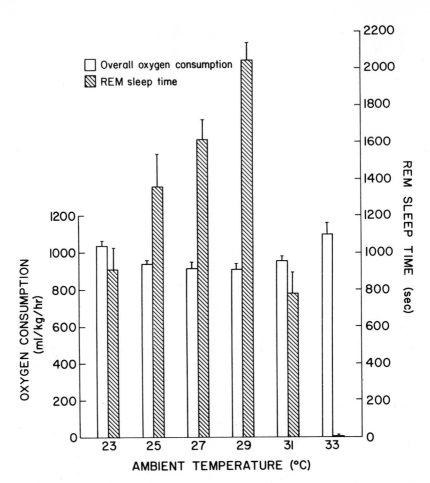

Figure 8-6. REM sleep time and overall oxygen consumption as a function of ambient temperature. REM sleep time at 29 and 33°C differed significantly from all other values. There were no significant differences in oxygen consumption between 25 and 31°C. (From Szymusiak & Satinoff, 1981.)

perature. Rats with such lesions have deranged thermoregulation, and their thermoneutral zones might well be different from normal.

We measured the amount of sleep in eight normal male rats before and after medial preoptic lesions for 2 hours at each of three different ambient temperatures—20, 25, and 30°C—on the same day. In the controls we found, as expected, that REM sleep time varied from a mean of 10% at 20°C to 14% at 25°C to 22% at 30°C. Twenty-four hours after the lesions, six out of eight rats had no REM sleep at any ambient temperature. However, by 5 days postlesion, REM sleep had clearly become ambient temperature-dependent. In one typical rat with small preoptic lesions (Figure 8-7), the ratio of REM sleep time to total sleep time was 1% at 20°C, 7% at 25°C, and on the same day, 20% at 30°C, the last being within the normal range (Satinoff & Szymusiak, 1981). Had we only tested the rats at 20°C, we might have concluded, as others have, that there is a basal forebrain system regulating REM sleep. However, for every rat there was an ambient temperature at which the ratio of REM sleep time to total sleep time was within control ranges, thus demonstrating that a large part of the REM sleep deficit in rats with basal forebrain lesions is secondary to their thermoregulatory disturbances and consequent altered thermoneutral zones.

This principle of looking for variables that affect subcomponents of behavior can be applied fruitfully at many levels of organization. Removal of the olfactory bulbs in mice results in deficits of social interactions. Bulbectomized mice do not mate (Rowe & Edwards, 1972), fight (Rowe & Edwards, 1971), or care for their young (Gandelman, Zarrow, Denenberg, & Myers, 1971). Huddling is a social behavior. It is also used in temperature regulation. Since social interactions are drastically affected, one might expect that bulbectomized mice would not huddle in the cold. This is in fact what happens. Other forms of thermoregulatory behaviors that are solitary, such as heat seeking and overeating in the cold, are not affected by the operation. Only that component of thermoregulatory behavior that is also a social behavior is affected by removal of the olfactory bulbs (Edwards & Roberts, 1972).

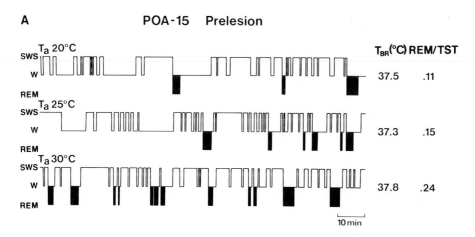

Figure 8-7a. Pattern of sleeping and waking in a normal rat. The rat was run for 2 hours at each of three ambient temperatures (T_a) on the same day during the 12-hour lights-on period. SWS is at the top, waking (W) in the middle, and REM sleep at the bottom (black bars) of each curve. (Abbreviations: T_{BR}, brain temperature; REM/TST, ratio of REM sleep time to total sleep time.)

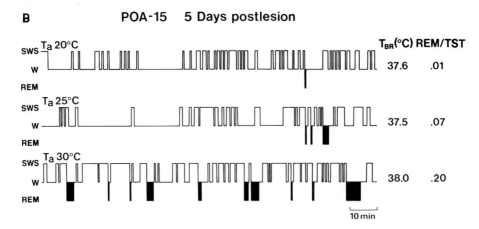

Figure 8-7b. Same rat 5 days after bilateral preoptic lesions that were not large enough to disturb thermoregulation. Note that REM/TST is normal at T_a 30°C but severely depressed at the other ambient temperatures.

Similarities Between Thermal and Sexual Behaviors

In trying to understand a single behavior pattern, one hopes that what is learned will be applicable to other behaviors—that general principles of neural organization will emerge. If this is true of the model proposed here for the neural control of thermoregulation, it ought to be useful in understanding the neural control of other complex behavior patterns. In this section similarities between thermoregulation and sexual behavior are described, with a view toward seeing whether these patterns are enough alike so that the same model can be used for both of them. I will concentrate on the following features:

1. Each pattern is made up of components that are separable after such treatments as brain transections, lesions, or drug administration. They are also separable after local thermal stimulation in the case of thermal regulation, or its sexual analogue, local injections of gonadal hormones.
2. Both patterns are hierarchically organized with alternating levels of inhibition and facilitation.
3. Temperature detectors and sex hormone receptors are found at several levels of the brain and spinal cord.
4. The individual components of each functional class were originally used for other purposes and are still components of several different behaviors.
5. There are species differences in both patterns.

Separation of Individual Components of Thermoregulatory and Sexual Patterns

One of the reasons it has taken so long to recognize that sexual behaviors are relatively independent (as is true for thermoregulation) is probably that (again, as in thermoregulation) one area of the brain is so overwhelmingly important in integrating the behaviors. After medial preoptic lesions, males of several species do not copulate (e.g., rats, Larsson & Heimer, 1964; cats, Hart, Haugen, & Peterson, 1973; dogs, Hart, 1974). Electrical stimulation of the preoptic area potentiates copulation in rats (Vaughan & Fisher, 1962; Merari & Ginton, 1975) and opossums (Roberts, Steinberg, & Means, 1967). Finally, copulatory behavior of castrated rats can be restored by preoptic implants of testosterone (Davidson, 1966; Lisk, 1967). These sorts of experiments were crucial in establishing the importance of the preoptic area in sexual behavior, but they were not designed to fractionate individual sexual responses. In fact, most experiments are not so designed. Instead, they measure either an end point or a single component.

One might consider a normal body temperature as an end point of successful thermoregulation. Similarly, an end point of successful copulation might be birth of young. The former is quick and simple to measure and the latter is expensive and time consuming, so some single component of the sexual pattern is generally measured instead and taken to represent the whole. Most often this is lordosis in females and intromission or ejaculation in males. In thermoregulation this would be analogous to measuring shivering or panting and not body temperature. On the other hand, a measure of body temperature alone is not sufficient to determine if an animal is thermoregulating normally. After a manipulation that increases heat loss by, for instance, preventing vasoconstriction, the animal may compensate by increasing shivering and the net effect might be a normal body temperature. Although a great deal has been learned by using these measures, neither an end point nor a single response is sufficient to enable us to understand how a system is organized because integration, by definition, consists of the appropriate elicitation of *all responses* with proper timing and magnitude and the simultaneous suppression of inappropriate ones. For instance, rats in the cold first vasoconstrict, then become immobile, then shiver. They do not first shiver and then vasoconstrict, nor do they shiver and vasodilate at the same time. However, measuring all responses in a particular pattern is not only impractical, it may be impossible, since at present we do not know what all the relevant responses in any given pattern are. (Furthermore, since the same responses are part of many subsystems, it would probably be necessary to understand the entire behavior, physiology, and evolutionary history of a species before one could completely characterize any particular subsystem such as thermoregulation or sexual behavior.) Nevertheless, from the work that does address the issues of integration we can see that the various components of each behavior are functionally and neuroanatomically separate from each other. Furthermore, some components of a normal pattern can be elicited independently of other components that would ordinarily appear in the sequence—a female rat may exhibit lordosis yet show no soliciting behaviors. This of course implies that the effector mechanisms are separately integrated; if there were one integrator for all sexual responses, they could never be isolated. This section presents some examples chosen to demonstrate fractionation of individual responses in male and female sexual patterns.

In male rats, sagittal knife cuts interrupting the medial–lateral connections between the medial preoptic area and the medial forebrain bundle greatly reduce the incidence of ejaculation (Szechtman, Caggiula, & Wulkan, 1978). This appeared to reflect a lowered probability of initiating mating rather than an inability to reach ejaculation because (1) the males did start to copulate on about 50% of the tests, and when they achieved their first intromission they continued on to ejaculation. (2) If they did ejaculate, they did not take longer to do so than did controls. (3) On the first test in which they achieved ejaculation, initial mount and intromission latencies were markedly extended. There were no impairments in genital reflexes or sensorimotor function.

Horizontal cuts dorsal to the preoptic/anterior hypothalamus that interrupted connections to several brain structures including the amygdala and hippocampus caused a very different copulatory pattern. Males with these cuts required more intromissions spaced at longer intervals to achieve ejaculation. But once they had ejaculated they were quicker than normal to resume copulating. The ejaculatory response appeared less intense—the males did not convulse to a normal extent, they dismounted more quickly, and they were not as quiescent afterward. Theoretically, with small enough knife cuts through the appropriate fibers, any or all of the components of these patterns could be differentiated from any others. Of course, this is not true for a response that depends for its appearance on a previous response. Obviously, if mounting is eliminated, so will be intromissions and ejaculation. But even this does not mean that sexual behavior disappears. Male monkeys with preoptic lesions lost all interest in copulating with receptive females but masturbated to ejaculation outside the test situation (Slimp, Hart, & Goy, 1978).

These results imply that the major function of the rostral hypothalamus in male sexual behavior may be to facilitate and inhibit the activity of lower level neural systems mediating different aspects of a complete copulatory pattern. Not surprisingly from this viewpoint, knife cuts differentially severing connections to these other areas lead to markedly different patterns of sexual impairments. The same is true in thermo-regulation. Bilateral parasagittal knife cuts that completely separated the preoptic/anterior hypothalamus from its lateral connections caused rectal temperature to fall in the cold, but had no effect in the heat (Lipton, Dwyer, & Fossler, 1974). Gilbert and Blatteis (1977) reported similar results and further found that the reason for the drop in body temperature in the cold was that, although the rats shivered normally, there was no cutaneous vasoconstriction. Hence, the rats were not con-serving the heat they were producing.

The components of female sexual behavior are equally separable. Caggiula, Herndon, Scanlon, Greenstone, Bradshaw, and Sharp (1979) found that large catecholamine depletion (by injecting 6-OHDA plus pargyline, a monoamine oxidase inhibitor) increased the intensity of lordosis and decreased soliciting behaviors. Furthermore, the nature of the soliciting changed. Before the drugs, darting (responses wherein the female takes several steps and travels more than a full body length before stopping) predominated over hopping (responses involving a single forward jump of less than a body length) in a ratio of 9/1. After treatment, 68% of soliciting responses were darts. (Vehicle-treated and unoperated controls showed 17% and 11% darts, respectively.) Thus, soliciting behavior, which can be thought of as one component of a female rat's sexual response, can itself be divided into hops and darts, and even these are not controlled by the same neural mechanisms.

Mating responses and the ovarian cycle are also independently con-trolled. Nance, Christensen, Shryne, and Gorski (1977) examined the effects of small hypothalamic and preoptic lesions on vaginal cyclicity, ovulation, and lordosis in gonadectomized hormone-primed rats. There was a clear dissociation between the neural control of cyclic gonado-tropin activity and sex-specific behaviors. Lesions in the dorsal preoptic area increased lordosis and had no effect on ovarian function. Lesions in the ventral preoptic area caused constant vaginal cornification (estrus), no ovulation, and more lordosis. Rats with lesions in the ven-tromedial nucleus had normal estrous cycles and ovulation, but lower levels of lordosis.

There are even different controls over the lordosis response within the same system. Mathews and Edwards (1977) reported that ventro-medial lesions induced much less lordosis than in controls when the rats were primed with estrogen. However, these females showed sig-nificant increases in lordosis when primed with estrogen and pro-gesterone (as was also seen in the study by Nance et al., 1977). As Mathews and Edwards suggest, the brain systems involved in the es-trogenic induction of lordosis may be quite different from those involved in inducing lordosis by the combined effects of estrogen and progesterone. Yanase and Gorski (1976) reached a similar conclusion based on their finding that crystalline progesterone implanted into the

medial reticular formation markedly increased lordosis in female rats
in whom estradiol benzoate had been implanted in the preoptic area
3 days earlier. From this and other experiments (see Gorski, 1976, for a
review) the authors concluded that estradiol benzoate acts at the level
of the preoptic area to facilitate lordosis and it also acts independently
at the level of the reticular formation, apparently by promoting responsiveness to progesterone.

One other line of research suggests that various aspects of female
sexual behavior are mediated by independent neural systems. Female
rats that were rendered sterile by neonatal adrogenization still showed
behavioral receptivity as adults (Barraclough & Gorski, 1961). Furthermore, in 60% of aged rats that were acyclic or had irregular cycles,
ovariectomy and hormone replacement led to good lordotic responding
(Peng, Chuong, & Peng, 1977). Thus, the systems for lordosis and gonadotropin regulation are dissociable in developing and in aging females.

In summary, experimental manipulations of the brain reveal that
there are miniature sexual behavior systems that are integrated separately. Malsbury and Pfaff (1974) reached a similar conclusion with respect to male sexual behavior: "The complicated sequence of responses
that make up the male behavior pattern can more fruitfully be considered to be the result of the interactions of several relevant neural
subsystems. . . . The individual response elements are not integrated
entirely by one particular neural area, but by interactions among all
relevant neural systems coordinated by changing sensory input."
Sachs (1978) similarly concluded that ". . . we are measuring a number
of relatively independent processes that contribute to the integrated
behavioral outcome."

Hierarchical Organization of Sexual Behavior

If all components of a complex behavior pattern are integrated separately in the brain, why do they normally appear so orderly, so smoothly
synchronized? Part of the answer is that the separate controllers for
each effector response, even if they have identical inputs, may have different thresholds of activation. Knife cuts, lesions, discrete hormone
injections, selective disruption of specific transmitter systems, and the
like are marvelous methods for studying central nervous system organization, but they are not normally encountered by an animal. Normally
the midbrain reticular formation is not stimulated by testosterone if the
hypothalamus is not. Normally the hypothalamus is coordinating and
adjusting the activity of lower level neural systems, but not when its
lateral connections have been cut while its dorsal connections are still
functioning.

In thermoregulation, when heat loss responses are inhibited and heat production is initiated, the animal is in a cold environment, or has a fever initiated by leukocytic pyrogen traveling through the bloodstream and affecting thermosensitive and other elements in the entire brain. Thus, in a normal animal in the cold or with a fever the progression from vasoconstriction to piloerection to shivering and their continued simultaneous occurrence can be explained by the external (noncentral) stimulus activating responses with successively higher thresholds. Similarly, in sexual behavior the sequence is activated by internal (hormonal) readiness to respond to appropriate external stimuli.

Another part of the answer to how orderly responses are obtained is that the separate systems, although they can act independently of each other, are normally not independent because they are hierarchically controlled.

It is more difficult to impose an overall hierarchical structure on sexual behavior because sexual behavior appears to be more complicated than thermoregulation in two major respects—the nature of the activating stimulus and the necessary early exposure to gonadal hormones. In the first case, a partner is involved, and a behaving other is an infinitely more complex stimulus than heat or cold. Second, neural mechanisms of sexual behavior are sensitized by exposure to gonadal hormones during a critical period around birth and they require these hormones later in life for their appropriate activation.

This latter difference may be more apparent than real. Cooper, Ferguson, and Veale (1980) reported that adult rabbits raised from birth in a warm environment ($33°C$) showed significant drops in colonic temperature when exposed to cold. Control animals reared at $20°C$ had no difficulty maintaining normal body temperatures. The warm-reared rabbits also had a reduced fever after endotoxin injection and a negligible rise in body temperature after intravenous noradrenaline infusion. Since these effects were not seen in adult rabbits that had been acclimated to warmth a few weeks before the tests were begun, the authors conclude that lack of specific types of thermal afferent inputs early in life may stimulate abnormal development of the thermoregulatory system. Thus, exposure to appropriate thermal information in early life may sensitize neural mechanisms of temperature regulation just as early hormone exposure is important for the development of adult sexual behavior.

The question of hierarchical organization is difficult to answer for another reason. Studies of di- and telencephalic lesions, at least with respect to sexual behavior, are not easy to compare with the effects of lower brain-stem or spinal transections. As Komisaruk (1978) aptly points out, in lower transection studies the implicit assumption is that sexual behavior will be abolished and the question is which, if any, components remain. In forebrain lesion studies the assumption is that copulation will be normal and the question is which components are abolished. These two assumptions lead to the odd results that components of sexual behavior persist after lower level damage but mating behavior is abolished by hypothalamic lesions.

Beach (1967) has reviewed evidence showing (1) that vertebrate copulatory reflexes are mediated by spinal and myencephalic mechanisms that can function independently after separation from more rostral areas of the brain, and (2) that in normal adults these lower centers are organized by higher neural areas. In 1967 Beach remarked that the evidence was disappointingly limited and the same is true today. The system that is best worked out and best illustrates a hierarchical organization is lordosis, and I will go into this in some detail. Certainly there are inhibitory and facilitatory controls over lordosis. The cortex is inhibitory, since neodecortication increased the range of stimuli to which female rats exhibited lordosis, and also increased the maintenance of the posture after the male had dismounted (Beach, 1944). Spreading cortical depression induced by potassium chloride similarly enhanced lordosis (Clemens, Wallen, & Gorski, 1967). The septal area is also inhibitory, since lesions there facilitated lordosis in hormone-primed rats (Nance, Shryne, & Gorski, 1975). Even without hormone priming septal-lesioned rats showed more intense lordosis than controls in response to vaginal and flank manipulation (Komisaruk, Larsson, & Cooper, 1972). In hamsters, electrical stimulation of the septal area suppressed lordosis responding (Zasorin, Malsbury, & Pfaff, 1975).

These results suggest that there is a forebrain lordosis-inhibiting system. Ovarian hormones affect the response, but it is not clear whether they inhibit the inhibitory systems, activate activating systems, or increase the sensitivity of the latter to hormonal or neurotransmitter stimuli (Komisaruk, 1978; Kow, Malsbury, & Pfaff, 1974).

Where are the activating systems? The anterior hypothalamus may be facilitatory (Singer, 1968; Rodgers & Schneider, 1979), as is part of the cuneiform nucleus of the mesencephalon (Pfaff & Sakuma, 1979). The role of the medial preoptic area is unclear. It has been reported to facilitate (Lisk, 1962; Gorski, 1976), inhibit (Rodgers & Schneider, 1979), or have no effect on (Singer, 1968; Gray, Sodersten, Tallentire, & Davidson, 1978) female mating behavior. However, two areas of the brain clearly facilitate lordosis—the ventromedial nucleus of the hypothalamus and the central grey of the mesencephalon. Lesions in the ventromedial nucleus eliminate estrogen-induced lordosis and reduce lordosis in estrogen/progesterone-primed rats (Mathews & Edwards, 1977; Pfaff & Sakuma, 1979). In the central grey lesions decrease and electrical stimulation facilitates lordosis in estrogen-primed ovariectomized rats (Sakuma & Pfaff, 1979a, b).

These two areas are hierarchically connected. After central grey lesions, electrical stimulation of the ventromedial nucleus no longer elicits lordosis. After ventromedial lesions, however, electrical stimulation of the central grey still can elicit lordosis (Sakuma & Pfaff, 1979a). Therefore, lordosis is facilitated at the hypothalamic level by action on the central grey but, in the absence of hypothalamic input, mesencephalic mechanisms are themselves capable of integrating the lordosis response (see Pfaff, 1980, for a complete discussion of neural pathways involved in lordosis).

There are differences between the two effects. Lordosis facilitation from the ventromedial nucleus requires a very long stimulus duration. Central grey stimulation elicits a very fast response. Thus, although the ventromedial axons are not essential for the integration of lordosis, hypothalamic impulses modulate the response, which is integrated at the mesencephalic level. This is entirely consonant with the hypothalamic influences on several different behavior patterns espoused throughout this chapter.

Temperature Detectors and Sex Hormone Receptors

If thermoregulation is organized at many different levels of the brain and spinal cord, then at all the levels there must be temperature-sensitive units able to transmit thermal information. Similarly, for sexual behavior separate neural systems must each have their own information as to their state of sexual readiness to respond. There must be gonadal hormone receptors at the various levels, and indeed there are.

Temperature-sensitive units are found throughout the central nervous system, from spinal cord to cerebral cortex (see Reaves & Hayward, 1979, for a review). There are two classes of temperature-sensitive units—thermodetectors and interneurons in thermoregulatory pathways. Although the distinction in individual cases is not always as clear as one might wish, in general it can be said that both classes of units change their firing rates with changes in their temperature, but only integrative units alter their firing rates with changes in the temperature of other parts of the brain or body (Hensel, 1973). The clearest distinction between them is the relationship between firing rate and temperature. With respect to primary thermodetectors, there is a linear relationship between impulse frequency and temperature. Thermointegrative units are nonlinear: They fire only when their threshold has been exceeded by the summation of impulses coming from primary units elsewhere (Eisenman & Jackson, 1967).

One technique for identifying detector units has been to record single-unit activity while locally heating or cooling various parts of the brain. Both warm-sensitive cells (firing rates increase with rising temperatures) and cool-sensitive cells (firing rates increase with falling temperature) have been found in the cortex (Barker & Carpenter, 1970), the preoptic and anterior hypothalamic area (Nakayama, Hammel,

Hardy, & Eisenman, 1963; Hardy, Hellon, & Sutherland, 1964), the posterior hypothalamus (Edinger & Eisenman, 1970), the rostral (Cabanac & Hardy, 1969) and caudal (Cronin & Baker, 1977) midbrain, the medullary reticular formation (Inoue & Murakami, 1976), and the spinal trigeminal nucleus (Poulos, Burton, Molt, & Barron, 1979).

Another method involves local thermal stimulation while measuring the degree of correspondence between the stimulation and evoked responses such as panting, shivering, vasomotor changes, and thermal behavior. In addition to demonstrating the thermosensitivity of the above-mentioned areas with this other method, the spinal cord (Simon, 1974) has also been shown to be thermally sensitive. In summary, thermosensitive structures are found throughout the nervous system, from cortex to spinal cord. There may well be temperature-sensitive areas in the brain other than those mentioned above, and the main reason they have not been found is simply that no one has looked. Single-unit recording is tedious, and unfortunately there is no way to radioactively label heat and cold, inject them, and see which areas of the brain concentrate them, a technique that has been used to great advantage in studying the neural substrates upon which sex hormones act.

After intraperitoneal injection of tritiated estradiol in female rats, Pfaff and Keiner (1973) found high concentrations of estrogen-containing cells in the medial preoptic, anterior, ventromedial, and arcuate nuclei of the hypothalamus, as well as in the medial and cortical nuclei of the amygdala, the lateral septal area, the ventral hippocampus, and other areas throughout the limbic system. Estradiol was also taken up by cells in the lateral and ventral portions of the mesencephalic central grey and the dorsal horns and intermediate grey of the spinal cord (Keefer, Stumpf, & Sar, 1973).

Using a similar technique, Sar and Stumpf (1973) autoradiographically localized sensitive areas of castrated male rats after injections of tritiated testosterone. Again, many areas of the brain were found to concentrate this steroid, including the medial preoptic area, ventromedial nucleus, arcuate nucleus, stria terminalis, lateral septum, hippocampus, and amygdala. The spinal cord of male rats also contains testosterone-concentrating cells (Sar & Stumpf, 1977). These localizations by autoradiographic techniques substantiate results found after using the other major tool for localizing brain areas involved in sexual behavior—that of local implants and injections of various sex steroids (analagous to local heating and cooling). Thus the areas of the brain that are involved in thermoregulation and sexual behavior as shown by lesion, transection, stimulation, unit recording, and pharmacological studies all contain the appropriate receptors. We do not know, of course, if all the receptors are components of their respective regulatory systems, but this seems a reasonable assumption for most of them, given the correlation between behavior, anatomy, and receptor sites.

Individual Components Were Originally and Still Are Used for Other Purposes

This issue has already been discussed with respect to the thermoregulatory responses of vasomotor changes and internal heat production. It is true for others as well. Rats build nests in the cold and in response to the presence of pups, and the quality of the nest is a joint function of both stimuli (Kinder, 1927). Rats salivate in the heat and also when they eat. Piloerection is a response both to cold and to emotionally disturbing stimuli. The question of which came first is debatable, and in some cases probably unanswerable, but it is self-evident that they could not have evolutionarily been integrated into several higher level complex patterns at the same time.

The components of sexual behavior are also used in other systems. Komisaruk (1978) has reviewed the evidence that the lordosis reflex is used in urination, defecation, and parturition and can be elicited in the absence of adrenal, ovarian, and/or pituitary hormones. With respect to voiding, Beach (1966) demonstrated that neonatal guinea pigs of both sexes assume the lordosis posture when their mother licks them. The licking stimulates the pups to void, which they cannot do by themselves at an early age.

The fact that male and female adults can and do perform the full copulatory pattern of the opposite sex (save, of course, for ejaculation in females) both in homosexual encounters and in dominance displays argues against the idea that sexual responses are limited to reproductive purposes.

Not only are the components of sexual behavior and thermoregulation used for other purposes now: It has been speculated that sexual reproduction might have evolved for nonreproductive purposes initially, and that thermoregulatory considerations were not the initial factor in the evolution of endothermy. Walker (1978) has proposed a model of sex that suggests that theoretically and originally it had nothing to do with reproduction aside from the possibility that individuals that were better able to repair themselves were also better reproducers. The argument is that if there is accidental damage to a unit that replicates itself asexually (a gene, a chromosome, a cell), the damage is faithfully reproduced. However, if there is sexual reproduction, by which is meant a process that allows two cells or two nuclei to align their homologous chromatids for repair, then the undamaged unit of one member can serve as a template to repair the damage in the other. Such a repair mechanism is known for chromosomes: In "excision repair" single-stranded DNA is excised and correctly resynthesized along the sister strand, which forms a template. Chromosomes contain information about cell structure and function. Therefore, fertilization results in cell repair. If multicellular organisms originate from repaired zygotes, sexual coupling between higher organisms results in repaired progeny. According to this theory, "Individuals on all levels of organization, from DNA strands to social animals and man, pair in order to repair their offspring."

Bennet and Ruben (1979) have suggested that thermoregulation was not the sole selective advantage behind the evolution of endothermy, nor did it necessarily provide the initial impetus. Endothermy comes at great cost: Birds and mammals require five to ten times more energy to maintain themselves than do ectotherms of similar size and body temperature. This energy could otherwise be used for growth or reproduction, which on the face of it seems more important to fitness. Why, then, evolve such high metabolic rates? Bennet and Ruben suggest that a major factor might have been an increase in aerobic (oxygen-based) capacity for the purpose of supporting sustained activity. An animal with greater stamina and increased running ability can avoid predators and capture food more readily than its slower relatives, which of course gives it a great selective advantage. Once this initial metabolic change had been established, thermoregulatory considerations could become important, whereas before they would not even have been feasible.

Species Differences

Species differences at any but the behavioral level are a variable that is generally not discussed openly in polite physiological psychology circles. Unless one specifically works on them, they are usually inserted in the discussion section of a paper when there is a discrepancy between results obtained and previous results of others. Even there, they are treated after differences in electrode or cannula placement, volume or dose of drug injected, age and sex of subjects, time of day, and anything else the experimenter can think of.

The reasons for this are obvious. Many of us (myself included) tend to think of a brain as "the brain," and to regard that brain, although varying in certain obvious ways, such as size and degree of cortical invaginations, as basically the same from rat to human. The reasons for this are also obvious. First, the most important facts are the most generalizable ones, and we all want what we find in rats and hamsters to be true also of guinea pigs, dogs, monkeys, and ultimately, humans. Second, parsimony demands the fewest number of underlying mechanisms for the greatest number of overt behaviors, and we are all taught to handle Occam's razor with respect. Nevertheless, species differences will not go away, and there is really no reason why they should. This final section gives some examples of species differences and then discusses how useful they can be in the understanding of complex behavior.

Species differences are particularly apparent in the work on the neurotransmitters involved in controlling thermoregulatory responses. (It may be more obvious in this field because so many species have been studied.) To give a single example, norepinephrine injected into the medial preoptic area causes (depending on the dose) falls in body temperature in monkeys and cats, rises in guinea pigs, rises or falls in rats and ground squirrels, and rises or no effect in rabbits (Satinoff, 1979; Clark & Clark, 1980). Even prostaglandins of the E series, which cause fever in many different species (Kluger, 1979) and are thought to be the causative agents in naturally occurring fevers, had no effect in echidnas (Baird, Hales, & Lang, 1974) and newborn lambs (Pittman, Veale, & Cooper, 1977), although both of these species develop fever after intravenous injection of natural pyrogenic substances. When all other obvious variables have been accounted for, a single model of the neuropharmacological control of heat-loss and heat-production responses at the neurotransmitter level will probably never be valid across species. As things stand now, it is impossible to predict the effect of any transmitter injected into the preoptic area on body temperature in an untested species.

The same considerations apply to sexual behavior. Progesterone had no effect on lordosis in guinea pigs when implanted in the anterior hypothalamic/preoptic area, and inhibited lordosis when implanted in the midbrain (Morin & Feder, 1974a). In rats, progesterone in both the preoptic area and midbrain appears to facilitate lordosis (Ross, Claybaugh, Clemens, & Gorski, 1971; Ward, Crowley, Zemlan, & Margules, 1975), although Powers (1972) found no effect of midbrain progesterone. In rats, rabbits, and hamsters estrogen acts at the median eminence to inhibit ovulation. However, the estrogen-sensitive sites that best mediate sexual receptivity are in the preoptic area in rats (Lisk, 1962), the premammillary nucleus in rabbits (Palka & Sawyer, 1966), the ventromedial–arcuate area in guinea pigs (Morin & Feder, 1974b), and the anterior hypothalamus–ventral filiform nucleus in hamsters (Ciaccio & Lisk, 1973/1974).

A most striking case of species differences is the demonstration that androgens, not estrogens, control sexual receptivity in female rhesus monkeys. After adrenalectomy, ovariectomy, and estrogen treatment, the monkeys were sexually unreceptive as measured by the number of invitations to the male to mount, the number of refusals to allow the male to mount, and the percentage of mounts initiated by the female. Small unilateral implants of testosterone propionate into the preoptic/ anterior hypothalamic area restored receptivity in seven out of eight monkeys. Implants of cholesterol or of testosterone propionate into the posterior hypothalamus or dorsal thalamus had no consistent effect on sexual behavior. Thus, although the site and mechanism of hormone action are similar in female primates and some nonprimates, "there is a clear difference between the two groups in the chemical structure required of a hormone if it is to be an effective stimulus" (Everitt & Herbert, 1975).

An organism's behavior at a particular time depends on the state of its nervous system, the stimuli in its immediate environment, its past individual history, and the evolutionary history of its species. It is only when the last variable is not taken into account that species differences become troubling. No one is upset that various species have diverse solutions to the problem of losing heat: Humans sweat, dogs pant, horses do both; pigs, elephants, and rats do neither, but rather wallow in mud, take showers with their trunks, or spread saliva on their fur, as the case may be. Why would anyone expect the same neurotransmitter to control all of these heat-loss responses?

Thermoregulatory sweating in horses is controlled by the apocrine glands, structures that are anatomically distinct from eccrine glands, through which humans sweat. The final common nervous pathway to the eccrine glands is cholinergic and to the apocrine glands it is adrenergic (Bligh, 1973). It would not be surprising, then, that the same neurotransmitter applied to the brain might have different effects in the two species. Species differences would be a problem only if one thinks in terms of generalized heat-loss rather than of individual species-specific heat-loss mechanisms.

A key feature of the model presented in this chapter is that a response that proves *accidentally* to be useful for purposes other than those for which it originally evolved may come to be taken over by the nervous system for those other purposes. Accidental takeovers may occur at any time, depending on what is available to be taken over, what else is competitively evolving, and what the constraints of the environment are. Clearly, all of these will vary with the species. The fastest way to a general theory of any particular complex behavior, then, may not be through a detailed analysis of a single species, but rather through a consideration of species differences in the patterns. With respect to sexual behavior, Dewsbury (1975) has made a valuable contribution by making order out of the extensive behavioral diversity in many species of muroid rodents. For instance, he has correctly predicted whether males of a species whose copulatory patterns had not been described would display locking (mechanical tie between penis and vagina), thrusting (repetitive intravaginal penetration), or both on the basis of anatomical differences in the penises of the species. These various patterns appear to have evolved repeatedly in response to particular selection pressures. If we start with behavioral differences between species and can analyze their adaptive significance and the evolutionary constraints that may have been placed on them, we may more rapidly understand the neurophysiological and neurochemical mechanisms that organize them.

Acknowledgments. The work described in this chapter was supported by Office of Naval Research Contract N00014-77-C-0465, National Science Foundation Grant 80-22468, and a grant from the Research Board of the University of Illinois. I thank C. S. Carter, E. J. Roy, and P. Teitelbaum for their critical reading of earlier versions of the chapter and Nancy O'Connell for typing them all.

References

Adelman, S., Taylor, C. R., & Heglund, N. Sweating in paws and palms: What is its function? *American Journal of Physiology*, 1975, *229*, 1400-1402.

Amini-Sereshki, L. Brainstem control of shivering in the cat, I: Inhibition. *American Journal of Physiology*, 1977, *232*, R190-R197.

Baird, J. A., Hales, J. R., & Lang, W. J. Thermoregulatory responses to the injection of monoamines, acetylcholine and prostaglandins into a lateral cerebral ventricle of the echidna. *Journal of Physiology*, 1974, *236*, 539-548.

Barker, J. L., & Carpenter, D. O. Thermosensitivity of neurons in the sensorimotor cortex of the cat. *Science*, 1970, *169*, 597-598.

Barraclough, C. A., & Gorski, R. A. Evidence that the hypothalamus is responsible for androgen-induced sterility in the female rat. *Endocrinology*, 1961, *68*, 68-79.

Beach, F. A. Effects of injury to the cerebral cortex upon sexually-receptive behavior in the female cat. *Psychomatic Medicine*, 1944, *6*, 40-55.

Beach, F. A. Ontogeny of "coitus-related" reflexes in the female guinea pig. *Proceedings of the National Academy of Sciences, U.S.A.*, 1966, *56*, 526-532.

Beach, F. A. Cerebral and hormonal control of reflexive mechanisms involved in copulatory behavior. *Physiological Reviews*, 1967, *47*, 289-316.

Bennett, A., & Ruben, J. Endothermy and activity in vertebrates. *Science*, 1979, *206*, 649-654.

Bligh, J. *Temperature regulation in mammals and other vertebrates.* Amsterdam: North-Holland, 1973.

Bullock, T. H. Operations analysis of nervous functions. In F. O. Schmitt (Ed.), *The neurosciences second study program.* New York: Rockefeller University Press, 1970.

Cabanac, M., & Hardy, J. D. Réponses unitaires et thermorégulatrices lors de réchauffements et réfroidissements localisés de la région préoptique et du mésencéphale chez le lapin. *Journal de Physiologie*, 1969, *61*, 331-347.

Caggiula, A., Herndon, J., Scanlon, R., Greenstone, D., Bradshaw, W., & Sharp, D. Dissociation of active from immobility components of sexual behavior in female rats by central 6-hydroxydopamine: Implications for CA involvement in sexual behavior and sensorimotor responsiveness. *Brain Research*, 1979, *172*, 505-520.

Carlisle, H. J. The effects of preoptic and anterior hypothalamic lesions on behavioral thermoregulation in the cold. *Journal of Comparative and Physiological Psychology*, 1969, *69*, 391-402.

Carter, C. S. Stimuli contributing to the decrement in sexual receptivity of female golden hamsters (*Mesocricetus auratus*). *Animal Behavior*, 1973, *21*, 827-834.

Chambers, W. W., Seigel, M. S., Liu, J. C., & Liu, J. C. Thermoregulatory responses of decerebrate and spinal cats. *Experimental Neurology*, 1974, *42*, 282-299.

Ciaccio, L., & Lisk, R. Central control of estrous behavior in the female golden hamster. *Neuroendocrinology*, 1973/1974, *13*, 21-28.

Clark, W. G., & Clark, Y. L. Changes in body temperature after administration of adrenergic and serotonergic agents and related drugs including antidepressants. *Neuroscience and Biobehavioral Reviews*, 1980, *4*, 281-375.

Clemens, L. G., Wallen, K., & Gorski, R. A. Mating behavior: Facilitation in the female rat following cortical application of potassium chloride. *Science*, 1967, *157*, 1208-1209.

Cooper, K. E., Ferguson, A. V., & Veale, W. L. Modification of thermoregulatory responses in rabbits reared at elevated environmental temperatures. *Journal of Physiology*, 1980, *303*, 165-172.

Cowles, R. B. Possible origin of dermal temperature regulation. *Evolution*, 1958, *12*, 347-357.

Crawford, E. Brain and body temperatures in a panting lizard. *Science*, 1972, *177*, 431-433.

Crawford, E., & Barber, B. Effects of core, skin, and brain temperature on panting in the lizard *Sauromalus obesus*. *American Journal of Physiology*, 1974, *226*, 569-573.

Cronin, M. J., & Baker, M. A. Thermosensitive midbrain neurons in the cat. *Brain Research*, 1977, *128*, 461-472.

Davidson, J. M. Activation of the male rat's sexual behavior by intracerebral implantation of androgen. *Endocrinology*, 1966, *79*, 783-794.

Dewsbury, D. Diversity and adaptation in rodent copulatory behavior. *Science*, 1975, *190*, 947-954.

Edinger, H. M., & Eisenman, J. S. Thermosensitive neurons in tuberal and posterior hypothalamus of cats. *American Journal of Physiology*, 1970, *219*, 1098-1103.

Edwards, D. A., & Roberts, R. L. Olfactory bulb removal produces a selective deficit in behavioral thermoregulation. *Physiology and Behavior*, 1972, *9*, 747-752.

Eisenman, J. S., & Jackson, D. C. Thermal response patterns of septal and preoptic neurons in cats. *Experimental Neurology*, 1967, *19*, 33-45.

Everitt, B. J., & Herbert, J. The effects of implanting testosterone propionate into the central nervous system on the sexual behaviour of adrenalectomized female rhesus monkeys. *Brain Research*, 1975, *86*, 109-120.

Gandelman, R., Zarrow, M. X., Denenberg, V. H., & Myers, M. Olfactory bulb removal eliminates maternal behavior in the mouse. *Science*, 1971, *171*, 210-211.

Gilbert, T. M., & Blatteis, C. M. Hypothalamic thermoregulatory pathways in the rat. *Journal of Applied Physiology*, 1977, *43*, 770-777.

Gorski, R. A. The possible neural sites of hormonal facilitation of sexual behavior in the female rat. *Psychoneuroendocrinology*, 1976, *1*, 371-387.

Gray, G., Sodersten, P., Tallentire, D., & Davidson, J. Effects of lesions in various structures of the suprachiasmatic-preoptic region on LH regulation and sexual behavior in female rats. *Neuroendocrinology*, 1978, *25*, 174-191.

Hamilton, C. L., & Brobeck, J. R. Food intake and temperature regulation in rats with rostral hypothalamic lesions. *American Journal of Physiology*, 1964, *207*, 291-297.

Hamilton, C. L., & Brobeck, J. R. Food intake and activity of rats with rostral hypothalamic lesions. *Proceedings of the Society for Experimental Biology and Medicine*, 1966, *122*, 270-272.

Hardy, J. D., Hellon, R. F., & Sutherland, K. Temperature-sensitive neurons in the dog's hypothalamus. *Journal of Physiology*, 1964, *175*, 242-253.

Hardy, J. D., Stolwijk, J., & Gagge, A. P. Man. In G. C. Whittow (Ed.), *Comparative physiology of thermoregulation* (Vol. 2). New York: Academic Press, 1971.

Hart, B. L. Medial preoptic–anterior hypothalamic area and sociosexual behavior of male dogs: A comparative neurophysiological analysis. *Journal of Comparative and Physiological Psychology*, 1974, *86*, 328–349.

Hart, B. L., Haugen, C. M., & Peterson, D. M. Effects of medial preoptic–anterior hypothalamic lesions on mating behavior of male cats. *Brain Research*, 1973, *54*, 177–191.

Heath, J. E. The origins of thermoregulation. In E. T. Drake (Ed.), *Evolution and environment*. New Haven: Yale University Press, 1968.

Hensel, H. Neural processes in thermoregulation. *Physiological Reviews*, 1973, *53*, 948–1017.

Ingram, W. R. Central autonomic mechanisms. In *Handbook of physiology*, Section 1: *Neurophysiology* (Vol. 2). Washington, D.C.: American Physiological Society, 1960.

Inoue, S., & Murakami, N. Unit responses in the medulla oblongata of rabbit to changes in local and cutaneous temperature. *Journal of Physiology*, 1976, *259*, 339–356.

Jackson, J. H. In J. Taylor (Ed.), *Selected writings of John Hughlings Jackson*. New York: Basic Books, 1958.

Keefer, D. A., Stumpf, W. E., & Sar, M. Estrogen-topographical localization of estrogen-concentrating cells in the rat spinal cord following ^{3}H-estradiol administration. *Proceedings of the Society for Experimental Biology and Medicine*, 1973, *143*, 414–417.

Keller, A. D. Separation in the brain stem of the mechanisms of heat loss from those of heat production. *Journal of Neurophysiology*, 1938, *1*, 543–557.

Keller, A. D., & McClaskey, E. B. Localization, by the brain slicing method, of the level or levels of the cephalic brainstem upon which effective heat dissipation is dependent. *American Journal of Physical Medicine*, 1964, *43*, 181–213.

Kinder, E. F. A study of the nest-building activity of the albino rat. *Journal of Experimental Zoology*, 1927, *47*, 117–125.

Kluger, M. J. *Fever*. Princeton: Princeton University Press, 1979.

Koizumi, K., & Brooks, C. M. The integration of autonomic system reactions: A discussion of autonomic reflexes, their control and their association with somatic reactions. *Ergebnisse der Physiologie*, 1972, *67*, 1–68.

Komisaruk, B. R. The nature of the neural substrate of female sexual behaviour in mammals and its hormonal specificity: Review and speculations. In J. B. Hutchinson (Ed.), *Biological determinants of sexual behavior*. New York: Wiley, 1978.

Komisaruk, B. R., Larsson, K., & Cooper, R. Intense lordosis in the absence of ovarian hormones after septal ablation in rats. *Society for Neuroscience, 2nd annual meeting*, 1972.

Kow, L. M., Malsbury, C. W., & Pfaff, D. W. Effects of progesterone on female reproductive behavior in rats: Possible modes of action and role in behavioral sex differences. In W. Montagna & W. A. Sadler (Eds.), *Reproductive behavior*. New York: Plenum Press, 1974.

Larsson, K., & Heimer, L. Mating behaviour of male rats after lesions in the preoptic area. *Nature*, 1964, *202*, 413–414.

Lipton, J. M. Effects of preoptic lesions on heat-escape responding and colonic temperature in the rat. *Physiology and Behavior*, 1968, *3*, 165–169.

Lipton, J. M., Dwyer, P. E., & Fossler, D. E. Effects of brainstem lesions on temperature regulation in hot and cold environments. *American Journal of Physiology*, 1974, *226*, 1356-1365.

Lisk, R. D. Diencephalic placement of estradiol and sexual receptivity in the female rat. *American Journal of Physiology*, 1962, *203*, 493-496.

Lisk, R. D. Neural localization for androgen activation of copulatory behavior in the male rat. *Endocrinology*, 1967, *80*, 754-761.

Liu, J. C. Tonic inhibition of thermoregulation in the decerebrate monkey (*Saimiri sciureus*). *Experimental Neurology*, 1979, *64*, 632-648.

Lucas, E. A., & Sterman, M. B. Effect of a forebrain lesion on the polycyclic sleep-wake cycle and sleep-wake patterns in the cat. *Experimental Neurology*, 1975, *46*, 368-388.

Malsbury, C., & Pfaff, D. W. Neural and hormonal determinants of mating behavior in adult male rats: A review. In L. V. DiCara (Ed.), *Limbic and autonomic nervous systems research*. New York: Plenum Press, 1974.

Mathews, D., & Edwards, D. The ventromedial nucleus of the hypothalamus and the hormonal arousal of sexual behaviors in the female rat. *Hormones and Behavior*, 1977, *8*, 40-51.

McGinty, D. J., & Sterman, M. B. Sleep suppression after basal forebrain lesions in the cat. *Science*, 1968, *160*, 1253-1255.

Merari, A., & Ginton, A. Characteristics of exaggerated sexual behavior induced by electrical stimulation of the medial preoptic area in male rats. *Brain Research*, 1975, *86*, 97-108.

Morin, L., & Feder, H. Hypothalamic progesterone implants and facilitation of lordosis behavior in estrogen-primed ovariectomized guinea pigs. *Brain Research*, 1974, *70*, 81-93. (a)

Morin, L., & Feder, H. Intracranial estradiol benzoate implants and lordosis behavior of ovariectomized guinea pigs. *Brain Research*, 1974, *70*, 95-102. (b)

Nakayama, T., Hammel, H. T., Hardy, J. D., & Eisenman, J. S. Thermal stimulation of electrical activity of single units of the preoptic region. *American Journal of Physiology*, 1963, *204*, 1122-1126.

Nance, D., Christensen, L., Shryne, J., & Gorski, R. Modifications in gonadotropin control and reproductive behavior in the female rat by hypothalamic and preoptic lesions. *Brain Research Bulletin*, 1977, *2*, 307-312.

Nance, D. M., Shryne, J., & Gorski, R. A. Facilitation of female sexual behavior in male rats by septal lesions: An interaction with estrogen. *Hormones and Behavior*, 1975, *6*, 289-299.

Nauta, W. J. H. Hypothalamic regulation of sleep in rats. An experimental study. *Journal of Neurophysiology*, 1946, *9*, 285-316.

Palka, Y. S., & Sawyer, C. H. The effects of hypothalamic implants of ovarian steroids on oestrous behaviour in rabbits. *Journal of Physiology*, 1966, *185*, 251-269.

Peng, M. T., Chuong, C. F., & Peng, Y. M. Lordosis response of senile female rats. *Neuroendocrinology*, 1977, *24*, 317-324.

Pfaff, D. W. *Estrogens and brain function*. New York: Springer-Verlag, 1980.

Pfaff, D. W., & Keiner, M. Atlas of estradiol-concentrating cells in the central nervous system of the female rat. *Journal of Comparative Neurology*, 1973, *151*, 121-158.

Pfaff, D. W., & Sakuma, Y. Deficit in the lordosis reflex of female rats caused by lesions in the ventromedial nucleus of the hypothalamus. *Journal of Physiology*, 1979, *288*, 203-210.

Pittman, Q., Veale, W., & Cooper, K. E. Effect of prostaglandin, pyrogen and noradrenaline, injected into the hypothalamus, on thermoregulation in newborn lambs. *Brain Research*, 1977, *128*, 473–483.

Poulos, D. A., Burton, H., Molt, J., & Barron, D. Localization of specific thermoreceptors in spinal trigeminal nucleus of the cat. *Brain Research*, 1979, *165*, 144–148.

Powers, J. B. Facilitation of lordosis in ovariectomized rats by intracerebral progesterone implants. *Brain Research*, 1972, *48*, 311–325.

Ranson, S. W. Regulation of body temperature. In *The hypothalamus and central levels of autonomic function (Proceedings of the Association for Research in Nervous and Mental Diseases)*. Baltimore: Williams & Wilkins, 1940.

Reaves, T. A., Jr., & Hayward, J. N. Hypothalamic and extrahypothalamic thermoregulatory centers. In P. Lomax & E. Schönbaum (Eds.), *Body temperature: Regulation, drug effects and therapeutic implications*. New York: Marcel Dekker, 1979.

Roberts, W. W., & Martin, J. R. Effects of lesions in central thermosensitive areas on thermoregulatory responses in rat. *Physiology and Behavior*, 1977, *19*, 503–511.

Roberts, W. W., Steinberg, M. L., & Means, L. W. Hypothalamic mechanisms for sexual, aggressive, and other motivational behaviors in the opossum, *Didelphis virginiana. Journal of Comparative and Physiological Psychology*, 1967, *64*, 1–15.

Rodgers, C. H., & Schneider, V. M. Inhibitory and facilitatory influences on mating in the female rat affected by lesions of the anterior hypothalamus or the preoptic area. *Psychoneuroendocrinology*, 1979, *4*, 127–134.

Ross, J., Claybaugh, C., Clemens, L. G., & Gorski, R. A. Short latency induction of estrous behavior with intracerebral gonadal hormones in ovariectomized rats. *Endocrinology*, 1971, *89*, 32–38.

Rowe, F. A., & Edwards, D. A. Olfactory bulb removal: Influences on the aggressive behaviors of male mice. *Physiology and Behavior*, 1971, *7*, 889–892.

Rowe, F. A., & Edwards, D. A. Olfactory bulb removal: Influences on the mating behavior of male mice. *Physiology and Behavior*, 1972, *8*, 37–41.

Ruch, T. C. Central control of the bladder. In *Handbook of physiology*, Section 1: *Neurophysiology* (Vol. 2). Washington, D.C.: American Physiological Society, 1960.

Sachs, B. D. Conceptual and neural mechanisms of masculine copulatory behavior. In T. McGill, D. Dewsbury, & B. Sachs (Eds.), *Sex and behavior*. New York: Plenum Press, 1978.

Sakuma, Y., & Pfaff, D. W. Facilitation of female reproductive behavior from mesencephalic central grey in the rat. *American Journal of Physiology*, 1979, *237*(5), R278–R284. (a)

Sakuma, Y., & Pfaff, D. W. Mesencephalic mechanisms for integration of female reproductive behavior in the rat. *American Journal of Physiology*, 1979, *237*(5), R285–R290. (b)

Sar, M., & Stumpf, W. Autoradiographic localization of radioactivity in the rat brain after the injection of 1,2-^{3}H-testosterone. *Endocrinology*, 1973, *92*, 251–256.

Sar, M., & Stumpf, W. Androgen concentration in motor neurons of cranial nerves and spinal cord. *Science*, 1977, *197*, 77–79.

Satinoff, E. Neural integration of thermoregulatory responses. In L. V. DiCara (Ed.), *Limbic and autonomic nervous systems research*. New York: Plenum Press, 1974.

Satinoff, E. Neural organization and evolution of thermal regulation in mammals. *Science*, 1978, *201*, 16–22.

Satinoff, E. Drugs and thermoregulatory behavior. In P. Lomax & E. Schönbaum (Eds.), *Body temperature, drug effects and therapeutic implications*. New York: Marcel Dekker, 1979.

Satinoff, E. Problems with the concept of homeostatic organization of temperature regulation and other motivated behaviors. In E. Satinoff & P. Teitelbaum (Eds.), *Motivation: Handbook of behavioral neurobiology*. New York: Plenum Press, 1982.

Satinoff, E., & Hendersen, R. Thermoregulatory behavior. In W. K. Honig & J. E. R. Staddon (Eds.), *Handbook of operant behavior*. Englewood Cliffs, N.J.: Prentice-Hall, 1977.

Satinoff, E., & Rutstein, J. Behavioral thermoregulation in rats with anterior hypothalamic lesions. *Journal of Comparative and Physiological Psychology*, 1970, *71*, 77–82.

Satinoff, E., & Shan, S. Loss of behavioral thermoregulation after lateral hypothalamic lesions in rats. *Journal of Comparative and Physiological Psychology*, 1971, *77*, 302–312.

Satinoff, E., & Szymusiak, R. Effects of ambient temperature on sleep in rats with basal forebrain lesions. Paper presented at the Association for the Psychophysiological Study of Sleep, Hyannis., Mass., June 1981.

Satinoff, E., Valentino, D., & Teitelbaum, P. Thermoregulatory cold-defense deficits in rats with preoptic/anterior hypothalamic lesions. *Brain Research Bulletin*, 1976, *1*, 553–565.

Schallert, T., Whishaw, I. Q., DeRyck, M., & Teitelbaum, P. The postures of catecholamine-depletion catalepsy: Their possible adaptive value in thermoregulation. *Physiology and Behavior*, 1978, *21*, 817–820.

Simon, E. Temperature regulation: The spinal cord as a site of extrahypothalamic thermoregulatory functions. *Review of Physiology, Biochemistry and Pharmacology*, 1974, *71*, 1–76.

Singer, J. J. Hypothalamic control of male and female sexual behavior in female rats. *Journal of Comparative and Physiological Psychology*, 1968, *66*, 738–742.

Slimp, J. C., Hart, B. L., & Goy, R. W. Heterosexual, autosexual and social behavior of adult male rhesus monkeys with medial preoptic-anterior hypothalamic lesions. *Brain Research*, 1978, *142*, 105–122.

Spotila, J. R., Terpin, K. M., & Dodson, P. Mouth gaping as an effective thermoregulatory device in alligators. *Nature*, 1977, *265*, 235–236.

Szechtman, H., Caggiula, A. R., & Wulkan, D. Preoptic knife cuts and sexual behavior in male rats. *Brain Research*, 1978, *150*, 569–591.

Szymusiak, R., & Satinoff, E. Maximal REM sleep time defines a narrower thermoneutral zone than does minimal metabolic rate. *Physiology and Behavior*, 1981, *26*, 687–690.

Szymusiak, R., Satinoff, E., Schallert, T., & Whishaw, I. Q. Brief skin temperature changes towards thermoneutrality trigger REM sleep in rats. *Physiology and Behavior*, 1980, *25*, 305–311.

Templeton, J. R. Reptiles. In G. C. Whittow (Ed.), *Comparative physiology of thermoregulation* (Vol. 1, *Invertebrates and nonmammalian vertebrates*). New York: Academic Press, 1970.

Thauer, R. Wärmeregulation und Fieberfähigkeit nach operativen Eingriffen am Nervensystem homoiothermer Säugetiere. *Pflügers Archiv*, 1935, *236*, 102–147.

Van Zoeren, J. G., & Stricker, E. M. Effects of preoptic, lateral hypothalamic, or dopamine-depleting lesions on behavioral thermoregulation in rats exposed to the cold. *Journal of Comparative and Physiological Psychology*, 1977, *91*, 989-999.

Vaughan, E., & Fisher, A. E. Male sexual behavior induced by intracranial electrical stimulation. *Science*, 1962, *137*, 758-760.

Walker, I. The evolution of sexual reproduction as a repair mechanism, Part I: A model for self-repair and its biological implications. *Acta Biotheoretica*, 1978, *27*, 133-158.

Ward, I. L., Crowley, W. R., Zemlan, F. P., & Margules, D. L. Monoaminergic mediation of female sexual behavior. *Journal of Comparative and Physiological Psychology*, 1975, *38*, 53-61.

Yanase, M., & Gorski, R. A. The ability of the intracerebral exposure to progesterone on consecutive days to facilitate lordosis behavior: An interaction between progesterone and estrogen. *Biology of Reproduction*, 1976, *15*, 544-550.

Zasorin, N. L., Malsbury, C. W., & Pfaff, D. W. Suppression of lordosis in the hormone-primed female hamster by electrical stimulation of the septal area. *Physiology and Behavior*, 1975, *14*, 595-599.

Chapter 9

Hormonal and Neural Mechanisms Underlying Maternal Behavior in the Rat

SUSAN E. FAHRBACH and DONALD W. PFAFF

Introduction

This chapter will survey current ideas on the physiological bases of maternal behavior in the rat. Maternal behavior is, of course, a characteristic of all mammals, and ethological descriptions of maternal care are on record for many species (Lehrman, 1961; Klopfer, McGeorge, & Barnett, 1973). However, only a few species have been the subjects of laboratory investigations of mother–young interactions. Included among these are the rat, mouse, hamster, gerbil, rabbit, and sheep, with the rat being the best studied in terms of physiological mechanisms. This fact has determined this chapter's emphasis, but one should not assume that the rat can serve as a general model for the regulation of maternal behavior in mammals. Striking interspecies differences, both in behavior and hormone profiles, have already been described; the significance of these differences is not yet clear.

In the rat, interest in and care for young are by and large confined to sexually mature females. Such behavior can be elicited from male rats in the laboratory, but in this species maternal-like behavior in males is otherwise rare, and we have chosen to use the adjective maternal as a reminder of this. In other mammalian species—mice, gerbils, or wolves, for example—and in many avian species this sex difference in behavior is much less pronounced under both natural and laboratory conditions (e.g., Elwood, 1975). These species' behavior toward their offspring is properly termed parental, although in turn the use of a gender-free label should not be taken to imply that the physiological bases of the behavior are the same in both sexes in species sharing parental duties. Concerning this interesting question, we have no information.

Stages of Investigation

The history of research on maternal behavior in the rat falls roughly into four eras if contemporary research is considered the modern era (Table 9-1). The first era includes studies from the final years of the 19th century through the 1920s. It can be named the descriptive era; in it the behavior we seek to understand today was first carefully recorded. Much attention was given to individual differences among subjects, and experimental interference was limited to environmental alterations. Small's 1899 paper in the *American Journal of Psychology* is a good example of the work of this era: It summarizes a wealth of accurate observations in a diary format.

The demarcation between the first and second eras should not be exaggerated, but it does signify a difference of approach. The concerns of research in the second era went beyond description to ask if maternal behavior is a motivated behavior—that is, does the maternal instinct influence animal behavior in a manner similar to the control exerted by the hunger and sex drives? Straightforward observation was not suited to answer such questions: It might reveal individual differences in vigor of performance of maternal behavior, but little else about the motivated aspects of the behavior. This led to the introduction of measures of drive using arbitrary responses to gauge the intensity of the maternal motivation. Typically, the mother was separated from her young at the start of testing, so that the incentive to perform a particular task was the opportunity for reunion with the litter. One of the most thorough of these studies was that by Nissen, published in 1930 in the *Journal of Genetic Psychology*.

Table 9.1. Research on Maternal Behavior in the Rodent

First Era: Descriptive
  Small (1899) Notes on the psychic development of the young white rat. *American Journal of Psychology*
Second Era: Is maternal behavior a "motivated" behavior?
  Nissen (1930) A study of maternal behavior in the white rat by means of the obstruction method. *Journal of Genetic Psychology*
Third Era: Transition to modern era
  Wiesner & Sheard (1933) *Maternal Behavior in the Rat*
  Riddle (1935) Aspects and implications of the hormonal control of the maternal instinct. *Proceedings of the American Philosophical Society*
  Beach et al. (1930s–1960s) Many studies on hormonal and neural substrates of maternal behavior

---

In the third era, roughly 1930–1960, the dependence of maternal behavior in the rat on both endogenous hormones and pup-related sensory stimuli was firmly established. The 1933 monograph of Wiesner and Sheard, *Maternal Behavior in the Rat*, remains the classic in the field. These researchers were the first to demonstrate that virgin female rats can be induced to behave maternally simply by housing them for several days in close quarters with young foster pups. Also, as did Riddle and his colleagues (Riddle, 1935; Riddle, Lahr, & Bates, 1935), Wiesner and Sheard began the exploration of hormonal facilitation of maternal behavior. Beach's many studies (Beach, 1937; Beach & Jaynes, 1956a, 1956b; Beach & Wilson, 1963) on the humoral and neural substrates of maternal behavior included the important demonstration that elimination of any particular sensory pathway does not abolish the successful performance of maternal behavior, even in inexperienced mother rats.

Contemporary research, with all the advantages of modern neurophysiological and endocrine techniques, has continued to pursue the twin themes of hormonal facilitation and sensory control, with much attention being paid to interactions of the two.

Description of Maternal Behavior

One task facing researchers in maternal behavior is the selection of behaviors for study. The behavioral changes of pregnancy, parturition, and lactation in the rat are many, and they are accompanied by a plethora of physiological changes. Tables 9-2 and 9-3 attempt to convey the

Table 9-2. Behavior Characteristic of Pregnant, Parturient, and Lactating Female Rats

Object-Directed	*Pup-Directed*
Nest building	Freeing from fetal membranes
Tail carrying	Licking, especially of anogenital region
Choice of safe nest location	Retrieval (carrying)
Consumption of fetal membranes and placenta	Crouching over (nursing posture)
	Attraction to pup-related stimuli (approach)
Self-Directed	Inhibition of cannibalism
Self-licking, especially of nipples	Eventual rejection of young
Ingestion of pup urine	
Alterations in food intake	*Directed toward Adult Conspecifics*
Decline in gross locomoter activity during pregnancy	Postpartum aggression
	Successful coordination of mating with maternal behavior during postpartum estrus

Table 9-3. Other Changes Characteristic of Pregnancy, Parturition, and Lactation in the Female Rat

---

Lower threshold for performance of thermoregulatory behavior during pregnancy (Wilson & Stricker, 1979)

Inhibition of sexual activity during pregnancy (Hardy, 1970)

Lactation

Rise in core body temperature during lactation (Thoman, Wetzel, & Levine, 1968)

Suppression of pituitary–adrenal response to stress during lactation (Thoman, Wetzel, & Levine, 1968)

Increase in serum PRL levels in response to the sight, smell, or sound of pups during lactation (Grosvenor, Marweg, & Mena, 1980)

Emission of a fecal maternal pheromone (Leon, 1974; Moltz & Lee, 1981)

Possible emission of a ventral surface attractant (Singh & Hofer, 1978)

---

richness of this behavior. Most experimentation in this field employs a considerably narrowed definition of maternal behavior that emphasizes a lack of cannibalism and the presence of nest building, pup carrying, pup licking, and crouching over the pups in the nursing posture. These activities are performed so repetitively by females with a litter that their presence or absence can be easily seen during brief observation periods; their presence is by and large taken as evidence that an animal is behaving maternally. The likelihood that a variety of items of maternal behavior will be seen during a brief observation period is often boosted by removing the nest and scattering the pups over the cage floor at the start of the test. The maternal animal will typically build a new nest, gather the pups to it, and lick and manipulate them before settling in for a nursing bout. The coappearance of these activities, however, is not necessarily a sign that they are jointly controlled. Slotnick (1967) has shown that during a 10-minute observation of 1-day postpartum rats, indices of nesting, nursing, and licking were only weakly positively correlated with one another; these were not related to the latency to initiate retrieval of scattered pups. Thus, if we wish to draw conclusions on the effects of a particular manipulation on an aspect of maternal behavior, it is essential that the incidence and quality of that behavior itself be measured.

A full description of maternal behavior in the rat would include object-directed behaviors such as nest building, tail carrying (a response related to nest building seen in the absence of nesting materials), choice of a safe nest site, and consumption of the fetal membranes and placenta at parturition. Pup-directed behaviors are numerous: The mother rat frees the newborn from its membranes and engages in vigorous licking of the pup, especially in the anogenital region. Mother rats carry pups without harming them, and once the pups are grouped together, crouch over them in a characteristic nursing posture, with the back arched upward and the outstretched limbs straddling the litter. Pups are rarely crushed. Mother rats show a strong attraction to all pup-related stimuli and an inhibition of cannibalism. These behaviors are directed full strength at young pups, begin to wane as the pups grow toward weaning (see Rosenblatt, 1965), and culminate in a rejection of the young characterized by active avoidance of their attempts to nurse. This phase sometimes occurs simultaneously with the demonstration of the full pattern of maternal behavior toward a new litter born as a result of mating during the postpartum estrus (Wiesner & Sheard, 1933). Self-directed changes in the behavior of the mother rat include those shown in Table 9-2, and postpartum aggression toward adult male conspecifics and the successful coordination of mating with care for the young during the postpartum estrus are current topics of investigation (e.g., Erskine, Barfield, & Goldman, 1978, 1980a, 1980b; Gilbert, Pelchat, & Adler, 1980).

Table 9-3 lists further changes characteristic of pregnancy, parturition, and lactation in the female rat. It is difficult to classify them as behavior proper, but they have an undoubted influence on mother-pup interactions and pup welfare. They are not typically measured in experimental studies of maternal behavior.

An essential feature of maternal behavior is the coordination of maternal care with pup development (Rosenblatt, 1965). As can be seen in Figure 9-1, during the typical 25 to 30-day lactation period, the mother rat appears to be exquisitely sensitive to the changing needs of her pups.

Is Maternal Behavior Motivated?

With the exception of those behaviors related to lactation, all the components of maternal behavior—carrying objects, building nests, licking—are part of the adult rat's normal repertoire of activities. Behaving maternally does not involve performance of a particular set of unique behaviors, but rather the application of already familiar behaviors to the afterbirth, pups, and nesting materials in meaningful sequences. As has already been mentioned, the tendencies to perform the component behaviors can vary independently. There is no fixed sequence of behaviors, such that eliminating one reliably prevents the performance of others (with the exception of the inhibition of cannibalism).

Because maternal behavior consists of new responsiveness to cues and not new actions, maternal behavior cannot be measured independently of pups. It is this goal-oriented nature of maternal behavior that most obviously claims it a place among other motivated behaviors. The goal object elicits approach: Mother rats alert to cues produced by the young (e.g., ultrasonic pup cries; Allin & Banks, 1971) and actively

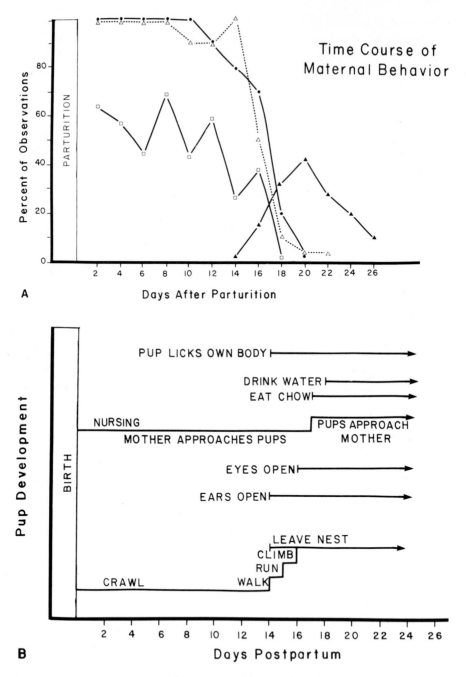

Figure 9-1. Interrelationship of maternal behavior and pup development. (A) Maternal behavior: △——△, retrieving; ●——●, nest building; □——□, nursing pups in nest; ▲——▲, nursing pups out of nest. Mother rat initiates nursing in the nest. Pups initiate nursing out of the nest. (B) Pup developmental landmarks. (Adapted from Rosenblatt, 1965, pp. 3–45.)

search for pups when the cues are distal, in doing so bringing themselves into a position to perform maternal activities. This sequence of approach followed by short-latency goal-directed activity is highly characteristic of other behaviors considered motivated, such as eating and drinking; willingness to approach pups is therefore one of our measures of maternal responsiveness.

Nissen utilized the Columbia Obstruction Apparatus, two cages separated by an electrified grid, to study maternal drive. The measure of drive was simply the number of times the animal crossed the electrified grid in order to approach its litter. Nissen's findings showed that, when compared with prior results also obtained using the Columbia Obstruction Apparatus, the maternal drive was greater in motivating value than the hunger, thirst, and sex drives purportedly measured at their maxima. Even if we do not accept Nissen's ranking (because of difficulties in defining equivalent incentives), such a finding offers compelling evidence that maternal behavior is indeed motivated.

Nissen's other findings are also of interest to the modern student of maternal behavior: His numbers show not only that maternal drive decreases as the age of the litter increases, but also that it decreases if the mother is separated from her litter for more than 4 hours immediately preceding the test. Here we have the first hint that the maternal drive is not strictly a result of the dramatic endocrine changes accompanying pregnancy and lactation, but that it is also dependent on the stimulation provided by the presence of young pups.

Since Nissen's (1930) early and important attempt to measure the maternal drive, there have been relatively few experiments involving arbitrary measures of willingness to respond to pups. Oley and Slotnick (1970) demonstrated that pregnant rats could be taught to bar press to obtain paper suitable for nest building; a dramatic increase in responding was seen immediately prior to parturition. Another type of test scores the readiness of the rat to leave the home cage and to enter a T maze in order to retrieve a pup from the end of one of its arms. Such a test can discriminate between types of maternally behaving rats (e.g., natural mothers and virgin females induced to become maternal by several days of being housed with foster pups; see below), even though the quality of care given in the home cage does not differ significantly (Bridges, Zarrow, Gandelman, & Denenberg, 1972). Yet another type of evidence that maternal behavior is motivated behavior is that, in addition to the changes in responsiveness to external cues that accompany its onset, maternally motivated animals show responsiveness both to suboptimal stimuli such as dead pups and to a broadened range of stimuli, including the young of other species (Wienser & Sheard, 1933). A further example of this heightened responsiveness is the tail carrying sometimes seen in rats near the time of parturition. Such rats, when lacking nest materials, may carry their own tails repeatedly to a corner of the cage (Sturman-Hulbe & Stone, 1929; Wiesner & Sheard, 1933).

When maternal behavior is compared with other motivated behaviors, the behaviors can be seen to differ in two important ways. First, there is no evidence that the concept of satiety can be applied to maternal behavior. Rats that have recently given birth and that have been exposed to young continuously since that time show an almost astounding capacity to respond to young. Le Blond (1940) has provided us with an account of a mother mouse who retrieved 50 foster pups to her nest during one test session. In the rat, the performance of maternal behavior can be extended in time by repeated presentations of foster pups of preweaning age. Wiesner and Sheard (1933) were able to maintain maternal behavior in rats for as long as 13 months postpartum by the litter replacement method. Thus, rats in a state of maternal responsiveness will apparently continue to perform as long as the proper eliciting cues are present. Behavior is turned off not by maternal changes but by changes in the stimulus characteristics of the pups, changes that mirror their decreasing need for attention (see Figure 9-1). This lack of satiety seems related to the diffuse and long-term nature of the ultimate maternal goal, pup survival, and the fact that the time course of pup development can vary. Undernutrition, for example, can cause pups to mature slowly. As long as they display characteristics of young pups, they will be provided with maternal care.

The second way in which maternal behavior differs from other behaviors that are also labeled motivated is that deprivation is not a useful means of intensifying performance of the behavior. As Rosenblatt (1965) has shown, pup responsiveness simply wanes, even in recently parturient rats, if mother and pups are separated for more than a few hours.

In summary, we can define the maternally motivated animal on the bases of (1) the motivated animal's immediate responsiveness to pup-related cues and nesting materials; (2) the willingness of such animals to approach the sources of such cues when they are at some distance or are separated from the mother by an obstacle such as an electrified grid; (3) the maternal animal's responsiveness to suboptimal stimuli.

Hormonal Mechanisms

Background and Approaches

In the rat the onset of maternal behavior is correlated with the birth of the pups (slight prepartum increases can be seen in the frequency of performance of some behaviors, e.g., nest building, but not in others such as placentophagia; see Rosenblatt, 1965; Slotnick, Carpenter, & Fusco, 1973; Kristal, 1980). Massive endocrine changes occur at the end of pregnancy (Shaikh, 1971; Amenomori, Chen, & Meites, 1970;

Morishige, Pepe, & Rothchild, 1973). As Figure 9-2 shows, the final days of gestation in the rat are marked by a decline from the elevated progesterone levels characteristic of pregnancy, accompanied by a gradual increase in the level of circulating estrogens. This rise in estrogen level begins around day 15 of pregnancy, before the drop-off in progesterone. A sharp increase in the level of circulating prolactin begins on day 21 (the rat gestation period is approximately 22 days). These dramatic endocrine changes are followed by the appearance of new and prominent stimuli—the pups themselves—in the rat's environment. A role for hormones in maternal behavior is suggested by the fact that only a small percentage of female rats not recently pregnant will behave maternally at first pup exposure (Wiesner & Sheard, 1933). The difference between these naive rats and mother rats is *not* that the mothers have given birth. Rats whose pups are delivered by caesarean section at term exhibit normal onset of maternal behavior (Moltz, Robbins, & Parks, 1966), so there is no critical need for rats to experience parturition-related stimuli before they will show immediate pup responsiveness.

Two important strategies have been used to explore the relationship between altered hormone levels and facilitated responsiveness to young.

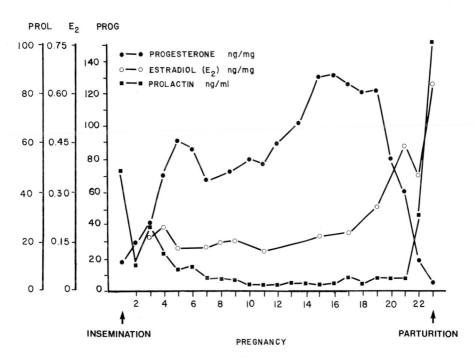

Figure 9-2. Circulating levels of progesterone, estradiol (E$_2$), and prolactin during pregnancy in the rat. (From Rosenblatt, Siegel, & Mayer, 1979, pp. 225–311.)

The first approach is to carry out experimental manipulations of hormone levels in female rats undergoing the normal cycle of pregnancy, parturition, and lactation. Alteration of the level or time of appearance of a hormone suspected to be critical should either disrupt or enhance maternal behavior. A second strategy of equal importance is to attempt the induction, by hormone treatments, of maternal behavior in animals, such as virgin females or males, that do not typically display maternal behavior. One feature of maternal responsiveness in the rat that contributes greatly to the feasibility of such experiments is the rat's willingness to accept foster pups of almost any preweaning age. This is not to imply that female rats are incapable of discriminating their own from other pups. When, for instance, her own pups are mixed with a group of foreign pups of the same age and scattered over the floor of the cage, the maternal rat readily retrieves all of the pups to the nest—but she reliably retrieves her own litter first (Beach & Jaynes, 1956a). This willingness of the rat to accept alien pups is strategically important, since many of the endocrine manipulations we will describe are incompatible with lactation, and the behavioral testing must be done with foster pups.

Are Any Hormones Necessary?

Gross manipulations of the endocrine systems of pregnant and lactating rats have suggested that although hormones almost certainly play some part in the normal onset and maintenance of maternal behavior, they are not indispensable. Postpartum ovariectomy does not alter the expression of maternal behavior (Moltz & Wiener, 1966); pre- or postpartum hypophysectomy does not have a deleterious effect (Le Blond & Nelson, 1937; Obias, 1957). Female rats ovariectomized during the final 2 days of pregnancy still behave normally toward neonatal pups (Moltz & Wiener, 1966; Catala & Deis, 1973). Adrenalectomized rats delivered of their young by caesarean section do not differ in their pup responsiveness from intact caesarean-delivered mothers (Thoman & Levine, 1970). Ergot derivative drugs such as ergocryptine, which severely diminish prolactin secretion, have no effect when given from day 1 postpartum onward (Numan, Leon, & Moltz, 1972). Apomorphine, another inhibitor of prolactin secretion, also has no impact on the quality or quantity of maternal care (Rodriguez-Sierra & Rosenblatt, 1977). These results suggest that the performance of maternal behavior postpartum does not *require* the postpartum presence of estrogens, progesterone, the adrenal steroids, or pituitary hormones.

One difficulty in interpreting these results is that, although these treatments may markedly reduce or nearly eliminate the hormones in question, small amounts of hormone capable of supporting the behavior may remain. For example, ovariectomy during late pregnancy certainly results in a reduction in circulating estrogen and progesterone and in an alteration in the balance between the two hormones, but under such conditions the rat placenta continues to produce at least small quantities of steroid hormones (Bulmer & Peel, 1979). Also, the hormonal events critical for maternal behavior might occur early in pregnancy—animals in the experiments summarized above have already had many days of hormonal stimulation before the surgical or pharmacological manipulations were begun. Another line of research, however, strongly supports these findings of experimental independence of hormonal changes and maternal behavior. These are studies in which maternal behavior is induced in virgin females or male rats simply by housing them with young pups. This phenomenon, known as *sensitization* or *concaveation*, was first described by Wiesner and Sheard in 1933. It is an extremely robust effect with a latency of 5–10 days, and it is exhibited by nearly all rats (Slotnick, 1975). Sensitized animals retrieve pups with the care of a natural mother, lick them, and even crouch over them in the nursing posture, though of course they do not lactate. Nest building is also present, although not quite to the same exaggerated degree seen in the lactating mother (for a detailed comparison of the behavior of natural and sensitized mothers, see Fleming & Rosenblatt, 1974a). One possible explanation for this phenomenon is that the sensory stimulation provided by the presence of pups elicits endocrine changes mimicking those which occur during the normal postpartum expression of maternal behavior. Such a hypothesis could account for the long latency to respond to pup presentation characteristic of the sensitized rat—time is required for the necessary endocrine changes to take place. Although it is now apparent that long-term exposure to pups of advancing age can cause endocrine changes such as raised serum prolactin even in virgin females (Marinari & Moltz, 1978), this is not an adequate account of the sensitization effect. In 1967 Rosenblatt published results of studies of sensitization carried out with ovariectomized and hypophysectomized females and with intact and castrate males. Nearly all of the females tested were successfully sensitized (the rats were scored for retrieving, crouching, nest building, and pup licking); the same was true for most of the males. The latencies to sensitize fell within the normal range for rats (5–10 days); they did not vary significantly among the groups tested. Subsequent studies have concentrated on reducing the latency to sensitize and contrasting the results with the zero latency shown by parturient females. The results of studies of the interaction of sensitization procedures (simply joint housing of the naive animal and several pups) and hormone supplements have yielded insight into the hormonal mechanisms facilitating the onset of maternal mechanisms that we presume are operative in the parturient rat.

Hormonal Facilitation of Short-Latency Maternal Behavior

In the 1930s, Riddle had claimed that a series of prolactin injections could induce short-latency (less than 24 hours of pup exposure) maternal behavior in rats (Riddle, Lahr, & Bates, 1935; Riddle, 1935). Such a result was satisfying in several ways: Similar results had been obtained in work on parental behavior in avian species (see Lehrman, 1956, 1961), and nature'e economy in using the same hormone to support milk production and maternal behavior would have been pleasing. However, Beach, in experiments published in the early 1960s, failed to replicate Riddle's results and concluded that the hormonal control of maternal behavior was unfortunately more complex than the prolactin story implied (Beach & Wilson, 1963). Nevertheless, hormonal means of shortening the sensitization latency have since been described.

At first, hormone combinations administered in regimens of long duration were used. Moltz and collaborators (Multz, Lubin, Leon, & Numan, 1970) demonstrated that a 10-day hormone treatment could reduce the sensitization latency of the ovariectomized virgin rat to between 35 and 40 hours. This treatment provided in a condensed format the endocrine changes characteristic of pregnancy and parturition. The successful treatment consisted of an 11-day course of estradiol benzoate (12 μg/day), 3 mg of progesterone twice daily on days 6-9 of the estrogen series, and 50 IU of prolactin on days 9 and 10. Pups were first presented on day 10. To be scored as "sensitized," a rat had to retrieve, build a nest, crouch over the young, lick them, and keep them warm. Such treatment not only dramatically reduced the latency to sensitize: It also produced a striking uniformity in time of onset of maternal behavior as measured from first pup exposure. None of the control groups, each of which received a vehicle substitute for one or more of the treatment hormones, did as well, although treatment with a combination of estrogen and progesterone minus the prolactin was the next best facilitator. (Note that progesterone was no longer present at the time the behavior was observed.) The role of prolactin in this study remains in question. It is certainly likely that in all cases the estrogen served to release endogenous prolactin (Chen & Meites, 1970), but only the animals given exogenous prolactin showed a strong facilitation effect. Zarrow, Gandelman, and Denenberg (1971) obtained similar results with a slightly different hormone administration protocol. Such an experiment is a demonstration that hormonal changes, particularly in the levels of circulating steroid hormones, *can* facilitate the expression of maternal behavior. An even more direct demonstration of the role of humoral factors is found in the work of Terkel and Rosenblatt (1972). These researchers studied the effects of cross-transfusion of large amounts of blood between freely moving rats with chronically implanted cardiac catheters connected via a pump system.

When blood from rats that had given birth less than 24 hours before the exchange was infused into intact virgins, the sensitization latency was reduced from the expected 5–10 days to a mere 14.5 hours. Only blood from newly parturient females was effective: Blood transferred from sensitized virgins to naive virgins had no impact on latency to respond to pups. None of these studies, however, specify the hormone events critical for the onset of maternal behavior, nor do they reveal the minimum hormonal stimulation that would result in responsiveness to young.

The Pregnancy-Terminated Model

The further study of the role of hormones in the onset of maternal behavior has been aided greatly by use of the experimental termination of pregnancy (Lott & Rosenblatt, 1969; Siegel & Rosenblatt, 1975c, 1978; Siegel, Doerr, & Rosenblatt, 1968; for a review see Rosenblatt, Siegel, & Mayer, 1979). These studies have used either the hysterectomized or the hysterectomized and ovariectomized pregnant rat. Such a preparation employs the termination of pregnancy under controlled conditions to simulate those occurring at the normal termination of parturition by pregnancy. The advantages are clear: The experimenter controls the starting point of the hormone changes and the time of the animal's first exposure to pups. The hormone changes following such surgery can be well defined. As predicted, experiments did show that pregnancy termination by hysterectomy shares some of the features of pregnancy termination by natural parturition with regard to the time of onset of maternal behavior after first presentation of pups. Maternal behavior is defined in these experiments as nest building, crouching over young, pup licking, and pup retrieving. (Foster young are used in the behavioral tests.) When pups are first introduced to a hysterectomized pregnant rat at 48 hours after surgery, nearly 100% of the rats behave maternally in less than 5 days (Rosenblatt & Siegel, 1975). As Figure 9-3 shows, the facilitatory effect is dependent upon how advanced the pregnancy is when the hysterectomy is performed. The later the operation, the more rapid is the onset of maternal behavior after exposure to pups.

Hysterectomy during pregnancy lowers levels of progesterone in the maternal circulation, both because the placental source is removed and because placental control over ovarian secretion is lost. A hysterectomy-induced decrease in circulating progesterone has been confirmed by radioimmunoassay (Bridges, Rosenblatt, & Feder, 1978a). The hysterectomized pregnant animal also experiences a rise in serum estrogen during the period when progesterone levels are declining (Rosenblatt et al., 1979). This change has been inferred from the appearance of the

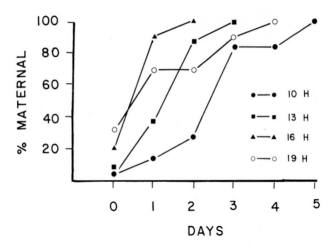

Figure 9-3. Cumulative percentage of females showing maternal behavior following hysterectomy (H) on the 10th, 13th, 16th, and 19th days of pregnancy. First test (0) at 48 hours after surbery. (From Rosenblatt, Siegel, & Mayer, 1979, pp. 225–311.)

vaginal smears of such animals; it is the posthysterectomy counterpart of the hormone changes accompanying the usual postpartum estrus. The timing of the progesterone decline has been studied in detail (Bridges et al., 1978a). After hysterectomy, serum progesterone levels decline starting 18–24 hours postoperatively. These animals typically show the rapid onset of maternal behavior 24 hours after the decline in progesterone levels begins. These results suggest that either the withdrawal of progesterone or the rise in estrogen levels (or both) is the event facilitating the onset of maternal behavior.

What happens if the ovaries are removed at the same time as the gravid uterus? This should also result in a decrease in progesterone, but an increase in estrogen is not possible following such surgery. When such animals are tested in the standard paradigm of first pup presentation at postoperative hour 48, they show much less of a facilitation than do comparable animals subjected only to hysterectomy (Rosenblatt et al., 1979). For example, the median latency to sensitize for animals hysterectomized on day 16 of pregnancy is 1 day, whereas 16-day pregnant rats hysterectomized *and* ovariectomized have a latency of 3 days. The primary difference between these two experimental groups is the lack of an estrogen rise before testing in the ovariectomized and hysterectomized animals. This suggests that giving estrogen to these females might render their latencies comparable to those of the hysterectomized-only group. This is exactly what happens: Giving estradiol benzoate in doses as low as 5 µg/kg to these animals results in short-latency maternal behavior like that shown by hysterectomized pregnant animals (Siegel & Rosenblatt, 1978). Figure 9-4 illustrates this estrogen effect.

It is not true, however, that ovariectomized and hysterectomized pregnant females are exactly the same as the hysterectomized animal but for estrogen. Radioimmunoassay studies (Bridges et al., 1978a) have shown that in the ovariectomized animals levels of circulating progesterone decline earlier—from 6 hours after surgery on—than those in the hysterectomized animal with intact ovaries (decline begins 18–24 hours after the uterus is removed). This reflects the fact that in the rat the corpus luteum is the major source of progesterone during the whole course of pregnancy (Turner & Bagnara, 1976).

Since facilitation of maternal behavior can occur at 24 hours after progesterone levels begin to decline, one might predict that ovariectomized and hysterectomized animals can show maternal behavior at this time. They do. If the first presentation of pups occurs at 24 and not at 48 hours after surgery, during the first hour of pup exposure approximately 25% of hysterectomized and ovariectomized 17-day pregnant females show maternal behavior, as opposed to 10% of hysterectomized females and 0% of intact pregnant animals (Bridges et al., 1978b). This effect wanes quickly, so that if testing is delayed until 48 hours post-surgery, it has already disappeared. Administering exogenous estrogen extends this period of progesterone withdrawal-dependent facilitated responsiveness.

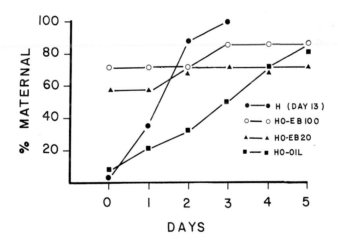

Figure 9-4. Cumulative percentage of 13-day pregnant rats showing maternal behavior after hysterectomy (H) or hysterectomy–ovariectomy (HO) plus estradiol benzoate (EB) treatment of 100 or 20 µg/kg. Maternal behavior tests started 48 hours after surgery and EB injection. (From Siegel & Rosenblatt, 1975c.)

This preparation has proved extremely useful for further studies of the role of hormones in the control of maternal behavior. The effects of estrogen have been found to be independent of any effect on prolactin release, since the pharmacological block of prolactin secretion does not disrupt the facilitatory effects of estrogen (Rodriguez-Sierra & Rosenblatt, 1977). The finding that ovariectomy very late in pregnancy, on either day 20 or 21, has no effect on the onset of maternal behavior suggests that it may be the earliest part of the estrogen rise, beginning on day 15 of pregnancy, that is of critical importance. This allows time for estrogen's effects to be mediated via changes in RNA and protein synthesis following nuclear binding in the brain, as opposed to short-latency effects on the excitability of neuronal membranes.

The importance of declining progesterone is emphasized in the pregnancy-terminated preparation. Not only do hysterectomized-ovariectomized pregnant female rats show a facilitation of maternal responsiveness approximately 24 hours after the decline in serum progesterone levels commences: Further experiments have shown that when rats ovariectomized and hysterectomized on day 17 of pregnancy are given subcutaneous silastic implants containing progesterone, the onset of maternal behavior is delayed (Bridges et al., 1978a).

Progesterone actions appear to depend on a rise in circulating estrogen levels. Maternal behavior is not facilitated in animals that have had silastic capsules containing progesterone removed after 12 or more days of implantation (Rosenblatt et al., 1979). Experiments on ovariectomized and hysterectomized virgin rats injected with estradiol benzoate (100 µg/kg) at the time of surgery have shown that the estrogen background need not be the normal 7 or 8 days for progesterone withdrawal effects to occur.

The work of Siegel and Rosenblatt (1975a) illustrates the impressive effects that can be achieved in hysterectomized and ovariectomized virgins with a single injection of estradiol benzoate. (Ovariectomy alone does not have this effect; the reason the uterus must also be removed is not clear, but is presumably related to its role as an estrogen target tissue. See Siegel, Andieh, & Rosenblatt, 1978.) Progesterone given 24 hours after the estradiol injection can block the effect, whereas progesterone given at the same time as the estradiol or 44 hours later has no such blocking effect (Siegel & Rosenblatt, 1975b).

There are differences, however, in hormonal sensitivity between the ovariectomized and hysterectomized pregnant rat and her virgin counterpart given the same surgical treatment. The pregnant female shows full maternal behavior at short latency with doses of estradiol benzoate as low as 5 or 20 µg/kg; the virgins require 100 µg/kg (Siegel, Doerr, & Rosenblatt, 1978). When CI-628, an antiestrogen, is administered simultaneously with the dose of estradiol given at the end of surgery, 2 mg will block estrogen's facilitatory effects in virgins, whereas a minimum of 10 mg of antiestrogen is required to have a similar effect in

Table 9-4. Effects of Hormonal Facilitation on Onset of Maternal Behavior

		Hormone events[a]			
Experiment		P↑	P↓	E↑	Short-latency maternal behavior?
I	Pregnant/H		+	+	yes (Rosenblatt & Siegel, 1975)
II	Pregnant/HO		+		no (Siegel & Rosenblatt, 1975c)[b]
III	Pregnant/HO + EB		+	+	yes (Siegel & Rosenblatt, 1975c)
IV	Pregnant/HO + EB + P	+		+	no (Numan, 1978)
V	Pregnant + P	+		+	no (Moltz et al., 1969)
VI	Virgin/HO + EB			+	yes (Siegel & Rosenblatt, 1975a)
VII	Virgin/HO + EB + P	+		+	no (Siegel & Rosenblatt, 1978)
VIII	Virgin/O + EB			+	no (Siegel & Rosenblatt, 1975a)
IX	Virgin − P		+		no (Rosenblatt et al., 1979)

[a] Abbreviations: P, progesterone; E, estrogens; H, hysterectomized; O, ovariectomized; EB, estradiol benzoate.
[b] Some pregnant/HO rats show a transient facilitation at 24 hours after surgery. See text.

pregnancy-terminated females (Siegel et al., 1978). The progesterone withdrawal that occurs in the former group is certainly likely to account for these differences. It is as if the declining levels of progesterone in some way permit the increase in estrogen to be more effective than it otherwise would be. These differences between the virgin and pregnancy-terminated animals could also be explained in terms of the duration of estrogen exposure, which is longer in the pregnancy-terminated group if surgery is performed after day 15 of pregnancy.

A chart displaying the results of experiments on the hormonal facilitation of the onset of maternal behavior is presented as Table 9-4. It shows clearly that the effects of estrogen on maternal responsiveness are always facilitatory. The presence of progesterone inhibits the effects of estrogen; both an absence of progesterone and its withdrawal interact with a rise in estrogen to promote short-latency maternal responsivness.

The role of hormonal changes in maternal behavior can be summarized as follows:

1. Behaviors classified as maternal, such as pup carrying, nest building, and pup licking, can be seen in the absence of any hormonal stimulation. The primary example of this is the phenomenon of *sensitization,* in which nonpostpartum rats respond to neonatal pups with a latency of 5 or more days.
2. A rise in estrogen levels is strongly associated with a significant reduction in the latency to show maternal behavior.
3. Progesterone withdrawal coupled with a rise in estrogen facilitates the display of maternal behavior. Maintained high levels of progesterone at the time of the estrogen rise inhibit maternal behavior.

4. Other hormonal changes seen near term, such as the sharp increase in prolactin levels, do not appear to be critical for the onset of maternal behavior.
5. A recent report has claimed that the peptide hormone oxytocin is capable of eliciting short-latency maternal behavior when injected into the cerebral ventricles of virgin rats (Pedersen, 1980). Oxytocin is certainly released during parturition and lactation, and it is now known that the magnocellular neurons of the hypothalamus staining for neurophysin project to sites other than the posterior pituitary (Swanson, 1977). Hence, a role for oxytocin in maternal behavior is plausible, although more evidence will be needed to strengthen its claims.

In almost every case, primiparous rats react more strongly than multiparous rats to experimental interference with endocrine function. How experience renders maternal behavior resistant to disruption is not yet understood. (Primiparous rats are typically used in the experimental study of maternal behavior. For examples of the advantage conferred by multiparity, see Moltz & Wiener, 1966; or Moltz, Levin, & Leon, 1969.)

The Onset–Maintenance Dichotomy

Up to this point we have considered solely the successful initiation of maternal behavior, yet its outstanding characteristic is its extension in time. Care is given over a preweaning period lasting 25–30 days. During this period the mother rat varies her activities to meet the changing needs of her quickly growing pups (see Figure 9-1). The hormonal pattern present during lactation is greatly different from that observed during pregnancy. A suspension of estrous cycling results from pup suckling. Suckling apparently exerts its effects through the inhibition of secretion of the anterior pituitary hormones, follicle-stimulating hormone (FSH) and luteinizing hormone (LH). After the postpartum estrus, prolactin levels are high, moderate levels of progesterone secretion are maintained, and estradiol levels are very low (Rosenblatt et al., 1979).

There is little evidence that, in the rat, display of maternal behavior is dependent upon the hormones of lactation. As was described above, many endocrine manipulations that disrupt lactation do not affect maternal responsiveness. Female rats subjected to total mammectomy at 21–30 days of age have normal maternal behavior when mated as adults (Moltz, Geller, & Levin, 1967). Further, there is no fixed postpartum time course for either lactation or maternal behavior. The duration of both can be greatly extended if the mother is continually resupplied with fresh young pups (Wiesner & Sheard, 1933). Finally, we know that sensitized rats, which do not lactate, display a convincing variety of behaviors considered maternal.

Since the hormonal state of sensitized rats does not become like that of natural mothers, it is possible that the converse relationship holds: Lactating mothers may be as dependent upon pup stimulation for the maintenance of behavior as are sensitized rats. A common neural mechanism could mediate both the normal postpartum maintenance of maternal behavior and sensitization. This would be consistent with the relative hormonal independence of this phase of mother–pup interaction, in contrast to the hormone dependence of the parturition–linked onset of maternal behavior.

The concept of a dichotomy between the mechanisms of the normal onset and maintenance of maternal behavior is not a new one. For example, in considering the results of studies on animals hypophysectomized postpartum, Le Blond and Nelson wrote in 1936: "The induction but not necessarily the maintenance of parental instinct may be dependent upon hormonal factors" (p. 30). In the modern era this widely held view has been clearly stated in the work of Rosenblatt (see Rosenblatt et al., 1979). It is an organizing concept rather than a dogma, and it offers at least a partial explanation why the phenomenon of sensitization should exist at all in the rat.

As the changing nature of the mother's responses to the growing pups indicates, lactating mothers are extremely sensitive to both the quantity and quality of pup stimulation they receive. The normal temporal development of the behavior is critically dependent upon the mother's interaction with pups of continually advancing age (Rosenblatt, 1965). Virgins show a similar sensitivity to pup age: Younger pups (1–2 days) are more effective stimulation than older pups for eliciting sensitization (Stern & MacKinnon, 1978). When sensitized virgins are exposed to pups of advancing age, like natural mothers they too show a decline in responsiveness to pups older than 10 days of age (in some cases the decline is slightly faster in the virgins than in the lactaters; Reisbick, Rosenblatt, & Mayer, 1975).

Only if the behavior of sensitized virgins could be shown to be exactly like that of lactating rats would we need to rule out the possibility of *any* hormonal influences on the maintenance phase. It is now becoming clear that an either/or position is not tenable. In most respects the behavior of the two types of animals is very similar, although earlier studies that relied heavily on simple measures of latency to behave maternally tended to deemphasize any difference. More recent studies have included a wider range of experimental situations and quantitative measures of behavior; they have also drawn a distinction between intact and gonadectomized sensitized animals. The results of some tests have demonstrated that sensitization does indeed have a general impact on the behavior of virgins. For instance, in contrast with nonmaternal virgins, both lactating and sensitized rats will choose a pup over a small toy in a retrieval preference test (Rosenblatt, 1975). Also, both sensitized virgins and primiparous rats show a shortened latency to respond to pups a month after their initial experience (Fleming & Rosenblatt, 1974a). The differences such studies have found are interesting but not overwhelming. Fleming and Rosenblatt (1974a), in a detailed study of the behavior of sensitized virgins provided with pups of advancing age, found that nest-building tendencies were weaker in sensitized animals but that they actually tended to lick their pups more frequently than do normal mothers. And, although sensitized animals are often seen to crouch over their foster young, it is harder for them to maintain this replica of the lactation posture for any length of time, perhaps due to lack of proper suckling stimulation. The striking postpartum aggression of the lactating rat is also not seen in the sensitized virgin, unless the pup exposure is of long duration (Erskine et al., 1978; Erskine et al., 1980b). T-maze tests have been used to compare the behavior of natural mothers and sensitized virgins; in such tests the natural mothers retrieve pups more frequently, even though the quality of care given by these two types of maternally behaving rats in the home cage does not differ significantly (Bridges et al., 1972).

Studies comparing sensitized castrates with sensitized intact subjects have shown that the castrates exhibit less nest building and less crouching than their intact counterparts (Krehbiel & Le Roy, 1979). Virgins with their gonadal hormones replaced by estradiol injections behaved as do natural mothers in a wide variety of tests, although they were characterized by a longer latency to retrieve scattered pups. Recently, Mayer and Rosenblatt (1980) have demonstrated that ovariectomy performed at any age increases the latency to sensitize in virgin rats, and, that even though they become sensitized, ovariectomized females build poorer nests, retrieve pups less consistently, and are less likely to retrieve pups in a T maze than are intact sensitized animals. Thus, it appears that even a hormonal background of normal cyclicity can enhance readiness to respond to pups and the quality of maternal behavior subsequently displayed. The relationship is in line with evidence showing a weak association between the onset of sensitized maternal behavior and the proestrous phase of the estrous cycle, the time at which circulating levels of estrogen are at their highest in the rat (Marinari & Moltz, 1978). There is other evidence that estrogen's facilitatory effects are not only short term. For example, when pregnancy-terminated hysterectomized and ovariectomized rats were given 200 μg/kg of estradiol benzoate, its effects on reducing the latency to respond to pups could still be detected 72 hours after the injection (Siegel, Doerr, & Rosenblatt, 1978). Such a holdover effect might explain how the hormonal fluctuations of the cycling rat produce subtle enhancement of maternal responsiveness.

In summary, while it seems likely that postpartum maternal behavior is controlled by nonhormonal mechanisms, it is also probable that parturition initiates a transition period during which the overlap between estrogen's actions on the onset of behavior and the potent stimulus effects of the neonatal pups ensures the emergence of maternal behavior.

Sensory and Neural Mechanisms

Sensory Control

Repeated emphasis on the importance of sensory control to maternal behavior leads very naturally to the question: "What senses are involved?" This is, of course, another way of asking which of the many cues produced by pups elicit maternal behavior. Beach's concept that maternal behavior in the rat is under multisensory control is still valid. For example, Beach (Beach & Jaynes, 1956a) demonstrated that even though the mother rat's ability to discriminate her own pups depends on an intact olfactory system, anosmic mothers can nevertheless retrieve their young. Blind rats and rats whose mouths and snouts have been deafferented also retrieve pups, as do deaf animals (Herrenkohl & Rosenberg, 1972). Combinations of these sensory losses do indeed impair behavior, but not to the point at which litter survival is threatened.

Effects of Central and Peripheral Anosmia

Anosmia may be produced in two ways, by ablation of the olfactory bulbs or by destruction of the peripheral sense organ. The effects of the two procedures are not always identical. The effects, for instance, of the anosmia produced by bilateral olfactory bulbectomy are generally mild in primiparous rats bulbectomized during pregnancy (Benuck & Rowe, 1975). There is no effect on nest building or time spent in the nusring position, but placentophagy is incomplete and pup retrieval is disrupted 24 hours postpartum. These relatively specific effects are not seen in rats with previous maternal experience or, rather surprisingly, in rats with peripheral anosmia produced by intranasal injections of zinc sulfate. Thus it is evident that in natural mothers the effects of central anosmia are probably due to the nonolfactory functions of the ablated bulbs (see Cain, 1974). The effect of either bulbectomy or zinc sulfate treatment on virgin females is quite different. Females rendered anosmic by bilateral bulbectomy either cannibalize or show a significantly reduced latency to retrieve (Fleming & Rosenblatt, 1974b); females treated with zinc sulfate show the reduction in latency without the cannibalism (Fleming & Rosenblatt, 1974c). Mayer and Rosenblatt (1975) have reported that the latter effect can be seen as early as during the first 15 minutes of pup exposure. This olfactory inhibition of virgin responses has been shown to be mediated by both the olfactory epithelium and the vomeronasal organ (Fleming, Vaccarino, Tambosso, & Chee, 1979). Aversiveness of pup-related stimuli accounts for the active avoidance of pups exhibited by virgins when they are first housed with the young. Contact with pup stimuli is necessary to produce the sensitized state: The facilitated responding of anosmic virgins can be explained in terms of the absence of this initial avoidance phase. Housing the females to be sensitized and their foster pups in very small cages, in which avoidance is physically impossible, has been shown to have similar facilitatory effects upon the latency to sensitize (Terkel & Rosenblatt, 1971). A more complete discussion of the role of olfaction in maternal behavior in the rat can be found in the review by Rosenblatt et al. (1979).

Neural Control

Lesions of many brain areas—for example, the neocortex, dorsal hippocampus, and septum—have been shown to impair the performance of maternal behavior in the rat (Beach, 1937, 1938; Fleischer & Slotnick, 1978; see reviews in Slotnick, 1975; Numan, in press). The broad effects of such lesions make interpretation of the role of these areas in maternal behavior nearly impossible at this time. Recent progress in the understanding of the neural mechanisms underlying maternal behavior has come from studies focusing on the role of the medial preoptic area of the rostral hypothalamus.

A strong case can be made that an intact medial preoptic area is essential to the performance of all of the commonly studied components of maternal behavior. Numan has shown that lesions of this region made 5 days postpartum severely disrupt maternal behavior in rats (Numan, 1974). The lesioned mothers, whose preoperative behavior was completely normal, no longer build nests, retrieve, or crouch over pups in the nursing posture. Although such females do not show an aversion to pups—they will occasionally approach, sniff, and lick young pups—they give them no care. The performance of these lesioned mothers does not improve significantly with continued exposure to pups.

Medial preoptic area lesions also prevent the sensitization of virgins housed with neonates (Numan, Rosenblatt, & Komisaruk, 1977), a finding that suggests that sensitization and the normal maintenance phase of maternal behavior do indeed share a common neural basis. That the medial preoptic area may also be involved in the onset of maternal behavior is indicated by Numan's finding that such lesions abolish the appearance of maternal behavior in ovariectomized and hysterectomized pregnancy-terminated rats injected with adequate doses of estradiol (Numan & Callahan, 1980).

Control studies have shown that knife cuts of the stria terminalis or the medial corticohypothalamic tract, the prominent fibers of passage of this region, do not reproduce the medial preoptic area deficits (Numan, 1974). The severe disruption caused by medial preoptic area lesions is mimicked by bilateral knife cuts severing the connections between the medial preoptic area and the lateral preoptic area (and the rostral part of the anterior hypothalamic area from the lateral hypothalamus). These findings suggest that the behavioral effects of medial preoptic area lesions are primarily the result of damage to medial preoptic area neurons and not to incidental damage to fibers of passage.

Numan and Callahan (1980) have used the knife cut technique to explore the importance of the connections of the medial preoptic area. Using the ovariectomized and hysterectomized 16-day pregnant preparation treated with estradiol benzoate, they have shown that only cuts defined as lateral relative to the medial preoptic area (severing most of the mediolateral connections throughout the entire preoptic region and the rostral anterior hypothalamic area) and anterior (placed rostral to the medial preoptic area from the level of the anterior commissure to the base of the brain) disrupt maternal behavior. Of animals given the lateral knife cuts, 5 out of 12 never displayed any maternal behavior. The remaining 7 never retrieved and showed depressed levels of the other behaviors assessed. Animals given the anterior cuts also did not retrieve, and they performed nursing and nest building very infrequently. Posterior and dorsal cuts had minimal effects on maternal behavior.

The lateral cuts produce a transient hyperthermia that does not seem to influence behavior unduly, and Numan has concluded that it is these lateral connections of the medial preoptic area which are of specific importance to maternal behavior. The effects of the anterior cuts are more difficult to interpret because these produce hypoactivity and a loss of body weight in addition to the disruption of maternal behavior. Numan suggests that these effects are at least in part due to the interruption of connections involved in the regulation of fluid balance, and that the effects seen during tests of maternal behavior are the result of a general debilitation. One qualification to such an interpretation is the possibility that the anterior knife cuts severed some of the connections between the medial preoptic area and the septal nuclei. Septal lesions have been shown to disorganize the performance of maternal behavior in rats, although they do not abolish it (Slotnick, 1975; Fleischer & Slotnick, 1978). It is therefore possible that medial preoptic area to septum connections are critical for maternal behavior, although the multiple effects of the anterior knife cuts prohibit us from concluding yet that this is so.

The lateral connections of the medial preoptic area are presumably with the medial forebrain bundle. Both neuroanatomical and behavioral evidence support this connection. Conrad and Pfaff (1976) have shown, using the tritiated amino acid autoradiographic tracing technique, that fibers from the medial preoptic area do descend in the medial forebrain bundle; others (Avar & Monos, 1967, 1969) have shown that lesions in the region of the medial forebrain bundle (rostral lateral hypothalamic area) produce behavioral deficits similar to those seen after medial preoptic area lesions.

The terminal areas of the efferents of the medial preoptic area important for maternal behavior remain to be defined. Conrad and Pfaff (1976) have shown that the lateral efferents of this region both ascend (to the septal nuclei) and descend (through the ventral tegmental area). As mentioned above, septal lesions have been shown to disorganize maternal behavior; it has also been shown (Gaffori & Le Moal, 1979) that lesions of the ventral tegmental area induce pup cannibalism and prevent the appearance of maternal behavior. A plausible explanation of the latter results is that such lesions interrupt the efferents of the medial preoptic area in their descent to the brain stem.

Brain Sites of Hormone Action

Another line of evidence supporting a critical role for the medial preoptic area in maternal behavior comes from studies involving the implantation of small amounts of crystalline estradiol benzoate directly into the brain (Numan, Rosenblatt, & Komisaruk, 1977). In ovariectomized and hysterectomized pregnant rats so treated, females receiving estrogen implants into the medial preoptic area had shorter latencies to sensitize than did animals with estrogen implanted into the hypothalamic ventromedial nucleus, into the mammillary bodies, or subcutaneously. Animals with cholesterol implants into the medial preoptic area showed no such facilitation as was seen in the estrogen implant group. The medial preoptic area contains a high density of cells that exhibit nuclear binding of estrogen (Pfaff & Keiner, 1973; see Figure 9-5). This finding strongly suggests that the medial preoptic area is a major site of action in the estrogen facilitation of maternal behavior. (It is not clear if the medial preoptic area mediates the inhibitory effects of progesterone; see Numan, 1978.) Although such evidence provides a means of combining the now separate research on the hormonal and neural bases of maternal behavior, we are lacking in our understanding of the nature of the hormone–brain interaction. This identification of so important a site of hormone action can be exploited by future experiments. However, there is no reason to assume that in the normal onset of maternal behavior, estrogen acts at only one site. This possibility has been raised by Fleming and colleagues (Fleming, Vaccarino, & Luebke, 1980) in their further investigations of the basis of olfactory inhibition in nonsensitized virgins. These researchers have found that the bimodal effects of bulbectomy—either cannibalism or

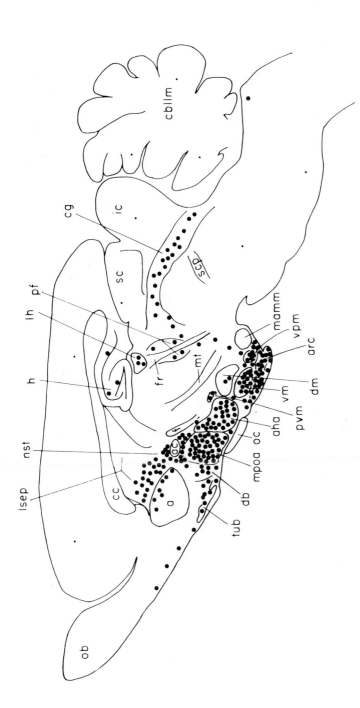

Figure 9-5. Distribution of estrogen-concentrating neurons in the brain of the female rat represented schematically in a sagittal plane. Locations of estradiol-concentrating neurons are represented by black dots. [Abbreviations: a, nucleus accumbens; ac, anterior commissure; aha, anterior hypothalamic area; arc, arcuate nucleus; cbllm, cerebellum; cc, corpus callosum; cg, central grey; db, diagonal band of Broca; dm, dorsomedial nucleus of the hypothalamus; f, fornix; fr, fasciculus retroflexus; h, hippocampus; ic, inferior colliculus; lh, lateral habenula; lsep, lateral septum; mamm, mammillary bodies; mpoa, medial preoptic area; mt, mammillothalamic tract; nst, bed nucleus of the stria terminalis; ob, olfactory bulb; oc, optic chiasm; pf, nucleus parafasicularis; pvm, paraventricular nucleus (magnocellular); sc, superior colliculus; scp, superior cerebellar peduncle; tub, olfactory tubercle; vm, ventromedial nucleus; vpm, ventral premammillary nucleus.] (From Pfaff, & Keiner, 1973.)

facilitated pup responsiveness—can be reproduced by lesions of the corticomedial amygdala. Both the lateral olfactory tract and the accessory olfactory tract project to the corticomedial amygdala (Scalia & Winams, 1975), which in turn projects to the medial preoptic area via the stria terminalis. That this connection of the corticomedial amygdala to the medial preoptic area is important is shown by Fleming et al.'s (1980) finding that lesions of the stria terminalis also facilitate the retrieving of pups by virgins (although such lesions have no effect on other aspects of maternal behavior; Numan, 1974). The corticomedial amygdala is another brain site known to concentrate estrogen (Pfaff & Keiner, 1973). It is possible that in addition to direct actions of estrogen on the medial preoptic area, estrogen bound at the corticomedial amygdala could also act, indirectly, to facilitate maternal responsivenes.

In summary:

1. Lesions of many brain regions have been shown to alter the rat's performance of various components of maternal behavior. Many of these effects are nonspecific (i.e., accompanied by other changes in behavior).
2. Lesions of the medial preoptic area have been shown to have relatively selective disruptive effects on all maternal behaviors tested (nursing, licking, nest building, and retrieving). Severing the anterior and lateral connections of the medial preoptic area reproduces these effects.
3. The medial preoptic area has been implicated as the major site of estrogen facilitation of maternal behavior, although actions of estrogen at other brain sites that influence maternal behavior are also likely.

Interaction with Other Motivated Behaviors

Although the relative specificity of effects of medial preoptic area lesions has been emphasized—for example, such lesions do not disrupt sexual behavior in the same rats who no longer behave maternally (Numan, 1974)—the proper conclusion is that medial preoptic area lesions do not produce a general debilitation or profound sensory deficits which would in themselves preclude maternal responses to pups, and not that the medial preoptic area is devoid of other functions. An intact medial preoptic area is also essential for the timing of ovulation (Clemens, Smalstig, & Sawyer, 1976), the performance of male sexual behavior (Malsbury & Pfaff, 1974), and thermoregulation (Hammel, 1968).

The potential for overlap of neural control mechanisms is especially striking in the cases of maternal behavior and thermoregulation. For example, Leon and his colleagues have recently shown that it is maternal temperature which determines the length of individual bouts of nursing in the rat (Leon, Croskerry, & Smith, 1978). Briefly, lactating mothers tend to overheat during nursing, and terminating a nursing bout by leaving the nest is a form of lactation-specific behavioral thermoregulation. Increases in both core temperature and ventral surface temperature produce this response, as does direct warming of medial preoptic area neurons via implanted electrodes (Woodside, Pelchat, & Leon, 1980). Moreover, nest building, a behavior highly characteristic of maternal animals, is also a thermoregulatory response to lowered ambient temperature (Kinder, 1927). Medial preoptic area lesions abolish nest building under cold conditions as well as in the presence of pups (Van Zoeren & Stricker, 1977). All rats build nests in the cold, but only a subgroup of animals—those in the physiological states of pregnancy or lactation—will build maternal nests. How this selective responsiveness is maintained and switched on and off remains an unexplored question. The mother rat's ingestion of pup urine during licking of pups is another component of maternal behavior that offers a potential intersection with a physiological regulatory mechanism (see Friedman, Bruno, & Alberts, 1981). Further study of the medial preoptic area offers both an opportunity to investigate how a small brain region coordinates diverse functions and possible insight into relationships, in terms of both current adaptations and evolutionary origins, among motivated behaviors.

References

Allin, J. T., & Banks, E. M. Effect of temperature on ultrasound production by infant albino rats. *Developmental Psychobiology*, 1971, *4*, 149-156.

Amenomori, Y., Chen, C. L., & Meites, J. Serum prolactin levels in rats during different reproductive states. *Endocrinology*, 1970, *86*, 506-510.

Avar, Z., & Monos, E. Effect of lateral hypothalamic lesion on maternal behavior and foetal vitality in the rat. *Acta Medica Academiae Scientiarum Hungaricae*, 1967, *23*, 255-261.

Avar, Z., & Monos, E. Biological role of lateral hypothalamic structures participating in the control of maternal behavior in the rat. *Acta Physiologica Academiae Scientiarum Hungaricae*, 1969, *35*, 285-294.

Beach, F. A. The neural basis of innate behavior, I: Effects of cortical lesions upon the maternal behavior pattern in the rat. *Journal of Comparative Psychology*, 1937, *24*, 393-436.

Beach, F. A. The neural basis of innate behavior, II: Relative effects of partial decortication in adulthood and infancy upon the maternal behavior of the primiparous rat. *Journal of General Psychology*, 1938, *53*, 109-148.

Beach, F. A., & Jaynes, J. Studies on maternal retrieving in rats, I: Recognition of young. *Journal of Mammology*, 1956, *37*, 177-180. (a)

Beach, F. A., & Jaynes, J. Studies of maternal retrieving in rats, III: Sensory cues involved in the lactating female's response to her young. *Behaviour*, 1956, *10*, 104-125. (b)

Beach, F. A., & Wilson, J. Effects of prolactin, progesterone, and estrogen on reactions of non-pregnant rats to foster young. *Psychological Reports*, 1963, *13*, 231-239.

Benuck, I., & Rowe, F. A. Centrally and peripherally induced anosmia: Influences on maternal behavior in lactating female rats. *Physiology and Behavior*, 1975, *14*, 439-447.

Bridges, R. S. Long-term effects of pregnancy and parturition upon maternal responsiveness in the rat. *Physiology and Behavior*, 1975, *14*, 245-249.

Bridges, R. S., Rosenblatt, J. S., & Feder, H. H. Serum progesterone concentrations and maternal behavior in rats after pregnancy termination: Behavioral stimulation following progesterone withdrawal and inhibition by progesterone maintenance. *Endocrinology*, 1978, *102*, 258-267. (a)

Bridges, R. R., Rosenblatt, J. S., & Feder, H. H. Stimulation of maternal responsiveness after pregnancy termination in rats: Effect of time of onset of behavioral testing. *Hormones and Behavior*, 1978, *10*, 235-245. (b)

Bridges, R. S., Zarrow, M. X., Gandelman, R., & Denenberg, V. H. Differences in maternal responsiveness between lactating and sensitized rats. *Developmental Psychobiology*, 1972, *5*, 123-127.

Bulmer, D., & Peel, S. The effects on the rat uterus and placenta of ovariectomy at day 10 of pregnancy. *Journal of Anatomy*, 1979, *128*, 185-194.

Cain, D. P. The role of the olfactory bulb in limbic mechanisms. *Psychological Bulletin*, 1974, *81*, 654-671.

Catala, S., & Deis, R. P. Effect of oestrogen upon parturition, maternal behavior, and lactation in ovariectomized pregnant rats. *Journal of Endocrinology*, 1973, *56*, 219-225.

Chen, C. L., & Meites, J. Effects of estrogen and progesterone on serum and pituitary prolactin levels in ovariectomized rats. *Endocrinology*, 1970, *86*, 503-505.

Clemens, J. A., Smalstig, E. B., & Sawyer, B. D. Studies on the role of the preoptic area in the control of reproductive function in the rat. *Endocrinology*, 1976, *99*, 728-735.

Conrad, L. C. A., & Pfaff, D. W. Autoradiographic study of efferents from the medial basal forebrain and hypothalamus in the rat, I: Medial preoptic area. *Journal of Comparative Neurology*, 1976, *169*, 185-220.

Elwood, R. W. Paternal and maternal behavior of the Mongolian gerbil. *Animal Behaviour*, 1975, *23*, 766-772.

Erskine, M. S., Barfield, R. J., & Goldman, B. D. Intraspecific fighting during late pregnancy and lactation in rats and effects of litter removal. *Behavioral Biology*, 1978, *23*, 206-213.

Erskine, M. S., Barfield, R. J., & Goldman, B. D. Postpartum aggression in rats, I: Effects of hypophysectomy. *Journal of Comparative and Physiological Psychology*, 1980, *94*, 484-494. (a)

Erskine, M. S., Barfield, R. J., & Goldman, B. D. Postpartum aggression in rats, II: Dependence on maternal sensitivity to young and effects of experience with pregnancy and parturition. *Journal of Comparative and Physiological Psychology*, 1980, *94*, 495-505. (b)

Fleischer, S., & Slotnick, B. M. Disruption of maternal behavior in rats with lesions of the septal area. *Physiology and Behavior*, 1978, *21*, 189-200.

Fleming, A. S., & Rosenblatt, J. S. Maternal behavior in the virgin and lactating rat. *Journal of Comparative and Physiological Psychology*, 1974, *86*, 957-972. (a)

Fleming, A. S., & Rosenblatt, J. S. Olfactory regulation of maternal behavior in rats, I: Effects of olfactory bulb removal in experienced and inexperienced lactating and cycling females. *Journal of Comparative and Physiological Psychology*, 1974, *86*, 221-232. (b)

Fleming, A. S., & Rosenblatt, J. S. Olfactory regulation of maternal behavior in rats, II: Effects of peripherally induced anosmia and lesions of the lateral olfactory tract in pup-induced virgins. *Journal of Comparative and Physiological Psychology*, 1974, *86*, 233-246. (c)

Fleming, A. S., Vaccarino, F., & Luebke, C. Amygdaloid inhibition of maternal behavior in the nulliparous female rat. *Physiology and Behavior*, 1980, *25*, 731-743.

Fleming, A., Vaccarino, F., Tambosso, L., & Chee, P. Vomeronasal and olfactory system modulation of maternal behavior in the rat. *Science*, 1979, *203*, 372-374.

Friedman, M. I., Bruno, J. P., & Alberts, J. R. Physiological and behavioral consequences in rats of water recycling during lactation. *Journal of Comparative and Physiological Psychology*, 1981, *95*, 26-35.

Gaffori, O., & Le Moal, M. Disruption of maternal behavior and appearance of cannibalism after ventral mesencephalic tegmentum lesions. *Physiology and Behavior*, 1979, *23*, 317-323.

Gilbert, A. N., Pelchat, R. J., & Adler, N. T. Postpartum copulatory and maternal behavior in Norway rats under seminatural conditions. *Animal Behaviour*, 1980, *28*, 989-995.

Grosvenor, C. E., Marweg, H., & Mena, F. A study of factors involved in the development of the exteroceptive release of prolactin in the lactating rat. *Hormones and Behavior*, 1970, *1*, 111-120.

Hammel, H. T. Regulation of internal body temperature. *Annual Review of Physiology*, 1968, *30*, 641-710.

Hardy, D. F. Behavior of the female rat during pregnancy, pseudopregnancy, lactation, and following ovariectomy. *Hormones and Behavior*, 1970, *1*, 235-245.

Herrenkohl, R. L., & Rosenberg, P. A. Exteroceptive stimulation of maternal behavior in the naive rat. *Physiology and Behavior*, 1972, *8*, 595-598.

Kinder, E. F. A study of the nest-building activity of the albino rat. *Journal of Experimental Zoology*, 1927, *47*, 117-161.

Klopfer, P. H., McGeorge, L., & Barnett, R. J. *Maternal care in mammals* (Addison-Wesley Module in Biology No. 4). Reading, Mass.: Addison-Wesley, 1973.

Krehbiel, D. A., & Le Roy, L. M. The quality of hormonally stimulated maternal behavior in ovariectomized rats. *Hormones and Behavior*, 1979, *12*, 243-252.

Kristal, M. B. Placentophagia: A biobehavioral enigma (or *De gustibus non disputandum est*). *Neuroscience and Biobehavioral Reviews*, 1980, *4*, 141-150.

Le Blond, C. P. Nervous and hormonal factors in the maternal behavior of the mouse. *Journal of Genetic Psychology*, 1940, *57*, 327-344.

Le Blond, C. P., & Nelson, W. O. Parental instinct in the mouse, especially after hypophysectomy. *Anatomical Record*, 1936, *64*, 29-30.

Le Blond, C. P., & Nelson, W. O. Maternal behavior in hypophysectomized male and female mice. *American Journal of Physiology*, 1937, *120*, 167-172.

Lehrman, D. S. On the organization of maternal behavior and the problem of instinct. In P. P. Grasse (Ed.), *L'Instinct dans le comportement des animaux et de l'homme*. Paris: Masson, 1956, pp. 475-520.

Lehrman, D. S. Hormonal regulation of parental behavior in birds and infrahuman mammals. In W. C. Young (Ed.), *Sex and internal secretions.* Baltimore: Williams & Wilkins, 1961, pp. 1268-1382.

Leon, M. Maternal pheromone. *Physiology and Behavior,* 1974, *13,* 441-453.

Leon, M., Croskerry, P. G., & Smith, G. K. Thermal control of mother-young contact in rats. *Physiology and Behavior,* 1978, *21,* 793-811.

Lott, D. F., & Rosenblatt, J. Development of maternal responsiveness during pregnancy in the rat. In M. B. Foss (Ed.), *Determinants of infant behavior* (Vol. 4). London: Methuen, 1969.

Malsbury, C., & Pfaff, D. W. Neural and hormonal determinants of mating behavior in adult male rats: A review. In L. Di Cara (Ed.), *Limbic and autonomic nervous systems research.* New York: Plenum Press, 1974, pp. 85-136.

Marinari, K. T., & Moltz, H. Serum prolactin levels and vaginal cyclicity in concaveated and lactating female rats. *Physiology and Behavior,* 1978, *21,* 524-528.

Mayer, A. D., & Rosenblatt, J. S. Olfactory basis for the delayed onset of maternal behavior in virgin female rats: Experiential effects. *Journal of Comparative and Physiological Psychology,* 1975, *89,* 701-710.

Mayer, A. D., & Rosenblatt, J. S. Hormonal interaction with stimulus and situational factors in the initiation of maternal behavior in nonpregnant rats. *Journal of Comparative and Physiological Psychology,* 1980, *94,* 1040-1059.

Moltz, H., Geller, D., & Levin, R. Maternal behavior in the totally mammectomized rat. *Journal of Comparative and Physiological Psychology,* 1967, *64,* 225.

Moltz, H., & Lee, T. M. The maternal pheromone of the rat: Identity and functional significance. *Physiology and Behavior,* 1981, *26,* 301-306.

Moltz, H., Levin, R., & Leon, M. Differential effects of progesterone on the maternal behavior of primiparous and multiparous rats. *Journal of Comparative and Physiological Psychology,* 1969, *67,* 36-40.

Moltz, H., Lubin, M., Leon, M., & Numan, M. Hormonal induction of maternal behavior in the ovariectomized nulliparous rat. *Physiology and Behavior,* 1970, *5,* 1373-1377.

Moltz, H., Robbins, D., & Parks, M. Caesarean delivery and maternal behavior of primiparous and multiparous rats. *Journal of Comparative and Physiological Psychology,* 1966, *61,* 455-460.

Moltz, H., & Wiener, E. Effects of ovariectomy on maternal behavior of primiparous and multiparous rats. *Journal of Comparative and Physiological Psychology,* 1966, *62,* 382-387.

Morishige, W. K., Pepe, G. J., & Rothchild, I. Serum luteinizing hormone, prolactin, and progesterone levels during pregnancy in the rat. *Endocrinology,* 1973, *92,* 1527-1530.

Nissen, H. W. A study of maternal behavior in the white rat by means of the obstruction method. *Journal of Genetic Psychology,* 1930, *37,* 377-393.

Numan, M. Medial preoptic area and maternal behavior in the female rat. *Journal of Comparative and Physiological Psychology,* 1974, *87,* 746-759.

Numan, M. Progesterone inhibition of maternal behavior in the rat. *Hormones and Behavior,* 1978, *11,* 209-231.

Numan, M. Brain mechanisms and parental behavior. In R. Goy & D. Pfaff (Eds.), *Neurobiology of reproduction.* In press.

Numan, M., & Callahan, E. C. The connections of the medial preoptic region and maternal behavior in the rat. *Physiology and Behavior,* 1980, *25,* 653-665.

Numan, M., Leon, M., & Moltz, H. Interference with prolactin release and the maternal behavior of female rats. *Hormones and Behavior*, 1972, *3*, 29-38.

Numan, M., Rosenblatt, J. S., & Komisaruk, B. R. Medial preoptic area and onset of maternal behavior in the rat. *Journal of Comparative and Physiological Psychology*, 1977, *91*, 146-164.

Obias, M. D. Maternal behavior of hypophysectomized gravid albino rats and the development and performance of their young. *Journal of Comparative and Physiological Psychology*, 1957, *50*, 120-124.

Oley, N. N., & Slotnick, B. M. Nesting material as a reinforcement for operant behavior in the rat. *Psychonomic Science*, 1970, *21*, 41.

Pedersen, C. A. Induction of maternal behavior by posterior pituitary hormones. *Eastern Conference on Reproductive Behavior*, June 22-25, 1980. The Rockefeller University, New York, p. 21 (Abstract).

Pfaff, D. W., & Keiner, M. Atlas of estradiol-concentrating cells in the central nervous system of the female rat. *Journal of Comparative Neurology*, 1973, *151*, 121-158.

Reisbick, S., Rosenblatt, J. S., & Mayer, A. D. Decline of maternal behavior in the virgin and lactating rat. *Journal of Comparative and Physiological Psychology*, 1975, *89*, 722-732.

Riddle, O. Aspects and implications of the hormonal control of the maternal instinct. *Proceedings of the American Philosophical Society*, 1935, *75*, 521-525.

Riddle, O., Lahr, E. L., & Bates, R. W. Maternal behavior induced in virgin rats by prolactin. *Proceedings of the Society for Experimental Biology and Medicine*, 1935, *32*, 730-734.

Rodriguez-Sierra, J. F., & Rosenblatt, J. S. Does prolactin have a role in estrogen-induced maternal behavior in rats: Apomorphine reduction of prolactin release. *Hormones and Behavior*, 1977, *9*, 1-7.

Rosenblatt, J. S. The basis of synchrony in the behavioral interaction between the mother and her offspring in the laboratory rat. In B. H. Foss (Ed.), *Determinants of infant behaviour* (Vol. 3). London: Methuen, 1965, pp. 3-45.

Rosenblatt, J. S. Selective retrieving by maternal and non-maternal female rat. *Journal of Comparative and Physiological Psychology*, 1975, *88*, 678-686.

Rosenblatt, J. S., & Siegel, H. I. Hysterectomy-induced maternal behavior during pregnancy in the rat. *Journal of Comparative and Physiological Psychology*, 1975, *89*, 685-700.

Rosenblatt, J. S., Siegel, H. I., & Mayer, A. D. Progress in the study of maternal behavior in the rat: Hormonal, nonhormonal, sensory, and developmental aspects. In J. S. Rosenblatt, R. A. Hinde, E. Shaw, & C. Beer (Eds.), *Advances in the study of behavior* (Vol. 10). New York: Academic Press, 1979, pp. 225-311.

Scalia, F., & Winams, S. S. The differential projections of the olfactory bulb in mammals. *Journal of Comparative Neurology*, 1975, *161*, 31-56.

Shaikh, A. A. Estrone and estradiol levels in the ovarian venous blood from rats during the estrous cycle and pregnancy. *Biology of Reproduction*, 1971, *5*, 297-307.

Siegel, H. I., Andieh, H. B., & Rosenblatt, J. S. Hysterectomy-induced facilitation of lordosis behavior in the rat. *Hormones and Behavior*, 1978, *11*, 273-278.

Siegel, H. I., Doerr, H. K., & Rosenblatt, J. S. Further studies on estrogen-induced maternal behavior in hysterectomized-ovariectomized virgin rats. *Physiology and Behavior*, 1978, *21*, 99-103.

Siegel, H. I., & Rosenblatt, J. S. Estrogen-induced maternal behavior in hysterectomized-ovariectomized virgin rats. *Physiology and Behavior*, 1975, *14*, 465-471. (a)

Siegel, H. I., & Rosenblatt, J. S. Progesterone inhibition of estrogen-induced maternal behavior in hysterectomized-ovariectomized virgin rats. *Hormones and Behavior*, 1975, *6*, 223-230. (b)

Siegel, H. I., & Rosenblatt, J. S. Hormonal basis of hysterectomy-induced maternal behavior during pregnancy in the rat. *Hormones and Behavior*, 1975, *6*, 211-222. (c)

Siegel, H. I., & Rosenblatt, J. S. Duration of estrogen stimulation and progesterone inhibition of maternal behavior in pregnancy-terminated rats. *Hormones and Behavior*, 1978, *11*, 12-19.

Singh, P. J., & Hofer, M. A. Oxytocin reinstates maternal olfactory cues for nipple orientation and attachment in rat pups. *Physiology and Behavior*, 1978, *20*, 385-389.

Slotnick, B. M. Intercorrelations of maternal activities in the rat. *Animal Behaviour*, 1967, *15*, 267-269.

Slotnick, B. M. Neural and hormonal basis of maternal behavior in the rat. In B. E. Eleftheriou & R. L. Sprott (Eds.), *Hormonal correlates of behavior*. New York: Plenum Press, 1975.

Slotnick, B. M., Carpenter, M. L., & Fusco, R. Initiation of maternal behavior in pregnant nulliparous rats. *Hormones and Behavior*, 1973, *4*, 53-59.

Small, W. S. Notes on the psychic development of the young white rat. *American Journal of Psychology*, 1899, *11*, 80-100.

Stern, J. M., & MacKinnon, D. S. Sensory regulation of maternal behavior in rats: Effects of pup age. *Developmental Psychobiology*, 1978, *11*, 579-586.

Sturman-Hulbe, M., & Stone, C. P. Maternal behavior in the albino rat. *Journal of Comparative Psychology*, 1929, *9*, 203-237.

Swanson, L. W. Immunohistochemical evidence for a neurophysin-containing autonomic pathway arising in the paraventricular nucleus of the hypothalamus. *Brain Research*, 1977, *128*, 346-353.

Terkel, J., & Rosenblatt, J. S. Aspects of nonhormonal maternal behavior in the rat. *Hormones and Behavior*, 1971, *2*, 161-171.

Terkel, J., & Rosenblatt, J. S. Humoral factors underlying maternal behavior at parturition: Cross transfusion between freely moving rats. *Journal of Comparative and Physiological Psychology*, 1972, *80*, 365-371.

Thoman, E. B., & Levine, S. Effects of adrenalectomy on maternal behavior in rats. *Developmental Psychobiology*, 1970, *3*, 237-244.

Thoman, E. B., Wetzel, A., & Levine, S. Lactation prevents disruption of temperature regulation and suppresses adrenocortical activity in rats. *Communications in Behavioral Biology*, 1968, *2*, 165-171.

Turner, C. D., & Bagnara, J. T. *General endocrinology* (6th ed.). Philadelphia: W. B. Saunders, 1976.

Van Zoeren, J. G., & Stricker, E. M. Effects of preoptic, lateral hypothalamic, or dopamine-depleting lesions on behavioral thermoregulation in rats exposed to the cold. *Journal of Comparative and Physiological Psychology*, 1977, *91*, 989-999.

Wiesner, B. P., & Sheard, N. M. *Maternal behavior in the rat*. Edinburgh: Oliver & Boyd, 1933.

Wilson, N. E., & Stricker, E. M. Thermal homeostasis in pregnant rats during heat stress. *Journal of Comparative and Physiological Psychology*, 1979, *93*, 585-594.

Woodside, B., Pelchat, R., & Leon, M. Acute elevation of the heat load of mother rats curtails maternal nest bouts. *Journal of Comparative and Physiological Psychology*, 1980, *94*, 61-68.

Zarrow, M. X., Gandelman, R., & Denenberg, V. H. Prolactin: Is it an essential hormone for maternal behavior in the mammal? *Hormones and Behavior*, 1971, *2*, 343-354.

Chapter 10

Neurobiological Mechanisms of Sexual Motivation

DONALD W. PFAFF

The Female

Lordosis Behavior in Female Rats

Lordosis Is a Motivated Behavior. From the reasoning that leads to the identification of "motivation" as an intervening variable, recounted in the first chapter of this book, it is clear that the occurrence of lordosis behavior reflects a motivational state. Ovariectomized female rats not given estrogen or progesterone treatment, though given large numbers of applications of behaviorally adequate somatosensory input through mounts by stud male rats or pressure on the skin by an experimenter, rarely do lordosis. A few days later (before maturational changes could occur), following a schedule of estrogen and progesterone treatment, the same females tested in the same behavioral context respond to the somatosensory stimuli with strong and frequent lordoses. Identifying the intervening variable "sexual motivation" contributes to the explanation of this behavioral change in an input–output manner.

Lordosis Circuitry and Mechanisms. In the female rat brain, neurons that bind estrogen can be found in the ventromedial nucleus of the hypothalamus, as well as in the anterior hypothalamus and medial preoptic area (Figure 10-1) (Pfaff & Keiner, 1973). Placement of local

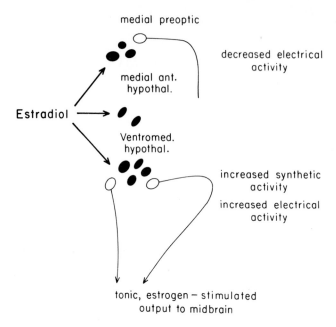

Figure 10-1. Estrogen increases biosynthetic and electrical activity among neurons in the ventromedial hypothalamus. The resulting increase in a tonic facilitating output to the midbrain central grey allows a heightened state of sexual motivation in the female rat and the occurrence of lordosis behavior. (From Pfaff, 1980.)

implants of estrogen in and near the ventromedial nucleus of the hypothalamus can facilitate lordosis in ovariectomized females (for a review see Pfaff, 1980). Electrical stimulation of this neuronal group at low frequencies leads to lordosis facilitation. In contrast, destructive lesions of these cells lead to a loss of lordosis. As a consequence of estrogen action, slowly firing neurons in the basomedial hypothalamus are activated, and electron microscopic evidence suggests increased synthetic activity (Cohen & Pfaff, 1981; for a review see Pfaff, 1980). All of these data are consistent with the theory that estrogen facilitates lordosis by increasing neuronal synthetic and electrical activity as a consequence of being bound by neurons in the ventromedial nucleus of the hypothalamus. The temporal characteristics of estrogen require that they act on lordosis behavior via a tonic output to the midbrain (Figure 10-1).

Effects of hypothalamic neurons on behavior are not necessarily separate from their effects on autonomic physiology. For example (Pfaff, 1980, pp. 118 and following; also see "Mating Behavior: Mechanisms" in the section on the male that follows), some effects of preoptic neurons on male mating behavior in rats may be secondary to their effects on the parasympathetic nervous system. Neurons from the basal forebrain and preoptic area important for male reproductive behavior and/or parasympathetic function descend to the midbrain via the medial forebrain bundle. Axons from the basomedial hypothalamus important for female reproductive behavior do not descend through the medial forebrain bundle; some follow a periventricular route while others loop laterally as they descend, eventually curving medially and dorsally to arrive at a position in and near the central grey of the midbrain (Krieger, Conrad, & Pfaff, 1979). Anatomically, therefore, the systems of masculine-typical behavior and parasympathetic function seem quite separate from those for female reproductive behavior and sympathetic function (see Figure 10-2). In turn, the overlap between the systems for female mating behavior and the sympathetic nervous system may not be coincidental. For example (see the subsection on "Systems Interpretations"), heightened sympathetic autonomic tone may be required for the muscular activity involved in precopulatory "courtship behaviors" in female rodents and for the axial muscular tenseness that facilitates lordosis.

Our current view of the entire circuit upon which hypothalamic influences play for the control of lordosis behavior has been documented at length (Pfaff, 1980). Briefly, cutaneous stimulus bilaterally on the flanks of the female followed by pressure against the posterior rump and perineal skin are necessary and sufficient for lordosis. Among the

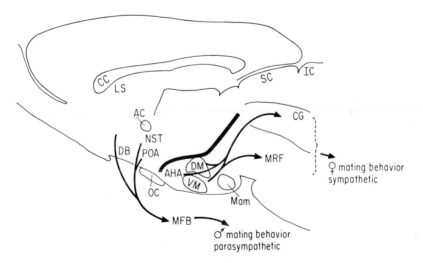

Figure 10-2. Neurons in the medial preoptic area (POA), with axons descending through the medial portion of the medial forebrain bundle (MFB) facilitate parasympathetic autonomic mechanisms and masculine mating behavior. Nerve cells with axons in the ventromedial hypothalamus (VM) have axons descending to the midbrain central grey (CG) which do not descend in the medial forebrain bundle. These ventromedial region neurons facilitate female mating behavior and sympathetic autonomic mechanisms. (From Pfaff, 1980.)

action potentials carried over dorsal root L_6 are those representing the activity of pressure receptors whose stimulus requirements closely fit those for lordosis behavior as a whole. They synapse in deep layers of the dorsal horn and intermediate grey in the lumbar spinal cord. Since female rats with this spinal tissue isolated from the brain have not been shown to perform normal lordosis behavior, supraspinal facilitation must be required. Ascending fibers carry information that could be relevant for lordosis behavior, terminating in the medullary reticular formation, dorsal caudal part of the lateral vestibular nucleus, and dorsal midbrain. Our current view, however, is that the major physiological impact of the sensory input from the required skin areas is at segmental levels. The main importance of supraspinal facilitation appears to be to translate and transmit hormone-dependent hypothalamic output such that midbrain (subcortical) "decision centers" are influenced and hindbrain postural control systems set so that lordosis-relevant motor neurons can be facilitated.

We know that midbrain neurons in and just lateral to the central grey receive output from the ventromedial hypothalamus over axon trajectories following periventricular routes and laterally running loops. Estrogen influences and ventromedial hypothalamic stimulation raise the excitability of neurons in the midbrain central grey that in turn project to the medullary reticulospinal region (Sakuma & Pfaff, 1979a, b). The two descending systems required for facilitation of spinal lordosis mechanisms are the lateral vestibulospinal tract and the medullary reticulospinal tract. Traveling back down to lumbar levels, these axons have the net effect of facilitating motor neurons, in the ventromedial and medial sides of the ventral horn, for the epaxial muscles lateral longissimus and transversospinalis. These two deep back muscle systems execute the vertebral dorsiflexion of lordosis (Figure 10-3).

Motivational Circuitry and Mechanisms. Since lordosis behavior has the logical status of a motivated response and since estrogen treatment is the crucial component operationally for the appearance of this behavior in ovariectomized female rats, the cellular mechanisms of estrogen action on lordosis behavior circuitry are in fact mechanisms of a motivational influence. Thus, reorganizing slightly the summary of the description of lordosis circuitry given above (and summarized previously by Pfaff, 1980), one can characterize the main physiological description of this motivational effect of estrogen as follows. Estrogen circulating in the blood is accumulated by nerve cells in and around the ventrolateral portion of the ventromedial nucleus of the hypothalamus. Receptors in the cytoplasm and then in the nucleus of these nerve cells concentrate the hormone. As a result, estrogen increases the biosynthetic capacity and electrical excitability of these nerve cells. Through

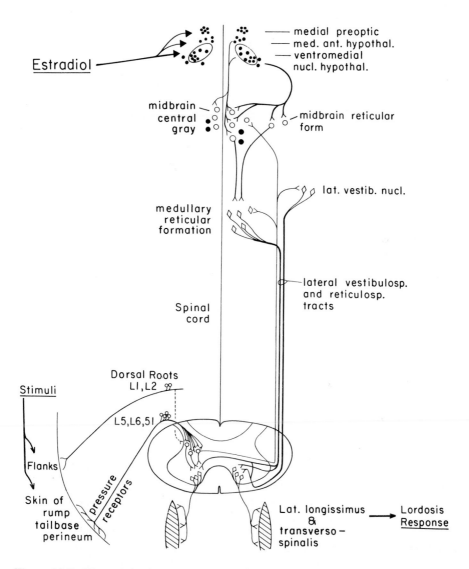

Figure 10-3. The minimal neural circuitry for lordosis behavior in the female rat, and estrogen effects upon it. In this behavior, stimuli, responses, circuitry, and hormone effects are all bilateral, and are shown here on just one side for convenience of presentation. (From Pfaff, 1980.)

their connections to the mesencephalon, these neurons prepare brainstem circuitry for lordosis to occur, given adequate somatosensory input.

Systems Interpretations of Manners in Which the Neural Circuitry Described Has Its Motivational Effects

Effects on behavioral responsivity to somatosensory input. Rats and other rodents are prey. In such animals, for which contact from other animals might signal immediate danger, the predominant behavioral reflex in a female not hormonally prepared for reproduction would be an avoidance response. Such somatosensory input can easily be understood to be "aversive." Similarly, with respect to population control limited by crowding in a species that can reproduce quickly and lives in burrows, somatosensory input from conspecifics might lead to behavioral responses denoting aversion even in otherwise safe circumstances.

In fact, the behavioral reactions of sexually unreceptive female rats that have not been handled frequently to somatosensory contact include escape, aggression, vocalization, and so forth. Similarly, unreceptive female hamsters show fierce aggression toward the male following even light cutaneous input (Floody & Pfaff, 1974, 1977a, 1977b; Floody, Pfaff, & Lewis, 1977).

When sexually receptive female rats control the timing of the somatosensory contact that the male rat will be allowed, regularities in their behavior show up as a function of the nature of the immediately foregoing response by the male (see references in subsection "Limitations on Approach Responses"). One point to note is that in those experiments and in recent work by Dr. Donna Emery at the State University of New York at Buffalo, female rats performed arbitrary responses either to approach the male or to allow the male to approach them, following which sexual contact will occur. This in itself is evidence for sexual motivation connected with lordosis behavior. In addition, however, Dr. Emery (Emery, 1981a) has used this kind of behavioral situation in a way that sheds light on the manner in which ventromedial hypothalamic output comprises part of a motivational mechanism.

Hypothalamic lesions destroying the ventromedial nucleus bilaterally can lead to failures of lordosis behavior, even with adequate estrogen and progesterone levels, in female rats (Mathews & Edwards, 1977; Pfaff & Sakuma, 1979; see Pfaff, 1980, for a review) and female hamsters (Malsbury, Kow, & Pfaff, 1977). When such females are subjected to cutaneous input by aggressive males or experimenters, with the females trapped in small arenas and the timing of somatosensory input not controlled by them, their responses are aversive, avoiding, violent, and "irritable," and may include attacking the male or the experimenter (Hetherington & Ranson, 1940; Mathews & Edwards, 1977; for hamsters, Malsbury et al., 1977). In dramatic contrast to those behavioral testing situations, Emery (Emery, 1981a) studied the effects of small ventromedial hypothalamic lesions in circumstances where test female rats could escape and reenter arenas containing stud males at times of their choosing. In these circumstances, small bilateral lesions allowed lordosis quotients to remain in the same range as those for unoperated controls and sham-lesioned animals. However, the hypothalamically lesioned females spent significantly more time in locations where the stud males could not contact them, and this resulted in the lesioned females allowing a significantly smaller number of copulatory attempts by the males. Thus, females with small ventromedial hypothalamic lesions behaved as though somatosensory input from the males was more aversive than is true for unoperated animals.

This interpretation received support from experiments on the central grey of the midbrain. It must be at least partly through their contact with central grey neurons that ventromedial hypothalamic axons have their effects on lordosis behavior (Sakuma & Pfaff, 1979a, 1979b; see Pfaff, 1980, for a review). In estrogen–progesterone-primed female rats with bilateral lesions on the central grey, responses to somatosensory input of the sort that can elicit lordosis manifest avoidance and aversion. For example, when manual cutaneous stimulation is applied five times by an experimenter, the central grey-lesioned animal's response to the first application may be as strong a lordosis as in unperated controls. On subsequent applications, however, such females may avoid contact vigorously as though the cutaneous input were aversive (Conrad & Pfaff, 1975, unpublished observations; Kow & Pfaff, 1980, unpublished observations). Here, as with ventromedial nucleus-lesioned animals, there are circumstances where it is clearly possible for the female to perform lordosis behavior, but the predominant responses show that the somatosensory input apparently is noxious.

In fact, a fair number of experimental manipulations that reduce noxious aspects of otherwise painful stimulation can improve lordosis behavior performance, and vice versa (Table 10-1). These are manipulations such as vaginal probing and electrical stimulation of the midbrain central grey (stimulation-produced analgesia), that reduce pain without anesthesia. In contrast, painful somatosensory input prevents or disrupts lordosis behavior in female rats and hamsters. Moreover, those manipulations which increase aversive responses to somatosensory input are correlated with reduced lordosis behavior (ventromedial hypothalamic lesions, central grey lesions). Obviously on a patch of skin, receptors specialized for nociception and the reception of cutaneous pressure that drives lordosis may both be found. Pain and lordosis sensory systems then share mixed cutaneous nerves heading toward the spinal cord, and both in peripheral sensory axons and in the spinal cord they may be distinct from each other for certain neurons only by spatiotemporal codes. The control over spinal reflexes to these two

Table 10-1. Opposite Effects of Manipulations on Lordosis Behavior and
Responses to Pain

Experiment	Effect on lordosis behavior	Effect on response to pain	Reference
Cutaneous pinch	↓	↑	
Vaginal probe	↑	↓	Komisaruk et al., 1976; Komisaruk, 1974
Ventromedial hypothalamic lesions			
female rats	↓	↑ ("irritability")	Mathews & Edwards, 1977; Hetherington & Ranson, 1943
female hamsters	↓	↑ (aggression)	Malsbury et al., 1977
Midbrain central grey			
lesions	↓	↑	Sakuma & Pfaff, 1979b
stimulation	↑	↓	Sakuma & Pfaff, 1979a; Mayer & Liebeskind, 1974; Geisler & Liebeskind, 1976
Septal lesions	normal, then ↑	↑, then normal	Nance et al., 1974, 1975; McGinnis et al., 1978; Nance et al., 1977

types of somatosensory input may share certain features when some
brain-stem sites are considered. Despite these various types of overlap,
however, it is clear that the coding for lordosis-relevant input must be
different from that for pain, that painful input interferes with reproductively relevant behavioral responses to lighter cutaneous input, and that
nerve cells in the ventromedial hypothalamus and midbrain central grey
can increase responses to one while decreasing responses to the other.

Thus, we hypothesize that one aspect of estrogen-influenced action
of ventromedial hypothalamic neurons is that these neurons cause somatosensory inputs that would otherwise have been treated as noxious
to be much less aversive. Thus, ventromedial neurons would militate
against competing responses (limb flexions, bilaterally asymmetric
trunk movements—Pfaff & Lewis, 1974; and other responses) that
would prevent the lordosis reflex from appearing. The effects of ventromedial hypothalamic output, translated through the central grey and
other dorsal midbrain neurons, must be registered on posture control

systems in the lower brain stem, including the medullary reticular formation.

During the estrous cycle of the female rodent and under experimental endocrinological conditions, progesterone magnifies the action of estrogen in facilitating reproductive behavior. With respect to the partial interpretation of estrogen-influenced hypothalamic output above, what might be the role of progesterone effects?

In a theory of progesterone facilitation of female reproductive behavior (Kow, Malsbury, & Pfaff, 1974), we hypothesized that progesterone inhibits activity in a midbrain–limbic loop that includes serotonergic fibers and that inhibits lordosis. Thus, progesterone action would facilitate lordosis behavior by disinhibition. Briefly, neuroanatomical and neurochemical data leading to the theory were as follows (see Kow et al., 1974, for references). Projections from midbrain raphe nuclei through serotonergic fibers in the medial forebrain bundle or through fibers in the fasciculus retroflexus–stria medullaris system reach the septum. Projections from the septum through the medial forebrain bundle or through the stria medullaris–fasciculus retroflexus route reach the midbrain raphe nuclei. A continued excitatory state of neurons in this loop clearly inhibits responses to somatosensory input, and we hypothesized that this included inhibiting lordosis responses to cutaneous input. Conversely, interruption of function in the loop by tissue destruction or neuropharmacological intervention facilitates responses to somatosensory input, including the facilitation of lordosis. Thus, if progesterone were to decrease the activity of neurons in this loop, it should facilitate lordosis.

At one level of discourse, this theory of progesterone action articulates with our approach to one aspect of estrogen action (stated above) in a traditional manner. Medial hypothalamic output, from the ventromedial nucleus, facilitates lordosis, while a system including fibers in the medial forebrain bundle opposes it. The theme of medial hypothalamic mechanisms "opposing" medial forebrain bundle mechanisms has been treated frequently, most prominently in the case of the control of feeding behavior.

Is there a problem, however, with the concepts of ventromedial hypothalamic output rendering somatosensory stimuli less aversive (decreasing the magnitude of certain avoidance responses) while a midbrain–limbic loop's decreased activity is supposed to make the animal more responsive, and both of these changes are supposed to facilitate the same reproductive behavior? If the various trains of experimental results leading to these two concepts (one for estrogen action, the other for progesterone) are all correct and if the reasoning is right, putting the two hypotheses side by side yields the following formulation. For maximal reproductive behavior, that is, following combined treatment with estrogen and progesterone, the female rat will not treat somatosensory input as noxious and in that sense will be partly analgetic; but she will be also aroused, motorically tense, and responsive to somatosensory input. If these two approaches must be crammed onto a single dimension (and there is no evidence that they must), we would speak of an "optimal level" of arousal, or motoric tenseness, or responsivity to somatosensory input. Another analogy that may be useful but does not seem required is to stress-produced analgesia (see the review by Mayer & Watkins, 1971). In this state, the animal is in fact stressed and can be tense and responsive, but analgetic.

In summary, one interpretation of the hypothalamic role of estrogen action on female reproductive behavior is to render somatosensory input less aversive even though the animal (partly via progesterone facilitation) is highly responsive to somatosensory input. These aspects of forebrain control over sexual motivation not only do not contradict the autonomic-motor interpretation in the subsection "Hypothalamic Effects . . ." below, but may be seen to converge with that interpretation.

Hypothalamic effects on female sexual arousal via autonomic-motor effects. The precopulatory "courtship" behaviors of estrous female rats include hopping and darting forms of locomotion with sudden starts and stops. We have hypothesized (Pfaff, Lewis, Diskow, & Keiner, 1973, p. 277ff.) that these forms of estrogen–progesterone-dependent precopulatory behaviors foster successful copulation by competent conspecifics (both proper mounting by the male and lordosis by the female) in at least three ways. The sudden stops, with the male rat following from the rear, encourage him to contact the female for a successful mount. The sudden stops also leave the female rat in a posture suited for braking a forward and downward force, as she will have to do when the male mounts. Third, the rapid whole-body accelerations are correlated with states of muscular tension in the female that facilitate the lordosis reflex.

The proven dependence of lordosis behavior on lateral vestibulospinal mechanisms gives additional force to this theory of the adaptiveness of female rodent precopulatory behavior. In fact, further thoughts (Pfaff, 1980, pp. 191–193) demonstrate how the exact forms of courtship behaviors of female rats could stimulate vestibulospinal mechanisms and thus set the stage for lordosis behavior.

Emphasizing the roles of the vigorous muscular activities in the locomotor aspects of precopulatory behavior fits well with an approach to hypothalamic output that includes controls of autonomic functions. It was clear (Pfaff, 1980, pp. 118 and following) that the involvement of preoptic neurons both in parasympathetic function and in male copulatory behavior might be causally related—that mechanisms of autonomic nervous system control over penile erection might be the routes by which preoptic manipulations would affect male mating-behavior responses. What about female mating behavior? The medial–posterior hypothalamus has been shown to activate the sympathetic portion of autonomic neural control. Elevating heart rate, blood pressure, and rate and depth of respiration all would provide the autonomic support for the vigorous locomotor activities in courtship behavior and the muscular tenseness that facilitates lordosis. Thus, the neuroanatomic overlap in the preoptic area between parasympathetic function and masculine mating behavior may find its parallel in a neuroanatomic overlap in the medial–posterior hypothalamus between sympathetic mechanisms and female mating behavior (Figure 10-2).

We would predict from this theory that disrupting sympathetic neural outflow would interfere with precopulatory locomotor activities. But if adequate somatosensory stimuli were forced upon the immobile female rat, lordosis could still occur if the animal were adequately estrogen and progesterone primed. In fact, preliminary data from the laboratory of Dr. Donna Emery (1981b) confirm the predictions. She achieved a decrease in sympathethic outflow in female rats by treatment with guanethidine sulfate. Both females in groups treated with this drug and control animals given the saline vehicle were adequately primed with estrogen and progesterone. The precopulatory behavior of the guanethidine-treated animals was deficient: They allowed significantly fewer copulatory acts because they stayed in an escape compartment. When they did allow males to mount, they were apparently less ready to do lordosis, because of a significant decrease in lordosis quotient. Yet, when adequate somatosensory input was forced upon them through manual stimulation by an experimenter, their lordosis performance was as good as the saline-treated controls. These preliminary results fit with the notion that sympathetic outflow would foster precopulatory behavior which fosters lordosis.

Thus, an aspect of output from neurons in and near the ventromedial hypothalamus which might show a mode in which these neurons have their motivational effects is through their autonomic connections: that activation of the sympathetic nervous system prepares the autonomic basis for the vigorous muscular activity of precopulatory behavior and the motor tenseness that facilitates lordosis (and within this chain of events, the precopulatory behavior itself fosters lordosis behavior). This approach is quite consistent with the "sensory" interpretation in the subsection "Effects on Behavioral Responsivity . . ." above, in which it seemed that the optimally prepared female would have to be aroused and responsive to somatosensory input though partly analgetic. For example, one analogy used, to stress-produced analgesia, would in fact involve autonomic reactions to stress and therefore would fit with the autonomic-motor aspect of ventromedial hypothalamic outflow mentioned here.

Summary. Estrogen, through its action on nerve cells in the ventro-lateral portion of the ventromedial nucleus of the hypothalamus, can achieve an increase in sexual motivation in female rats. In doing this it raises the biosynthetic and electrical activity of some neurons in the ventromedial hypothalamus. As a result, these neurons send an elevated output to cells in the midbrain central grey, tonically preparing brain-stem neurons to send facilitating descending signals such that, following adequate somatosensory input, lordosis behavior will occur. Thus, a large part of the neuronal circuitry and mechanisms for a mammalian motivational change have been described.

Descriptions of the behavioral modes in which this physiological motivational mechanism might operate are less clear. It appears that lordosis-relevant output from the ventromedial hypothalamus reduces the aversiveness of somatosensory input. It also appears that medial posterior hypothalamic output could prepare the autonomic basis for the motor tenseness and activity of reproductively important courtship behaviors. Combining these two possibilities, behaviorally speaking, we can theorize that the female rat that is endocrinologically and hypothalamically well prepared to reproduce is aroused and active, but analgetic.

Converging Operations to Demonstrate Motivational State

We hope that an intervening variable such as motivation can be defined in each case not just by one empirical relation but by hypotheses bear-ing on sets of "converging operations" (Miller, 1959, 1967). This ap-proach was elaborated in the first chapter of this book. Therefore, although variations in the occurrence of lordosis behavior have seemed to establish estrogen as a bona fide motivational variable, approach responses by female rats under a variety of experimental situations (and estrogen effects upon them) have helped secure the motivational status of female rodent reproductive behavior.

Limitations on Approach Responses: Natural Pacing of Contacts by the Females. Experimental designs must be planned and results inter-preted knowing that female rats pace sexual contact naturally according to their recent experience. Peirce and Nuttall (1961) experimented to document the impression that periods of resistance by female rats to contacts from males accounted for some aspects of the timing of repro-ductive behavior sequences. They gave estrous female rats free access to sexually active male rats and to compartments without males, in order to find out how the females would pace their contacts with the males. Indeed, all females paced their contacts with male rats according to the nature of the immediate foregoing contact. While females went to the escape compartment after only 37% of mounts without intromission, they left the mating compartment on 95% of the intromissions and following 100% of ejaculations. The amount of time for which they prevented access with the male was also an orderly function of the intensity of the foregoing somatosensory contact with the male: after no contact, only 7 sec; after a simple mount, 27 sec median; after an intromission; 60 sec median, while after an ejaculation females prevented contact with the male for a median 218 sec. Peirce and Nuttall concluded that the sexual motivation of the female rat to approach the male (or to allow approach by him) is conditioned by those times where contact with the male apparently would be aversive.

Similarly, Bermant (1961) showed that estrous female rats performing an operant response to allow entry by the male will time the performance of that response according to the type of previous contact with the male. Delays before performance of that response were shortest following simple mounts, compared, for example, to the delays following intromissions, whose delays in turn were shorter than those following ejaculations.

What is the nature of the somatosensory stimulation that accounts for these delays by the female? Bermant and Westbrook (1966) found that following ejaculations females showed shorter response intervals when the formation of the vaginal plug was prevented than when it was allowed to remain. Similarly, treatment of the vaginal and perineal epithelium with a local anesthetic reduced delays of response for simple mounts, intromissions, and ejaculations. Finally, when contacted by males that could not intromit, females showed short delays of response to readmit males, even throughout long tests. In summary, the absence of vaginal contact, the reduction of it through anesthetic, and the prevention of its maintenance following contact with the male (by prevention of plug deposition) all had the predicted effects: that the female would wait less time before reintroducing the male.

We note that in all of these experiments and in recent work by Emery (1981a) female rats did actually perform arbitrary responses to approach males or admit males in experimental circumstances firmly connected with sexual contacts. This in itself is further verification of sexual motivation in these females, and the natural temporal requirements by the female are superimposed upon this motivational state.

Demonstrations of Approach Responses in Arbitrary Conditions. In the first good study attempting to measure sex drive under objective experimental conditions, Warner (1927) used apparatus in which the test rat had to get from an entrance compartment to an "incentive compartment" by crossing a chamber whose floor was an electrified grid.

Frequency of crossing this grid, from which the test rats would receive
60-cycle electric shocks, was taken as an index of sexual motivation.
Warner measured the number of times female rats would cross the electrified grid when a male rat was in the incentive compartment as a function of the female's estrous condition. Clearly (Figure 10-4) the number
of grid crossings was greatest during the period of the cornified vaginal
smear, reflecting high estrogen levels. Significant relationships between
histological characteristics of the estrogen-dependent smear and grid-
crossing behavior were noted by Warner. For example, during meta-
estrous types of smears, none of the 32 female rats crossed more than
five times, whereas among the cornified smear group, only 3 of 21
crossed as few as five times. As a control, when there was no male in
the incentive compartment, crossings were only about one third of the
frequency seen when there was a male there. In summary, female rats
were willing to cross electrified grids to get to stud male rats. During
the stage of a cornified vaginal smear, frequency of grid crossing was
maximum; that is, approaches to male rats were almost rigidly confined
to the period of estrus. From this, one can infer that high levels of
ovarian hormones increased female rat sex drive.

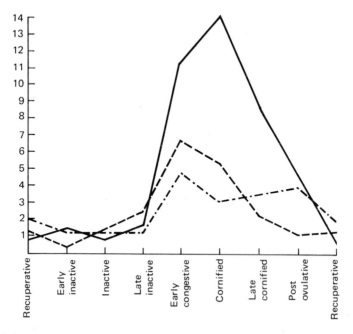

Figure 10-4. The number of times a female rat would cross an electric grid to
achieve contact with a male rat (solid line) was greatest in and about the time that
the vaginal smear was cornified. This histological characteristic of the vaginal smear
reflects high estrogen levels. (From Warner, 1927.)

Nissen's experiments (1929) also used the Columbia Obstruction Apparatus, in which animals had to cross an electrified grid to get to the incentive compartment. Test procedures were generally the same as for previous uses of this apparatus: The test rat was allowed to make four crossings from the entrance to the incentive box with no shock. This established the incentive. On the last preliminary crossing (the fifth) the circuit was closed while the animal was on the grid but after the door leading back to the entrance compartment had been closed so that the test rat was forced to pass from a place where it was being electrically shocked to the incentive compartment. Then the tests began. All tests were 20 minutes and the following behaviors were scored: approach, the animal brings its head into the shock compartment; contact, the test rat steps on the grid but goes back into the entrance compartment; crossings, the rat crosses the grid and reaches the incentive.

From Nissen's results (Figure 10-5) it was clear that ovariectomized uninjected female rats and cycling diestrous females would hardly ever cross the grid to get to the male. In contrast, unoperated cycling females with cornified smears, including those that had had control sham

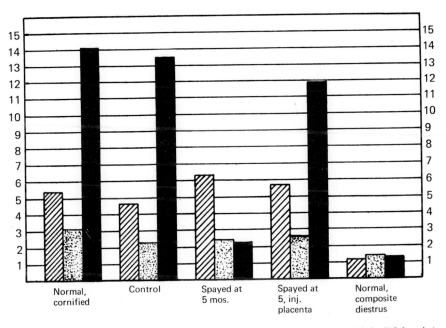

Figure 10-5. The willingness of female rats to cross an electric grid (solid bars) to reach a male was high in normal animals with cornified smears including those given control sham operations. It was low in normal diestrous animals and in ovariectomized females. Following ovariectomy, it was partly restored by injections of placental extract. (From Nissen, 1929.)

operations, crossed the grid significantly more often. Experimental females that had been ovariectomized but then injected with placental extract crossed frequently, like the normal estrous animals. All of these results are consistent with the interpretation that estrogens increase the female's motivation to approach the male.

Jenkins (1928) used the Columbia Obstruction Apparatus to verify the specificity of the requirement for the incentive animal. Female rats crossed the electrified grid for incentive males significantly more frequently than if a receptive female was in the incentive compartment.

Meyerson and Lindstrom (1971, 1973) extended their studies of the effects of ovarian hormones on the brain from analyses of copulatory behavior to analyses of sexual motivation as such. In these experiments, their experimental females were required to seek contact with another animal. Their most important experimental questions dealt with whether ovarian hormones would increase the frequency with which female rats would perform arbitrary responses or cross obstructions in order to reach males.

In Meyerson and Lindstrom's open-field tests, the amounts of time females spent in the vicinities of incentive males or incentive females

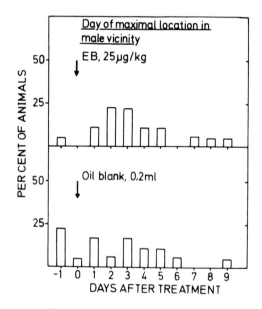

Figure 10-6. In an open-field test, in females given estradiol benzoate (EB) treatment, those days on which the female spent the greatest time in the vicinity of a male followed estrogen treatment with about the same latency that high sexual receptivity scores would. In contrast, in control females given the oil vehicle, there was no synchronization of this behavior measure with the injection. (From Meyerson & Lindstrom, 1973.)

were recorded. They found (Figure 10-6) that estradiol benzoate treatment clearly increased the percentage of observations in which the female was located close to a sexually vigorous male. This effect developed shortly after estradiol benzoate injection (Figure 10-6) and lasted for several days. The magnitude of the effect was a function of estradiol benzoate dose (Figure 10-7).

In another type of experiment, Meyerson and Lindstrom found that estradiol benzoate significantly increased the number of crossings over an electrified grid that ovariectomized females would perform to get to an incentive male (Figure 10-8). The same dose of estrogen did not affect grid crossings to get to an incentive female or to an empty incentive compartment (Figure 10-8). Once again, larger and longer effects were seen with higher doses of estradiol benzoate (Figure 10-9). As a side point, Meyerson and Lindstrom noted that neonatally androgen-treated female rats, who are sexually unresponsive, similarly failed to show an effect of estradiol benzoate on this method of measurement of sexual motivation.

Finally, in runway-choice experiments, Meyerson and Lindstrom found that preference for an intact male over a castrated male by ovariectomized female rats was unaffected by a vehicle control injection. But in ovariectomized females given estradiol benzoate, 2–4 days following injection the test females showed a significantly greater preference for intact male incentive animals (Figure 10-10). The degree of preference in these runway experiments for an incentive male over an incentive female rat was a function of the dose of estradiol benzoate

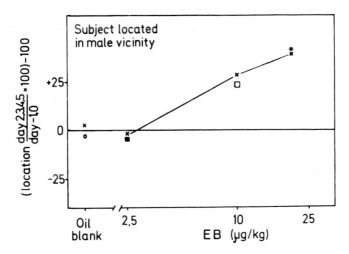

Figure 10-7. The magnitude of the estrogen effect on the tendency of the female rat in an open-field test to be located in the vicinity of the male was a function of the dose of estradiol benzoate (EB). (From Meyerson & Lindstrom, 1973.)

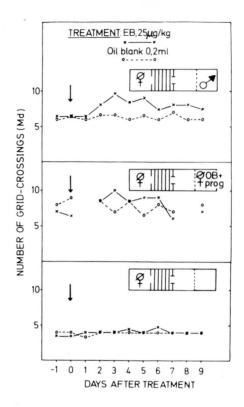

Figure 10-8. Estradiol benzoate (EB) increased the frequency with which ovariectomized female rats crossed an electrified grid to get to an incentive male rat (top
panel), but had no effect when the incentive compartment contained a female or
was empty (middle and bottom panels). (From Meyerson & Lindstrom, 1973.)

given the test female rat (Figure 10-11). Thus, with all three behavioral
methods, Meyerson and Lindstrom's results indicated that estrogen
injections of an ovariectomized female rat increase the frequencies
of arbitrarily chosen responses that result in contact with a vigorous
male rat.

   Meyerson and Lindstrom concluded that estrogen induced a drive to
seek contact with a sexually vigorous male. Because the arbitrarily
chosen responses in the three types of experiments were much different from each other, the results are unlikely to be an artifact of one
particular behavioral technique. In those experiments where different
types of incentive animals were used, the most striking results always
involved seeking contact with a male rather than other types of rats,
suggesting that the motivation was specifically sexual rather than generally social.

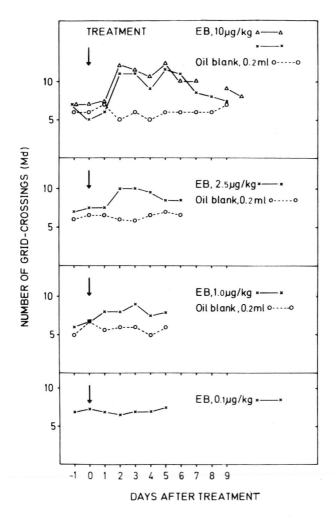

Figure 10-9. The largest and longest increases in the frequency with which ovariectomized female rats would cross electrified grids to reach a sexually active male were caused by the highest doses of estradiol benzoate (EB) (e.g., see top panel). (From Meyerson & Lindstrom, 1973.)

Summary. Implications from experiments in which female rats perform arbitrary responses to approach males or to admit males to their vicinity fit perfectly with the inferences about motivation from studies of lordosis behavior itself. Reproductive behavior in the female rat has the status of a motivated set of responses, and estrogen increases the level of sexual motivation.

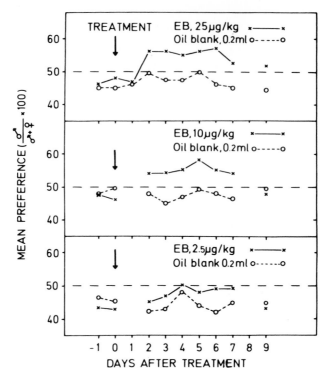

Figure 10-10. After 25 μg/kg of estradiol benzoate (top panel), ovariectomized rats showed a significant tendency to choose the goal cage containing a sexually active male as opposed to one containing another female. (From Meyerson & Lindstrom, 1973.)

The Male

Mating Behavior: Concepts

Because the male rat that is reproductively competent searches for and pursues estrous females, there has been little doubt that sexual mounting and subsequent mating responses by the males reflect a sexual motivational state. Nevertheless, it has been important to remember constraints on the definitions of motivated responses, as mentioned in the first chapter of this book and as noted in the treatment of female sexual motivation. First, it has been important to identify molar behavioral responses and link motivational definitions to their gross occurrence or large changes in their quantitative aspects, so as not to be in the position of misidentifying "noise" in a simple reflex mechanism. Second, investigators must attempt heuristic definitions of motivated

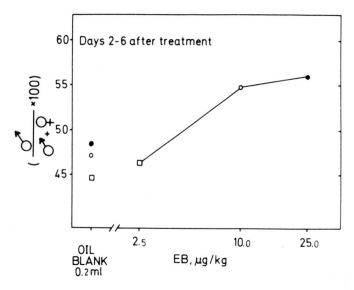

Figure 10-11. The tendency of estrogen-treated female rats to choose the goal box containing a sexually active male versus one containing an estrous female was an increasing function of the estradiol benzoate (EB) dose given the test ovariectomized females. (From Meyerson & Lindstrom, 1973.)

responses, such that their quantitative relations will reflect the hypothetical intervening variable.

Following two decades of distinguished endocrine, neural, and behavioral research on mating behavior, Beach (1956) theorized about the underlying nature of sexual motivation in male organisms. Here he was concerned with explaining natural sequences of masculine copulatory behavior.

In particular, Beach's concepts were intended to identify motivational mechanisms that would account for the temporal patterning of a male rat's sexual performance. Beach postulates that initial approaches to the female by the male are accounted for by a *sexual arousal mechanism* (SAM). When this is high, the male's sexual excitement is increased to a point that a copulatory threshold is reached. This results in mounting and intromission. Intromission, requiring erection and insertion, demands hypothesis of a second mechanism, the *intromission and ejaculatory mechanism* (IEM). Finally, the sensory input from intromission eventually brings the male to the ejaculatory threshold.

Quantitative behavioral measures thought to reflect the sexual arousal mechanism include the latency for the male to mount the female and the latency for the male to perform an intromission.

Striking manifestations of high sexual arousal can be seen, for ex-

ample, in the sexually inexperienced male rat who thoroughly investi-
gates the female, which leads naturally to his following the female
excitedly. Approaching from the rear, when the female displays a typical hopping and darting sequence of locomotion, he will mount. Sexual
arousal is thought to cause the generalized excitement by these sexually
naive males, accounting for the continued exploration, following responses, and mounting. Then, when mounting results in an intromission, the excited behavior due to the sexual arousal mechanism can be
contrasted to the rather methodical sequence of intromissions by the
male, which will proceed at regular intervals until ejaculation occurs.
This sequence of behavior is postulated by Beach (1956) to be under
control of the intromission and ejaculatory mechanism.

Beach's views of male rat temporal patterning were updated most
substantially by the experiments and theory of Sachs and Barfield.
They (Sachs & Barfield, 1970) were able to describe accurately the
mating behavior of male rats in terms of the duration of "mount bouts"
(series of mounts of the females separated by short periods of time)
and intermount-bout intervals. The stability of this measure and the
fact that its temporal characteristics did not depend on intromission
suggested that during an ejaculatory series the mount bout, rather than
the intromission, might be the basic unit to be considered as regulated
by underlying variables such as sexual arousal or ejaculatory potential.
In fact, female rats neonatally treated with testosterone so that they
would exhibit high levels of male copulatory behavior demonstrated
numbers of mount bouts, durations of mount bouts, and intermount-
bout intervals remarkably similar to genetic male rats (Sachs, Pollak,
Krieger, & Barfield, 1973). This reinforced the authors' conviction that
mount bouts represent a useful measure for the analysis of mechanisms
of sexual arousal.

It is important, therefore, that the role of nonspecific arousal contributing to the concept of sexual arousal was demonstrated powerfully
by Barfield and Sachs' (1968) experiment in which electric shock was
delivered periodically to the skin of male rats in the presence of receptive female rats. Shortly after each electric shock to the skin, males
initiated mounting or intromission. Here, the usefulness of the mount-
bout interval measure was shown by the fact that intermount-bout
intervals were remarkably shortened by electric shocks to the skin. A
sudden increase in apparent general arousal hastened the pacing of an
underlying sex behavior controlling mechanism. In subsequent experiments, Barfield and Sachs (1970) replicated their demonstration that
general arousal (as presumed to be caused by electric shock to the skin)
could increase the rate of copulatory behavior. Here their measure was
the rate and nature of the decline of mating behavior following castration. Cutaneous shock slowed the decline in numbers of ejaculations,
intromissions, and simple mounts. This presumably showed the input

from this nonspecific arousing stimulus to the sexual arousal mechanism. However, mating behavior did eventually disappear even in animals receiving electric shock. Thus, the nonspecific stimulus did not entirely substitute for androgen administration, suggesting either that electric shock is not an omnibus activator of the sexual arousal mechanism or that androgen does something other than initiate a simple arousing effect.

Finally, in this extensive series of experiments, Sachs and Barfield (1974) showed big effects of cutaneous electric shock in reducing the postejaculatory latencies to the next mount, postejaculatory latencies to the next intromission, and interintromission intervals.

From their work on the temporal patterning of masculine sex behavior in general, and on the effects of arousing electric shock in particular, Sachs and Barfield (1974) developed a model of sexual arousal in the male rat that built upon Beach's (1956) sexual arousal mechanism and intromission–ejaculatory mechanism concepts. Their new model differed in that the interval between intromissions, for example, previously ascribed to an intromission–ejaculatory mechanism, may be understood in terms of changes in simple sexual arousal. As usual, mounting activity is assumed to reflect the level of the intervening variable, "sexual arousal." Sexual arousal falls following ejaculation and its recovery over time is reflected by the postejaculatory mount and intromission latencies. It also falls following each intromission and recovers with time. Electric shock, which can speed the recovery of mounting and intromissions following ejaculation and can reduce intervals between intromissions, is assumed to act directly by increasing sexual arousal. For all measures it is assumed that the mount will occur in the presence of a receptive female as soon as the level of sexual arousal exceeds a mount threshold.

Convering Operations to Demonstrate Motivational State

Because of the natural approach behaviors by male rats to females, including responses in which the male seems to be searching for the female, it seems clear that the initiation of male mating behavior reflects a state of high sexual motivation. For example, in experimental circumstances, male rats will sniff avidly at a bottle with odors of urine from estrous female rats, and spend significantly more time at such odor sources than near the odors from anestrous female rats or blank control bottles (Pfaff & Pfaffmann, 1969). Significantly, testosterone when injected into castrated male rats increased the amount of time spent sniffing at the estrous odor. By this measure, then, testosterone increases sexual motivation.

Still, it has been useful to analyze the response of male rats in a variety of experimental situations in which predictions about arbitrarily chosen responses could be taken to confirm the interpretation that their mating responses reflect a motivational state and that testosterone increases sexual arousal. Warner (1927) found that male rats with normal testicular hormone levels would cross electrified grids to reach estrous females significantly more often than if no female was in the goal box. The frequency of grid crossings was a function of time since the last exposure to the female, peaking about 1 day following such an exposure and remaining high (Figure 10-12).

Nissen (1929) also used the Columbia Obstruction Apparatus to measure male sex drive. Normal unoperated male rats and sham-operated control animals crossed 10–13 times per test to reach a goal box containing a receptive female rat. Castration significantly reduced this frequency (Figure 10-13). When placental extract was injected over 2–3 days into castrated animals there was an increase in the average number of crossings. When normal uncastrated males were given injections of placental extract, no effects were seen. Similarly, extracts from male accessory organs injected into castrated males had no effect.

Later, Kagan (1955) was able to teach male rats to make a correct

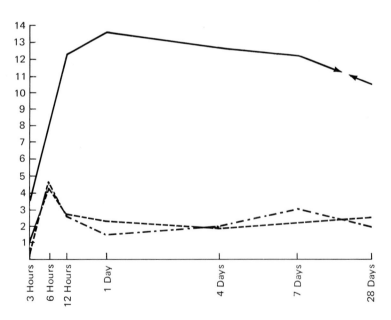

Figure 10-12. Male rats were willing to cross an electrified grid (solid line) to gain access to a receptive female rat. The frequency of grid crossings (ordinate) was a function of the number of hours females were withheld from the test males (abscissa). The number of grid crossings increased markedly after 12 hours or 1 day of deprivation and stayed high for several days. (From Warner, 1927.)

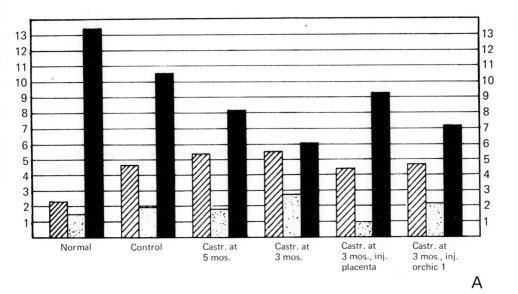

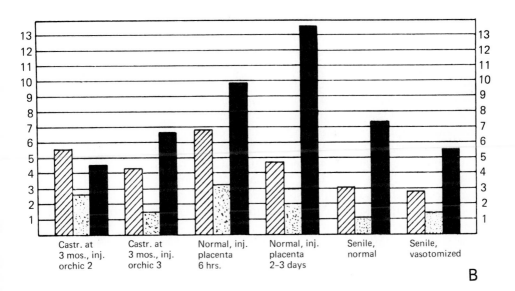

Figure 10-13. Normal and control sham-operated male rats crossed an electric grid (solid bars) with a high frequency to reach an estrous female. Castrated uninjected males had a significantly reduced frequency of grid crossings. Castrated males with injections of placental extracts showed a somewhat elevated number of crossings, while normal males injected with placental extracts showed their usual high sexual motivation. (From Nissen, 1929.)

turn in a T maze when the reward was defined as mating with a receptive female, including ejaculation. There was even a reward value in the opportunity to mount the female without ejaculation, but performance was better when ejaculation was allowed. Beach and Jordan (1956) found that castrated male rats that were running slowly or not at all in an alley to enter a goal box containing a receptive female responded to daily injections of testosterone propionate by increased running speed toward the goal box and, in parallel, increased sexual activity with the estrous female in the goal box. Thus, rate of approach to the female was increased by the androgenic hormone, and (from Kagan's experiment) we see that male rats are willing to learn an arbitrary response to reach a female.

All of these experimental results are consistent with the interpretation that the male rat's approach to the female and subsequent mating behavior reflect a state of sexual motivation. Testosterone elevates the level of this motivation.

Mating Behavior: Mechanisms

A detailed account of our current knowledge on the neuroendocrine mechanisms and neural circuitry for masculine mating behavior is outside the scope of this chapter. An excellent recent review was written by Hart (1981). In one of the earlier attempts to conceptualize neural mechanisms for male mating behavior, Beach (1967) tested the propositions that lower nervous centers for reproductive behavior are under inhibitory control by more anterior neural centers, and that steroid sex hormones operate on the more anterior centers to release lower reflexive mechanisms from inhibition. Evidence for this type of mechanism was found in research on male amphibia, but no clear lines of experiments forced this conclusion for male rats. Instead, many results have emphasized the facilitating role of preoptic tissue.

In male rats, electrical stimulation of the medial preoptic area facilitates copulatory behavior (Malsbury, 1971; see Malsbury & Pfaff, 1974, for a review). Lesions of the preoptic area disrupt it (Heimer & Larsson, 1966). Transections, placed in such a way as to cut axons of preoptic neurons that would join the fibers of the medial forebrain bundle (Conrad & Pfaff, 1976) also disrupt male mating behavior.

Local implants of testosterone have favored the interpretation that androgenic hormones operate on preoptic neurons so as to facilitate male mating responses. In the first experiment of this sort, Davidson (1966) found that the most effective site for restoring male sex behavior of castrated male rats by testosterone propionate implants was in the medial preoptic area. Other, hypothalamic sites had some effects but quantitatively, the facilitation was not as strong as after medial preoptic implants. A later series of testosterone implant experiments confirmed these conclusions (Johnston & Davidson, 1972). Independently, Lisk (1967) showed that implants of testosterone in the anterior hypothalamic–preoptic region can increase male sex behavior scores in castrated male rats, while control implant sites had little or no effect.

The preeminence of medial preoptic tissue in facilitating masculine mating behavior and, apparently, mediating at least some of the androgen effects on this behavior has tremendous zoological generality, in that comparisons across species over a wide phylogenetic range among vertebrates keep leading to the same conclusions. In a variety of mammals, birds, amphibia, and fish, destruction of medial preoptic tissue leads to decrements in male mating behavior, or electrical stimulation of medial preoptic neurons facilitate it, or application of testosterone directly into the preoptic area facilitates it (see Kelley & Pfaff, 1978, for a review). Since testosterone is accumulated by preoptic neurons in a wide variety of vertebrates (Morrell & Pfaff, 1978), we have hypothesized that a phylogenetically stable mechanism is for circulating testosterone to arrive at preoptic neurons and by facilitating their electrical or biosynthetic activity to cause them to send increased output to the midbrain, for the facilitation of male copulatory and courtship behaviors.

Preoptic area neurons facilitate parasympathetic mechanisms in the autonomic nervous system. Thus, it was interesting to note that some of the behavioral changes in male mating following preoptic lesions could be attributed to the failure of penile erection, involving autonomic changes (see Pfaff, 1980, for a review). Thus, we hypothesized that part of the way in which preoptic neurons have their effects on masculine mating behavior might be through their connections with autonomic mechanisms in general and the parasympathetic nervous system in particular (Figure 10-2).

The brain-stem and spinal cord circuitry on which signals from hormone-influenced preoptic neurons could play are unknown. However, one fascinating end point for neuroanatomical and electrophysiological work in this regard is likely to be the control of motoneurons for penile muscles. Their cell bodies are located in a distinct part of the spinal cord and are sexually dimorphic in their appearance (Breedlove & Arnold, 1980).

Summary

Testosterone injections facilitate male mating behavior. From the intrinsic nature of this behavior and the willingness of male rats to perform a variety of arbitrary responses to reach estrous females, we conclude that the occurrence of the behavior reflects a state of high sexual motivation. Therefore, testosterone has the status of a chemically identified biological variable that raises sexual motivation. This androgen or its metabolites are likely to increase this motivational state by facilitating the activity of medial preoptic neurons.

References

Barfield, R. J., & Sachs, B. D. Sexual behavior: Stimulation by painful electrical shock to skin in male rats. *Science*, 1968, *161*, 392-395.

Barfield, R. J., & Sachs, B. D. Effect of shock on copulatory behavior in castrate male rats. *Hormones and Behavior*, 1970, *1*, 247-253.

Beach, F. A. Characteristics of masculine "sex drive." In M. R. Jones (Ed.), *Nebraska Symposium on Motivation 1956*. Lincoln: University of Nebraska Press, 1956, pp. 1-32.

Beach, F. A. Cerebral and hormonal control of reflexive mechanisms involved in copulatory behavior. *Physiological Reviews*, 1967, *47*, 289-316.

Beach, F. A., & Jordan, L. Effects of sexual reinforcement upon the performance of male rats in a straight runway. *Journal of Comparative and Physiological Psychology*, 1956, *49*, 105-110.

Bermant, G. Response latencies of female rats during sexual intercourse. *Science*, 1961, *133*, 1771-1773.

Bermant, G., & Westbrook, W. H. Peripheral factors in the regulation of sexual contact by female rats. *Journal of Comparative and Physiological Psychology*, 1966, *61*(2), 244-250.

Breedlove, S. M., & Arnold, A. P. Hormone accumulation in a sexually dimorphic motor nucleus of the rat spinal cord. *Science*, 1980, *210*, 564-566.

Cohen, R., & Pfaff, D. W. Electron microscopic observations of cells in the ventromedial nucleus of the hypothalamus in estrogen-treated and control ovariectomized female rats. *Cell and Tissue Research*, 1981, in press.

Conrad, L. C. A., & Pfaff, D. W. Efferents from medial basal forebrain and hypothalmus in the rat, I: An autoradiographic study of the medial preoptic area. *Journal of Comparative Neurology*, 1976, *169*, 185-220.

Davidson, J. M. Activation of the male rat's sexual behavior by intracerebral implantation of androgen. *Endocrinology*, 1966, *79*, 783-794.

Emery, D. Effects of hypothalamic lesions in female rats. To be submitted. 1981. (a)

Emery, D. Effects of chemical sympathectomy in female rats. To be submitted. 1981. (b)

Floody, O., & Pfaff, D. W. Steroid hormones and aggressive behavior: Approaches to the study of hormone-sensitive brain mechanisms for behavior. *Research Publications, Association for Research in Nervous and Mental Disease*, 1974, *52*, 149-185.

Floody, O. R., & Pfaff, D. W. Aggressive behavior in female hamsters: The hormonal basis for fluctuations in female aggressiveness correlated with estrous state. *Journal of Comparative and Physiological Psychology*, 1977, *91*, 443-464. (a)

Floody, O. R., & Pfaff, D. W. Communication among hamsters by high-frequency acoustic signals, III: Responses evoked by natural and synthetic ultrasounds. *Journal of Comparative and Physiological Psychology*, 1977, *91*, 820-829. (b)

Floody, O. R., Pfaff, D. W., & Lewis, C. D. Communication among hamsters by high-frequency acoustic signals, II: Determinants of calling by females and males. *Journal of Comparative and Physiological Psychology*, 1977, *91*, 807-819.

Giesler, G. J., Jr., & Liebeskind, J. C. Inhibition of visceral pain by electrical stimulation of the periaqueductal gray matter. *Pain*, 1976, *2*, 43-48.

Hart, B. Neural mechanisms of male reproductive behavior. In R. Goy & D. Pfaff (Eds.), *Neurobiology of reproduction.* New York: Plenum Press, 1981, in press.

Heimer, L., & Larsson, K. Impairment of mating behavior in male rats following lesions in the preoptic-anterior hypothalamic continuum. *Brain Research*, 1966, *3*, 248-263.

Hetherington, A., & Ranson, S. Hypothalamic lesions and adiposity in the rat. *Anatomical Record*, 1940, *78*, 149-172.

Jenkins, M. The effect of segregation on the sex behavior of the white rat as measured by the obstruction method. *Genetic Psychology Monographs*, 1928, *3*(6), 455-568.

Johnston, P., & Davidson, J. M. Intracerebral androgens and sexual behavior in the male rat. *Hormones and Behavior*, 1972, *3*, 345-357.

Kagan, J. Differential reward value of incomplete and complete sexual behavior. *Journal of Comparative and Physiological Psychology*, 1955, *48*, 59-64.

Kelley, D. B., & Pfaff, D. W. Generalizations from comparative studies on neuroanatomical and endocrine mechanisms of sexual behavior. In J. Hutchison (Ed.), *Biological determinants of sexual behavior.* Chichester, England: Wiley, 1978, pp. 225-254.

Komisaruk, B. R. Neural and hormonal interactions in the reproductive behavior of female rats. In W. Montagna & W. A. Sadler (Eds.), *Reproductive behavior.* New York: Plenum Press, 1974.

Komisaruk, B. R., Ciofalo, V., & Latranyi, M. B. Stimulation of the vaginal cervix is more effective than morphine in suppressing a nociceptive response in rats. In J. J. Bonica & D. Albe-Fessard (Eds.), *Advances in pain research and therapy* (Vol. 1). New York: Raven Press, 1976, pp. 439-443.

Kow, L.-M., Malsbury, C., & Pfaff, D. W. Effects of progesterone on female reproductive behavior in rats: Possible modes of action and role in behavioral sex differences. In W. Montagna & W. Sadler (Eds.), *Reproductive behavior.* New York: Plenum Press, 1974, pp. 179-210.

Krieger, M. S., Conrad, L. C. A., & Pfaff, D. W. An autoradiographic study of the efferent connections of the ventromedial nucleus of the hypothalamus. *Journal of Comparative Neurology*, 1979, *183*, 785-816.

Lisk, R. D. Neural localization for androgen activation of copulatory behavior in the male rat. *Endocrinology*, 1967, *80*, 754-761.

Malsbury, C. W. Facilitation of male rat copulatory behavior by electrical stimulation of the medial preoptic area. *Physiology and Behavior*, 1971, 7, 797-805.

Malsbury, C. W., & Pfaff, D. W. Neural and hormonal determinants of mating behavior in adult male rats. A review. In L. V. DiCara (Ed.), *Limbic and autonomic nervous systems research.* New York: Plenum Press, 1974, pp. 85-136.

Malsbury, C., Kow, L.-M., & Pfaff, D. W. Effects of medial hypothalamic lesions on the lordosis response and other behaviors in female golden hamsters. *Physiology and Behavior*, 1977, *19*, 223-237.

Mathews, D., & Edwards, D. A. Involvement of the ventromedial and anterior hypothalamic nuclei in the hormonal induction of receptivity in the female rat. *Physiology and Behavior*, 1977, *19*, 319-326.

Mayer, D. J., & Liebeskind, J. C. Pain reduction by focal electrical stimulation of the brain: An anatomical and behavioral analysis. *Brain Research*, 1974, *68*, 73–93.

Mayer, D. J., & Watkins, L. R. The role of endorphins in endogenous pain control systems. In *Modern problems of pharmacopsychiatry: The role of endorphins in neuropsychiatry.* 1981.

McGinnis, M., Nance, D. M., & Gorski, R. A. Olfactory, septal and amygdala lesions alone or in combination: Effects on lordosis behavior and emotionality. *Physiology and Behavior*, 1978, *20*, 435–440.

Meyerson, B. J., & Lindstrom, L. Sexual motivation in the estrogen treated ovariectomized rat. In V. H. T. James & L. Martini (Eds.), *Hormonal steroids.* (Proceedings of the Third International Congress on Hormonal Steriods, Hamburg, 7–12 September 1970.) Amsterdam: Excerpta Medica, 1971, pp. 731–737.

Meyerson, B. J., & Lindstrom, L. H. Sexual motivation in the female rat: A methodological study applied to the investigation of the effect of estradiol benzoate. *Acta Physiologica Scandinavica* (Suppl. 389), 1973, 1–80.

Miller, N. E. Liberalization of basic S–R concepts: Extensions to conflict behavior, motivation and social learning. In S. Koch (Ed.), *Psychology: A study of a science* (Study 1, Vol. 2). New York: McGraw-Hill, 1959, pp. 196–292.

Miller, N. E. Behavioral and physiological techniques: Rationale and experimental designs for combining their use. In C. F. Code & W. Heidel (Eds.), *Handbook of physiology*, Section 6: *Alimentary canal* (Vol. 1, *Food and water intake*). Baltimore: Williams & Wilkins, 1967, pp. 51–61.

Morrell, J. I., & Pfaff, D. W. A neuroendocrine approach to brain function: Localization of sex steroid concentrating cells in vertebrate brains. *American Zoologist*, 1978, *18*, 447–460.

Nance, D. M., Shryne, J. E., Gordon, J. H., & Gorski, R. A. Examination of some factors that control the effects of septal lesions on lordosis behavior. *Pharmacology, Biochemistry and Behavior*, 1977, *6*, 227–234.

Nance, D. M., Shryne, J., & Gorski, R. A. Septal lesions: Effects on lordosis behavior and pattern of gonadotropin release. *Hormones and Behavior*, 1974, *5*, 73–81.

Nance, D. M., Shryne, J., & Gorski, R. A. Effects of septal lesions on behavioral sensitivity of female rats to gonadal hormones. *Hormones and Behavior*, 1975, *6*, 59–64.

Nissen, H. W. Experiments on sex drive in rats. *Genetic Psychology Monographs*, 1929, *5*, 451–548.

Peirce, J. T., & Nuttall, R. L. Self-paced sexual behavior in the female rat. *Journal of Comparative and Physiological Psychology*, 1961, *54*, 310–313.

Pfaff, D. W. *Estrogens and brain function: Neural analysis of a hormone-controlled mammalian reproductive behavior.* New York: Springer-Verlag, 1980.

Pfaff, D. W., & Keiner, M. Atlas of estradiol-concentrating cells in the central nervous system of the female rat. *Journal of Comparative Neurology*, 1973, *151*, 121–158.

Pfaff, D. W., & Lewis, C. Film analyses of lordosis in female rats. *Hormones and Behavior*, 1974, *5*, 317–335.

Pfaff, D. W., Lewis, C., Diakow, C., & Keiner, M. Neurophysiological analysis of mating behavior responses as hormone-sensitive reflexes. In E. Stellar & J. M. Sprague (Eds.), *Progress in physiological psychology* (Vol. 5). New York: Academic Press, 1973, pp. 253–297.

Pfaff, D. W., & Pfaffmann, C. Behavioral and electrophysiological responses of male rats to female rat urine odors. In C. Pfaffmann (Ed.), *Olfaction and taste*. New York: Rockefeller University Press, 1969, pp. 258-267.

Pfaff, D. W., & Sakuma, Y. Deficit in the lordosis reflex of female rats caused by lesions in the ventromedial nucleus of the hypothalamus. *Journal of Physiology*, 1979, *288*, 203-210.

Sachs, B. D., & Barfield, R. J. Temporal patterning of sexual behavior in the male rat. *Journal of Comparative and Physiological Psychology*, 1970, *73*(3), 359-364.

Sachs, B. D., & Barfield, R. J. Copulatory behavior of male rats given intermittent electric shocks. *Journal of Comparative and Physiological Psychology*, 1974, *86*(4), 607-615.

Sachs, B. D., Pollak, E. I., Krieger, M. S., & Barfield, R. J. Sexual behavior: Normal male patterning in adrogenized female rats. *Science*, 1973, *181*, 770-772.

Sakuma, Y., & Pfaff, D. W. Facilitation of female reproductive behavior from mesencephalic central grey in the rat. *American Journal of Physiology*, 1979, *237*(5), R278-R284. (a)

Sakuma, Y., & Pfaff, D. W. Mesencephalic mechanisms for integration of female reproductive behavior in the rat. *American Journal of Physiology*, 1979, *237*(5), R285-R290. (b)

Warner, L. H. A study of sex behavior in the white rat by means of the obstruction method. *Comparative Psychology Monographs*, 1927, *4*, 1-66.

Part Four

Approach vs. Avoidance in Motivation and Emotion

Chapter 11

The Opponent Processes
in Acquired Motivation

RICHARD L. SOLOMON

Mammals come equipped with a variety of species-specific motivation systems. With amazingly little experience, they appropriately eat food, drink liquids, become fearful in the presence of predators, or copulate with conspecifics. The stimuli that control such behaviors are decidedly different from species to species, but these differences are relatively independent of the widely differing life histories of the individual conspecifics. The controlling stimuli, as Epstein (Chapter 7, this volume) has so lucidly pointed out, may function as releasers of fixed action patterns or as elicitors of reflexes or as arousers of affect. If they are arousers of affect, they have a motivational function; they induce affective states that energize large arrays of behavior and create the conditions for what the psychologist calls *reinforcement*. If they merely elicit fixed action patterns or reflexes without affect, they have no motivational significance: They do not create persisting affective states, and they sometimes will have no capacity to reinforce behaviors. Epstein has described examples of motivating and nonmotivating stimuli that can control innately organized behaviors.

The perfected, innately organized motivation systems are crucial to the survival of the individual and the species. It is not sufficient that some organisms have reflexive ingestive reactions to specified stimuli. They also have to become hungry. This seems to be true even of the lowly blowfly (Dethier, 1978). When we identify such a motivational system in a mammal, we are also able to modify the functional significance of some of the stimuli surrounding the motivated behaviors. Sometimes these modifications lead to what are called *acquired* motives, a vast array of motives that animals can *acquire through experience* with repeated environmental stimuli and events, motives that do *not* seem to have an intimate connection with survival. Indeed, some of these acquired motives can lead to destruction of the individual animal. A few examples of acquired motives are addiction to certain drugs, arbitrary social attachments, and seemingly masochistic tendencies to deliver unpleasant stimuli to oneself. Such acquired motives are unnecessary, and they do not have to eventuate at all during a given individual life history. But often they do, and in humans most of the important social motives are of this acquired, rather than innate, type.

It is quite remarkable that psychologists have so far discovered only three ways to create acquired motives in the laboratory:

1. By the first method, we discover a stimulus that innately arouses an affective state, such as fear. Then we precede each presentation of that stimulus with a neutral stimulus or event (one that innately cannot arouse fear). After several such pairings, the neutral stimulus is no longer neutral: It now can arouse fear all by itself, in the absence of the original, innately given arouser. Once this happens, the *removal* of the new arousing stimulus will have a *reinforcing* function in that many kinds of behavior that precede the removal will be learned or will increase in probability of occurrence in the same environment. Stimuli that have acquired fear-arousing properties through experience, not through innately given properties, are called *conditioned fear stimuli*. The laws of their acquisition are believed to be much as Pavlov described the process of acquisition of conditioned salivary reflexes (for a review of these striking similarities, see Maier, Seligman, & Solomon, 1969, pp. 306–316.) A conditioned fear stimulus has acquired a novel control over an affective reaction with motivational properties. Thus the presence or absence of that stimulus now controls a state of the organism. Originally it could *not* do so. Organisms will work hard to remove or get away from such new stimuli that arouse the fear state.
2. A second way we can establish an acquired motive is to identify a stimulus that is an innate reinforcer and then associate with it in space or time some neutral stimulus that originally is *not* a reinforcer. We can often thereby create a new *conditioned* or *secondary* reinforcer for which the animal will work (see Hendry, 1969, for a review of the properties of such conditioned reinforcers).
3. The third way one can establish an acquired motive is by mere repetition of a reinforcer. Sometimes when we do that the organism seems to become dependent on the incessant repetition of the reinforcer. This can happen even if the reinforcer is an arouser of unpleasant affect initially.

This chapter emphasizes the last phenomenon at the expense of the first two. It does so because the first two ways of establishing acquired motives have received a great deal of attention (see Brown, 1979, pp. 231–272), but the third way has not (see Solomon, 1980).

Usually, when we have identified an acquired motive system that does not depend on a conditioning or associative process (in contrast to the first two ways), a system built up by repetition of a reinforcer rather than the pairing of a neutral stimulus with a reinforcer, we will also observe three highly correlated affective phenomena. These are (1) affective contrast, (2) affective habituation or tolerance, and (3) affective withdrawal symptoms or the abstinence syndrome.

Affective contrast is a term referring to the fact that the sudden removal of a reinforcer can induce an affective state quite unlike that induced by the presence of the reinforcer. If we show a newly hatched duckling a moving object, we will see excitement and signs of positive affect. The stimulus is a positive reinforcer, as evidenced by the fact that the duckling can be trained to perform an arbitrary response, like pecking at a pole, in order to make the moving object appear. In contrast, removal of the moving object after it has been present for a while causes signs of negative affect. The duckling emits cries and the crying lasts a lot longer than did the prior exposure to the moving object. Removal of the moving object is a negative reinforcer, as is evidenced by the fact that ducklings will learn an arbitrary response, like pecking at a pole, in order to prevent the moving object from being removed. These are the facts evidencing affective contrast. Removal of the reinforcer does not return the duckling to its original affective neutrality. Instead, it plunges the duckling into a contrasting state from which it eventually recovers, given the passage of time.

Affective habituation (or tolerance) may occur if the reinforcer is frequently repeated with relatively short time intervals between presentations. The affective reaction of the animal to the onset and maintenance of the reinforcing stimulus appears to diminish gradually with successive presentations. In addition, if one wishes to maintain a large-magnitude affective reaction, it then becomes necessary to increase the intensity and/or quality of the reinforcing stimulus. Of course, the best example of this is the affective reaction (the "high" or the "low," etc.) produced by certain reinforcing drugs during the development of drug tolerance. However, many species-specific reinforcers share this tolerance feature with affect arousing drugs.

The *affective withdrawal syndrome* often appears after habituation or tolerance has developed. It, too, depends on the frequent repetition of the reinforcer with relatively short time intervals between presentations. It is characterized by the emergence of a new affective experience whenever the reinforcer is terminated or omitted. The experience can be pleasant or unpleasant, depending on whether the presence of the reinforcer was positively or negatively reinforcing. The relation of con-

trast or oppositeness holds here. Thus, if the presence of the reinforcer
was initially aversive, but now as a result of constant repetition is no
longer especially so, the removal of that reinforcer will cause a positive
affect, one that functions as a positive reinforcer. The runner's "high"
is a good example. So are the sauna bather's exhilaration and the sport
parachutist's elation.

We are dealing here with those cases wherein the affective reaction to
the presence of a reinforcing stimulus declines with repetition, whereas
the contrasting or emergent afterreaction intensifies with repetition. It
is as though the affect system becomes more and more tolerant of the
presences of stimuli while it becomes more and more intolerant of the
absences of stimuli. We will see that such occurrences are lawful. They
generally follow closely the deductions from an opponent-process
theory of acquired motivation.

The opponent-process theory is the simplest model we could devise
to account for the facts of affective contrast, tolerance, and withdrawal
syndrome. It is portrayed as a flowchart in Figure 11-1.

The model is a negative feed-forward control system designed to

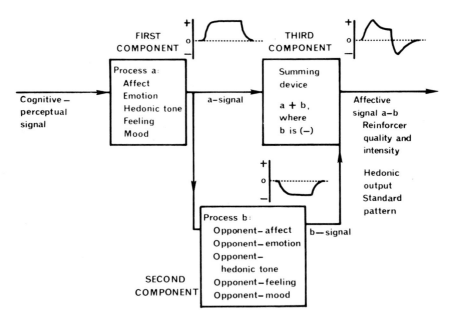

Figure 11-1. Flowchart of processes postulated for an opponent-process theory of
motivation. The affect-arousing input activates its primary a-process, which in turn
sends out two messages, one to a summator and one to its opponent process, or
b-process. The b-process then sends its message to the summator, where the sum
a − b is computed. The resultant reinforcement attributes of stimulation follow the
standard pattern of affective dynamics, as shown in the upper right-hand corner of
the diagram. (From Solomon & Corbit, 1973.)

keep affect in check while stimulation is occurring. Two opponent processes control a summator, and the summator determines the controlling affect, motivation, or reinforcement magnitude at any moment. It is assumed that the onset and maintenance of a reinforcing stimulus sets into action the primary affective process, the a-process. It is quick and so tracks the stimulus intensity, quality, and duration quite faithfully. Arousal of the a-process eventually will lead to arousal of the opponent process, the b-process, whose action feeds into the summator just as does the a-process. However, the b-process, unlike the a-process, is sluggish and inertial. It has a relatively long latency, a slow recruitment, and a generally lower asymptote, as well as a longer decay time after stimulation ceases. The summator will therefore produce the *standard pattern of affective dynamics* as shown in Figure 11-2. There will be a peak value of the sum |a − b| during the early seconds of stimulation by a reinforcer or affect arouser. Because a > b, the subject will be in State A, an affect mainly produced by the a-process. Then, as the stimulation continues, the b-process will become more active, thus reducing the sum |a − b| or producing a less intense A-state. Finally, when the stimulation is suddenly terminated, the value of the a-process quickly goes to zero, leaving the slowly decaying b-process to control the affective state. The subject will then be in State B, because b > a.

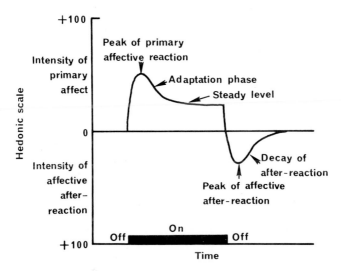

Figure 11-2. The standard pattern of affective dynamics. Note the five labeled distinctive features of the complex affective outcome produced by a simple square-wave stimulus input. (From "An Opponent Process Theory of Motivation, I: Temporal Dynamics on Affect" by R. L. Solomon and J. D. Corbit, *Psychological Review*, 1974, *81*, 119–145. Copyright 1974 by the American Psychological Association. Reprinted by permission.)

The pattern of affective reaction shown in Figure 11-2 derives from the simple assumptions of the model. However, it requires *one more postulate* in order to account for the three affective phenomena we have emphasized: The b-process will be strengthened through use and weakened by *disuse*. This postulate, when imposed on the opponent-process model, enables us to deduce the occurrence of habituation or tolerance, as well as the emergence of the withdrawal syndrome. The patterns of affective dynamics shown in Figure 11-3 serve to contrast the affective state of the experimental animal during the first few exposures to a reinforcer with that during later reinforcements. The stimulus input remains invariant, but the b-process is strengthened by frequent repetitions (its latency becomes shorter, its rise time becomes less sluggish, while its decay time is now increased), so that the A state is weak and the B state is strong and enduring.

Do the facts fit the theory? We have used a variety of approaches and settings in order to test the model. They focus on three major variables: (1) the frequency of *use* or exercise of the putative opponent process; (2) the degree of *disuse* of the putative opponent-process system; and (3) the *duration* and *quality* of the stimuli which arouse the opponent-process systems. Frequency of *use* is easy to vary; all one needs to do is get a measure of an opponent affect after differing num-

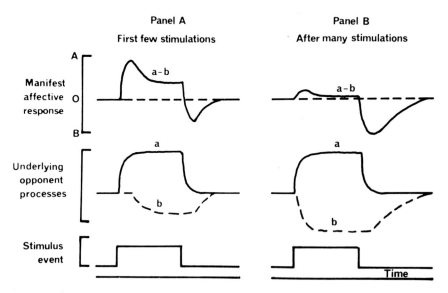

Figure 11-3. The standard pattern of affective dynamics when a reinforcing stimulus is relatively novel compared to the standard pattern after the stimulus has been repeated many times. The change in the sum a − b is brought about by the increase in the magnitude of the opponent or b-process as it is strengthened by use. (From Solomon, 1980.)

bers of exposures to a reinforcing stimulus. Amount of *disuse* is easy to vary; all one needs to do is measure the opponent affect, with frequency of exposure held constant, but with the time intervals between stimulations being varied across groups of subjects. Finally, quality of stimulation can easily be varied by establishing preference hierarchies for different reinforcers and then determining whether high-preference stimulation generates a bigger opponent process than does low-preference stimulation.

Repeated Stimulations (Use)

Hoffman, Eiserer, Ratner, and Pickering (1974) exposed ducklings to an imprinting object repeatedly. Each exposure duration was 1 minute, as was each separation period. With this 1-minute on, 1-minute off regime repeated 15 times, there was a gradual increase of separation distress during the off periods. We can consider separation distress to be the b-process aroused by presentation of the positively reinforcing imprinting object (a moving object). Level of distress was indexed by the amount of time, in a 1-minute observation period, filled with distress calls (a distinctive vocalization of ducklings). As Figure 11-4 shows, the growth of distress calling was an orderly function of repeated presentation and removal of the reinforcing stimulus.

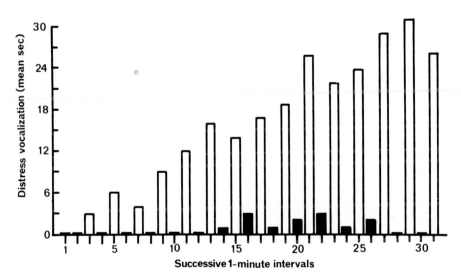

Figure 11-4. The growth of the opponent process (indexed by intensity of distress calling) for the action of an imprinting unconditioned stimulus. This growth function was produced by alternating 1-minute presentations of the unconditioned stimulus with 1-minute absences of it. (From Hoffman et al., 1974. Reprinted by permission.)

Interstimulus Interval (Disuse)

Starr (1978) used the techniques of Hoffman et al., but he varied across several experimental groups the time interval between successive constant-duration presentations. Figure 11-5 shows Starr's findings for (1) a control group that received 6 minutes of continuous exposure to the imprinting object prior to a 1-minute test of distress calling; (2) an experimental group receiving 30-sec exposures separated by a 1-minute interstimulus interval; (3) an experimental group receiving 30-sec exposures separated by a 2-minute interstimulus interval; and (4) an experimental group receiving 30-sec exposures separated by a 5-minute interstimulus interval. Because the three experimental groups received a total of 12 successive exposures, the total familiarity with the imprinting object (the reinforcer) was 6 minutes, the same as that for the control group. Yet, despite this, the distress-calling data varied considerably across the three interstimulus intervals. The 1-minute group approached an asymptote of distress calling very similar to that in the Hoffman et al. (1974) experiment and practically identical to that of Starr's control group, which had received 6 minutes of continuous exposure to the imprinting object. The 2-minute group showed a slow growth of distress calling, but approached an asymptote significantly lower than that for the 1-minute group. Finally, the 5-minute group showed *no growth* of distress calling: their distress remained at the level it was after the first exposure.

From these findings, Starr (1978) inferred the existence of a "critical decay duration of the b-process," defined as that interstimulus interval just long enough to provide sufficient disuse to allow the b-process to decay almost completely after each reinforcement. Thus one could repeat reinforcements frequently, but if they were sufficiently separated in time, the b-process would not be strengthened. As a general principle, this would imply that for any reinforcer, the growth of the strength of an opponent process is not an inevitability. The significance of this conclusion for drug use is obvious: the aversive withdrawal syndrome can be avoided by a judicious choice of interdose interval.

Seaman (1980) asked whether the critical decay duration was ascertainable for morphine tolerance in the rat. The growth of the b-process or opponent process for morphine reinforcement can be indexed either by a tolerance measure or by a withdrawal-syndrome intensity measure. This is true because an increased magnitude of the b-process will render the sum $|a - b|$ small *during* stimulation, so the A state will be small (tolerance), and it will render the B state large directly *after* stimulation is terminated. Seaman inserted indwelling catheters in the carotids of rats. Boluses of morphine were injected via the catheters at preset intervals, and during the period of time right after the injection, when the morphine is an effective analgesic, the rats were given a standard hot-plate analgesia test. One group of rats received their morphine every 8 hours, a second group every 24 hours, a third every 48 hours, and a fourth every 120 hours. The 8-hour group developed tolerance very rapidly, the 120-hour group very slowly, and the other two groups were intermediate. The function relating morphine tolerance to inter-dose time interval is shown in Figure 11-6. In interpreting this graph, remember that the analgesic index is inversely related to tolerance to

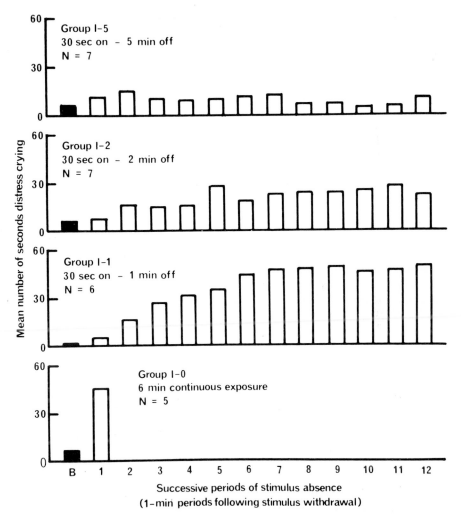

Figure 11-5. The results of Starr's (1978) experiment on distress calling (an index of the b-process) in ducklings as a function of the length of time intervals between presentations of the effective reinforcer (a mother duck). Note that distress calling fails to increase in intensity when the interreinforcer interval is as long as 5 minutes.

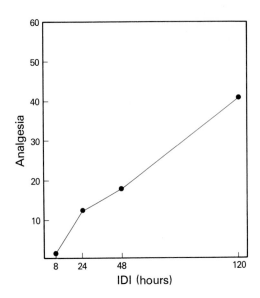

Figure 11-6. The analgesic effect in rats of a single dose of morphine following six previous doses given at different interdose time intervals. Note that tolerance is least for long interdose intervals (IDI). (From Seaman, 1980.)

morphine, because the more tolerant the subject is to the effects of morphine, the less analgesic effect there will be from a dose of morphine.

Seaman also varied dose size, and measured the effect of this variable on morphine tolerance. Four groups of rats received doses of 5 mg/kg, 10 mg/kg, 20 mg/kg, and 40 mg/kg, respectively. Then, after 6 repeated doses at a constant interdose interval the analgesic effect of morphine was measured by the hot-plate test. Tolerance was established more quickly with the larger doses than with the smaller doses. Thus, the rats were more analgesic on the hot plate after 5-mg/kg doses than they were after 40-mg/kg doses, because the morphine was having less of an analgesic effect for the 40-mg/kg condition. We can conclude that dose size as well as interdose interval are crucial in determining the growth of tolerance. By inference, these variables control the growth of the b-process.

Quality of Reinforcement

This variable has not been studied extensively for tolerance or for withdrawal symptoms in drugs. In studies of separation distress in ducklings, Starr (1978) tried to enhance the effectiveness of the imprinting object by adding a honking sound whenever the visual object was presented.

Such a procedure increased the amount of distress calling produced by removal of the imprinting object as compared with the procedure using visual stimulation alone. The interaction of reinforcement quality with interstimulus interval has not been studied either for tolerance or for withdrawal symptoms.

Quality of reinforcement has been shown to be an effective variable in the growth of an opponent process in a very puzzling area of investigation, the so-called adjunctive behaviors. If a hungry rat is given a small pellet of food only once every minute, and a water spout is available during the interpellet interval, gradually, over many sessions and hundreds of reinforcements, postpellet drinking will develop. This slow growth of a tendency to drink will gradually result in hyperdipsia, the consuming of quantities of water far beyond the needs of the rat subject (it is water satiated before each pellet session), far in excess of normal prandial drinking. Such behavior is usually called adjunctive, because it is a motivationally irrelevant or unnecessary addition to the adaptive behavior of the subject. It is a poorly understood behavioral adjunct. The opponent-process model suggests a possible explanation. Suppose that the period directly following each consummation of the tiny food pellet is considered to be a taste-termination event. Because the taste is a positive reinforcer, then its termination should be aversive. Such aversiveness might energize *any* other behaviors made possible by, or potentially elicitable by, contextual features of the eating situation. One such feature is the water spout, which would elicit some, but not much, prandial drinking under the usual conditions of consuming a meal. But with 1-minute interreinforcement intervals, if there were a new source of aversiveness, drinking might be elicited. If an opponent process were the motivation, we would expect it to have its peak effect right after each pellet was consumed and definitely not toward the end of the interpellet interval. Furthermore, the opponent-process magnitude should be greater for high-quality reinforcers (i.e., the more preferred ones). Finally, there should be a limit to how long the interreinforcer interval could be and still support the development of the b-process, a limit suggested by the critical decay duration concept.

Rosellini and Lashley (1980) have tested these predictions in the hyperdipsia experiment. First, they determined the preference hierarchy for four types of food pellets, using a paired-comparisons method. The pellet types were sucrose flavored, a standard flavor called Formula A, peanut flavored, and quinine flavored, preferred in that descending order. When separate groups of rats were exposed to one of these pellet types at 1-minute interpellet intervals, the rate of growth of hyperdipsia was highly predictable on the basis of pellet preference order. The results of two separate pellet-comparison experiments are shown in Figures 11-7 and 11-8. There we have plotted the amount of water drunk during the interpellet intervals for each of the four pellet flavors.

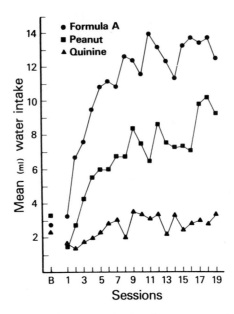

Figure 11-7. A comparison of the growth of and asymptote of hyperdipsic drinking in the rat as a function of the preference value of the food pellets. Here, the most preferred pellet was Formula A, next was the peanut-flavored pellet, and least preferred was the quinine-flavored pellet. The growth of the hyperdipsic drinking was followed over 19 sessions of 30 minutes each. Pellets were presented every 60 sec. The baseline drinking for each flavor, labeled B, was determined by measuring the amount drunk after a full meal of pellets, so-called prandial drinking. (Data taken from Rosellini & Lashley, 1980.)

Note that Formula A and quinine were replicated across the two experiments, and there was a high degree of reproducibility of the absolute amounts of water consumed as well as the rates of growth of the drinking over experimental sessions (compare Figures 11-7 and 11-8). It seems clear that reinforcer quality is importantly involved in hyperdipsic drinking. Rosellini also determined that the hyperdipsic drinking did not develop if the interpellet interval was as long as 5 minutes, using standard pellets. Finally, Rosellini determined that the peak of hyperdipsic drinking occurred during the early seconds of the interpellet interval.

Although hyperdipsic drinking is a strange type of acquired motivation, it certainly does seem to act like many of the opponent-process systems we have studied.

So far, we have discussed a theory of acquired motivation that is strictly psychological in nature. It deals with environmental variations and their consequent behaviors, explained by appeal to psychological (emotional, hedonic, affective) states. It is, however, possible to shift

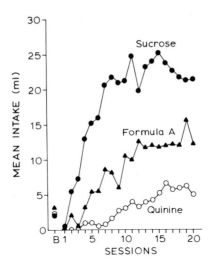

Figure 11-8. Another comparison of the growth of and asymptote of hyperdipsic drinking in the rat as a function of the preference value of the food pellets. Here, the most preferred was the sucrose-flavored pellet, next was Formula A, and least preferred was the quinine-flavored pellet. Note that the absolute asymptote for Formula A for this group of rats was almost identical to that for the rats in Figure 11-7. The same is true for the quinine-flavored pellets. The sucrose-flavored pellets caused enormous water intakes. (Data taken from Rosellini & Lashley, 1980.)

the level of analysis to physiology or to neurochemistry, at the same time retaining the features of the opponent-process system. We can manipulate physiological variables and we can measure either behavioral or physiological dependent variables. Or we can manipulate environmental variables and observe physiological dependent variables. Two examples of the employment of an opponent-process analysis with a physiological variable will illustrate this point.

Schull (1980) studied the effect of naloxone, an opiate receptor blocker, on reported unpleasantness of ischemic pain and cold pressor pain in human subjects. It had been previously determined (Grevert & Goldstein, 1978) that naloxone did not change pain thresholds in human subjects. However, Schull allowed enough experience with the sources of pain to produce some tolerance to them. In that circumstance, naloxone enhanced the unpleasantness judgments. Schull concluded that the opponent process intimately concerned the endogenous opiate system—that it functioned to produce pain tolerance.

Another physiological example is described by Solomon (1980), in analyzing previously gathered data of Church, LoLordo, Solomon, and Turner (1966) and Katcher, Solomon, Turner, LoLordo, Overmier, and Rescorla (1969). The experimenters recorded heart rates of dogs exposed to frightening shocks of 10-sec duration in naive dogs and in "veteran" dogs. The heart rate reactions are shown in Figures 11-9 and 11-10. In Figure 11-9 we see in the upper panel the heart rate increase induced by shock onset. We see that heart rate starts to decline before the shock is terminated. In the bottom panel, we see the heart rate decrease below the baseline rate when the shock is terminated. If we put together in temporal sequence the upper and lower panels, the result is strikingly like the manifest affective response graphed on the left side of Figure 11-3. In Figure 11-10, we see a typical dog who has

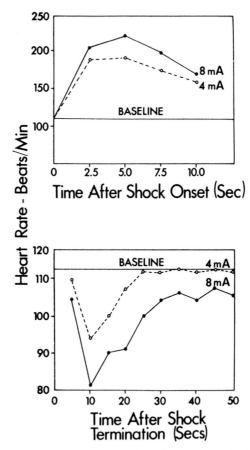

Figure 11-9. In the upper panel are plotted the heart rates of naive dogs stimulated by 10-sec shocks. Note the quick rate increase followed by a decrease even though the shock is still on. Note the larger increase with the more intense stimulus. In the lower panel are plotted the heart rates of the same naive dogs during the time interval directly following shock termination. Note that the rate decline falls below the baseline or resting rate, then it slowly returns to baseline. Note also that the peak of the decline is lower after the termination of the more intense stimulus, thus showing the contrast phenomenon. (These data are adapted from Church et al., 1966.)

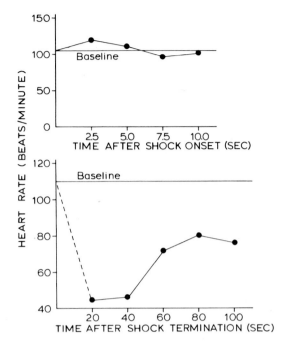

Figure 11-10. Here we see the heart rates of a typical dog from the group represented in Figure 11-9, but after the dog had become a veteran of the shock experience. In the upper panel we see the heart rates during 4-mA shocks. In the lower
panel are the rates during the recovery from shocks. Note that the heart rate increases during the 10-sec shocks were negligible. Note also that the poststimulation
decrease in heart rate was much greater for this veteran dog than it was for the
naive dogs of Figure 11-9. (These data are adapted from the work of Katcher et al.,
1969.)

experienced hundreds of shocks over many daily sessions. The heart
rate acceleration is minimal, as shown in the top panel. The heart rate
decrease is well below the baseline, and it lasts a long time. If we put
together the two panels of Figure 11-10 in temporal sequence, the
result is strikingly like that for the manifest affective response on the
right-hand side of Figure 11-3. These data are strongly in harmony with
the expectations of an opponent-process model of affect.

   The generality of the opponent-process theory of acquired motivation should be tested in a variety of experimental settings. Both positive
and negative reinforcers should be used, and then motivational consequences carefully explored. The theory suggests a standard strategy for
doing this, emphasizing measures of tolerance to stimulus onset and
measures of withdrawal-syndrome quality and intensity when stimuli
are terminated, both measures to be looked at as a function of reinforcer intensity, quality, and duration, and of interreinforcer interval.

Acknowledgments. This research was supported by Grant MH29187, the National Institutes of Health, USPHS.

References

Brown, J. S. Motivation. In E. Hearst (Ed.), *The first century of experimental psychology.* Hillsdale, N.J.: Lawrence Erlbaum Associates, 1979.

Church, R. M., LoLordo, V., Overmier, J. B., Solomon, R. L., & Turner, L. H. Cardiac responses to shock in curarized dogs: Effects of shock intensity and duration, warning signal, and prior experience with shock. *Journal of Comparative and Physiological Psychology*, 1966, *62*, 1-7.

Dethier, V. G. *The hungry fly.* Cambridge, Mass.: Harvard University Press, 1978.

Grevert, P., & Goldstein, A. Endorphins: Naloxone fails to alter experimental pain or mood in humans. *Science*, 1978, *199*, 1093-1095.

Hendry, D. P. *Conditioned reinforcement.* Homewood, Ill.: Dorsey Press, 1969.

Hoffman, H. S., Eiserer, L. A., Ratner, A. M., & Pickering, V. L. The development of distress vocalization during withdrawal of an imprinting stimulus. *Journal of Comparative and Physiological Psychology*, 1974, *86*, 563-568.

Katcher, A. H., Solomon, R. L., Turner, L. H., LoLordo, V. M., Overmier, J. B., & Rescorla, R. A. Heart-rate and blood pressure responses to signaled and unsignaled shocks: Effects of cardiac sympathectomy. *Journal of Comparative and Physiological Psychology*, 1969, *68*, 163-174.

Maier, S. F., Seligman, M. E. P., & Solomon, R. L. Pavlovian fear conditioning and learned helplessness. In B. A. Campbell & R. M. Church (Eds.), *Punishment and aversive behavior.* New York: Appleton-Century-Crofts, 1969.

Rosellini, R. A., & Lashley, R. L. 1980. An opponent-process theory of motivation, VIII: Pellet preference and adjunctive behavior. *Learning Motivation*, 1980,

Schull, J. I. Pain, pleasure and the effects of opiate receptor blockade in humans. Unpublished PhD thesis, University of Pennsylvania, 1980.

Seaman, S. F. Dose size and interdose interval effects on morphine tolerance in the rat. Unpublished PhD thesis, University of Pennsylvania, 1980.

Solomon, R. L. The opponent-process theory of acquired motivation. *American Psychologist*, 1980, *35*, 691-712.

Solomon, R. L., & Corbit, J. D. An opponent-process theory of motivation, II: Cigarette addiction. *Journal of Abnormal Psychology*, 1973, *81*, 158-171.

Starr, M. D. An opponent-process theory of motivation, VI: Time and intensity variables in the development of separation-induced distress calling in ducklings. *Journal of Experimental Psychology: Animal Behavior Processes*, 1978, *4*, 338-355.

Chapter 12

Brain-Stimulated Reward and Control of Autonomic Function: Are They Related?

RONNIE HALPERIN and DONALD W. PFAFF

Intracranial self-stimulation (ICSS) was originally believed to be the result of activation of a *forebrain* reward mechanism. However, since its initial discovery, ICSS has been shown to be a more ubiquitous phenomenon, occurring at virtually every level of the brain, and at brain sites associated with a variety of functions. Thus, the hope of understanding ICSS as a unitary brain phenomenon related to a naturally occurring event or set of events seems even further from reach. In this chapter, we treat ICSS as a homogeneous entity and, as such, try to relate it to the organizing principles derived from the understanding of brain control of autonomic function (Hess, 1954). In the first section we provide a brief historical review of the literature relating ICSS to other brain and/or behavioral events. In the second section we review the organization of forebrain control of autonomic function, regulatory behaviors, and behavior controlled through the autonomic nervous system. Finally, we entertain a hypothesis that relates brain control of ICSS and autonomic function. Although our simple and straightforward attempt to link these two areas does not provide a simple answer, it suggests experiments that would shed light on the question of whether a known functional system is the mediating mechanisms underlying brain-stimulated reward.

Intracranial Self-Stimulation

In 1954 Olds and Milner discovered that rats would learn an operant response if electrical brain stimulation were made contingent upon that response. Initially, they and others (Caggiula & Hoebel, 1966; Herberg,

1963; Hoebel & Teitelbaum, 1962; Margules & Olds, 1962; Olds, 1958a) explained this phenomenon by suggesting that the neural tissue activated by the electrical stimulation was similarly excited in other learning situations in response to naturally occurring reinforcers such as food, water, and an appropriate mate. The phenomenon of intracranial self-stimulation (ICSS) held the promise of providing a way to directly study the neural mechanisms mediating learning and motivation.

Reinforcement Theories of ICSS

ICSS was first studied in the context of experimental paradigms previously used to study responding contingent upon other reinforcers. Using this framework, investigators attempted to explore ICSS response parameters during a variety of stimulus conditions. Initial comparisons of brain stimulation to other reinforcers revealed that according to most criteria brain stimulation was a potent reinforcer. Animals exhibited rapid acquisition and maintained high rates of responding (Olds & Milner, 1954). In addition, they preferred brain stimulation to other reinforcers (Falk, 1961; Spies, 1965), and would respond for long periods of time without exhibiting satiation (Olds, 1958c). Paradoxically, animals did not maintain rapid response rates when placed on more demanding work schedules (Sidman, Brady, Conrad, & Schulman, 1955; Brady, 1960), and they exhibited rapid extinction when responding was no longer followed by brain stimulation (Olds, 1955; Seward, Uyeda, & Olds, 1959). Figure 12-1 demonstrates the high response rate, relative insatiability, and rapid extinction observed in response to electrical brain stimulation. In contrast to observations with other reinforcers, when a neutral stimulus was paired with electrical brain stimulation, that stimulus did not acquire secondary reinforcing properties (Seward, Uyeda, & Olds, 1959; but see also Mogenson, 1965; Stein, 1958). Finally, when animals were placed in the test chamber, after repeated test sessions they often did not initiate responding unless they were "primed" with a few noncontingent trains of brain stimulation (Gallistel, 1964; Lilly, 1958). Early research on ICSS was based on theoretical models focused on explaining deviations in the way animals responded to electrical brain stimulation as compared to natural reinforcers. This was accomplished by adapting already existing explanations of learning to the special circumstances of ICSS.

We will discuss two predominant theoretical approaches that incorporate the basic mechanisms utilized by most of the ICSS theorists at that time. Gallistel (1973) provides a comprehensive review of this subject. The hedonic or incentive model proposed that stimulus conditions exert total control over responding, a view that is traceable to reinforcement theories of Skinner (1938) and Thorndike (1911). Specifically, it hypothesizes the existence of a reinforcement system that

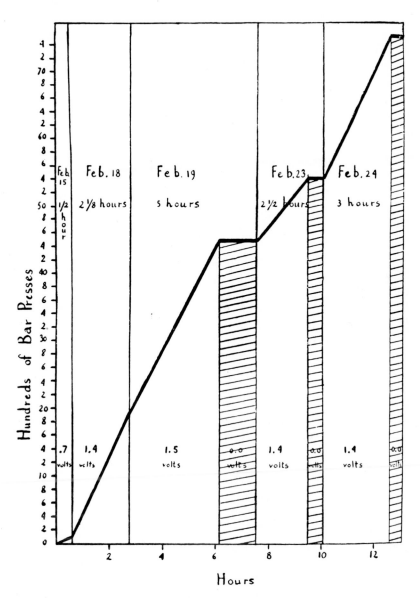

Figure 12-1. Cumulative response curve exhibited by one rat during acquisition, maintenance on continuous reinforcement, and extinction. (From Olds & Milner, 1954.)

is responsive to rewarding stimuli. Further, the reward signal is channeled through a positive feedback loop, so that when a response is followed by a rewarding stimulus, the probability of that response recurring is increased (see Figure 12-2). Olds and Olds (1965) and Stein (1964) applied this model to explain ICSS by proposing that

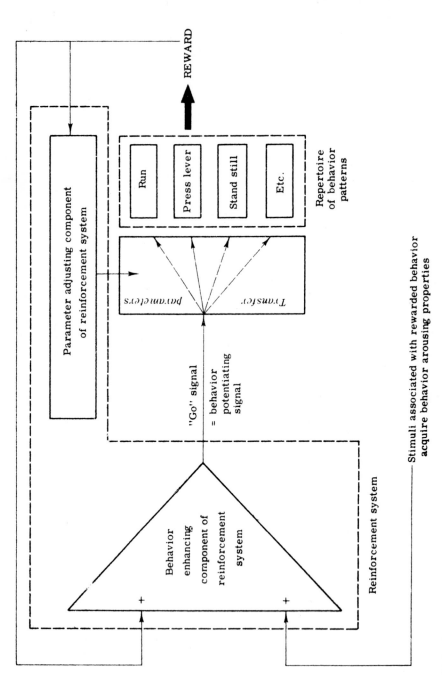

Figure 12-2. Schematic of hedonic model described by Gallistel (1973). Behavior is determined by a reinforcement system that detects reward and detects the behavior upon which reward is contingent. The occurrence of reward increases the amount of behavior exhibited. (From Gallistel, 1973.)

electrical brain stimulation is activating the neural tissue ordinarily excited by other reinforcers (see Figure 12-3). Therefore, since a particular operant response is always followed by brain stimulation, the probability of that response occurring is continually increased. Although this model provides a parsimonious explanation of the acquisition and maintenance of reinforced operant responding, Gallistel (1973) has pointed out that it has been classically associated with certain difficulties. Specifically, it is not clear why an animal ever terminates responding once it has begun, and why, once terminated, a response would ever be initiated again. Furthermore, it is not clear to us how the reinforcement system determines which response is rewarded. As regards the application of this model to the ICSS phenomenon, these very limitations in explaining behavior associated with natural reinforcers become assets in explaining the anomalies associated with the ICSS response. For example, this theory explains why animals needed to be primed, why the response is insatiable, the failure of animals to respond to demanding schedules of reinforcement, and rapid extinction. However, it does not explain ICSS in a manner that sheds new light on behavior in response to natural reinforcers.

The homeostatic model of ICSS, proposed by Deutsch and Howarth (1963), applied concepts used by "drive" theorists who attempted to explain motivated behavior (Hull, 1943; Miller, 1961; Deutsch, 1960). Unlike the hedonic model, behavior according to this theory is under the control of both stimulus conditions (i.e., reward) and biological variables. Thus, a drive mechanism energizes behavior when certain biological conditions deviate from a homeostatic set point. In addition, a reinforcement mechanism is proposed to be responsive to stimulus conditions and to exert control over response strength. Thus, according

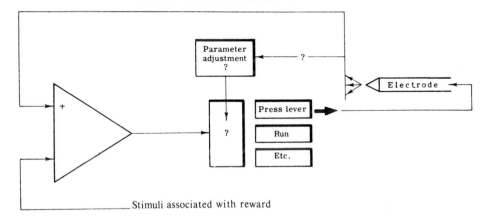

Figure 12-3. Schematic depicts the application of the hedonic model in explaining brain-stimulated reward. Components of the system are identical to those in Figure 12-2. (From Gallistel, 1973.)

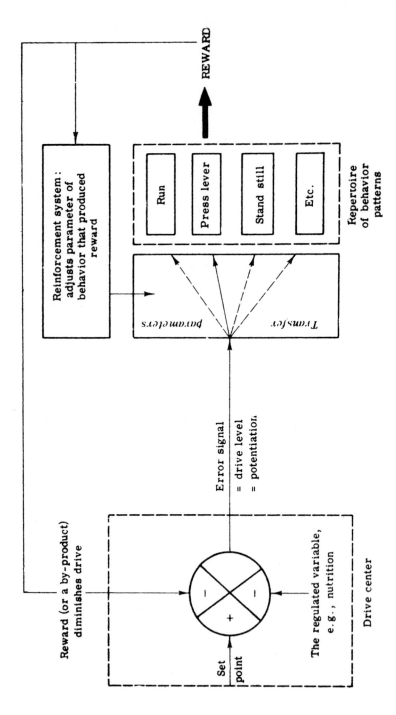

Figure 12-4. Schematic depicts the homeostatic model of reinforcement proposed by Deutsch and Howarth (1963) as described by Gallistel (1973). According to this model the drive center energizes behavior and the reinforcement system selects the behavior upon which reward is contingent. The output of the drive center is a function of the existing deviation from the homeostatic set point. The occurrence of reward reduces the output of the drive system but increases the output from the reinforcement system. (From Gallistel, 1973.)

to this model, reward has the dual effect of bringing biological conditions closer to the homeostatic set point, and increasing the probability of the response with which it is temporally associated (see Figure 12-4). Deutsch and Howarth (1963) proposed that during ICSS electrical brain stimulation activates the neural substrates of the drive and the reinforcement mechanisms (see Figure 12-5). Therefore, during electrical brain stimulation and natural reward, the reinforcement mechanism is activated in the same way, but the drive mechanism is affected in exactly the opposite direction by brain stimulation and natural reinforcers. Thus, while natural reinforcers decrease drive, ICSS increases drive. This explains the paradoxes encountered in trying to determine the potency of brain stimulation as a reinforcer in comparison to other reinforcers. Most important, the homeostatic model explains ICSS in a context that is applicable to other motivated behavior.

We find two problems inherent in this model. First, as in the case of the hedonic model, it is not clear how the reinforcement system determines which response is rewarded. The second problem involves the fact that the reward signal is channeled independently to the drive and

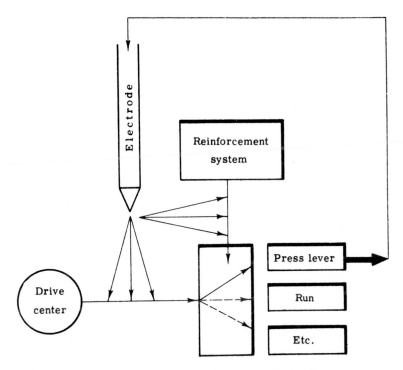

Figure 12-5. Schematic represents the application of Deutsch's homeostatic model to ICSS. The stimulation electrode excites both the drive and reinforcement systems. (From Gallistel, 1973).

reinforcement mechanisms (see Figure 12-4). Our understanding of reward according to this model is that it is defined as a stimulus that reduces drive. Since the power of this model in explaining the anomalies of ICSS rests upon the independence of the drive and reward mechanisms, we feel that it falls short of reaching its intended goal.

The hedonic and homeostatic models are representative of the attempt to understand the neural substrate of motivated behavior by studying response parameters to electrical brain stimulation and presuming its equivalence to natural reinforcers. This approach to studying ICSS waned in the early 1970s when it became apparent that this presumption may not be valid. Trowill, Panksepp, and Gandelman (1969) reviewed data demonstrating the significance of variables such as magnitude and delay of reinforcement and level of pretraining deprivation in determining the response parameters investigators were measuring. For example, they cite studies by several investigators (Gibson, Reid, Sakai, & Porte, 1965; McIntyre & Wright, 1965; Pliskoff, Wright, & Hawkins, 1965; Terman & Kling, 1968) which demonstrated that by varying the delay of presentation of natural reinforcers one can account for the puzzling phenomenon of rapid extinction observed during ICSS. Beninger, Bellisle, and Milner (1977) have recently shown that rats will perform under demanding work schedules, and that priming is not needed to initiate responding. Thus, it appeared difficult to equate brain stimulation reward with other reinforcers. Furthermore, evidence for a physiological basis of the mechanisms hypothesized in these models was not forthcoming.

Neurotransmitter Theories of ICSS

Further investigation of the ICSS phenomenon focused on testing whether already known neural systems mediated ICSS. Initially, this approach took the form of testing the role of various neurotransmitters in the mediation of ICSS. The first, and most extensively studied, neurotransmitter system was the ascending norepinephrine (NE) system (Arbuthnott, 1976; Crow, 1972, 1973; Poschel & Ninteman, 1963; German & Bowden, 1974; Stein, 1969). The hypothesis that reward is mediated by the release of NE into the synapse was based, initially, on the correspondences of ICSS-sensitive brain sites and brain sites at which NE could be found (German & Bowden, 1974). Figure 12-6 illustrates the brain sites that support ICSS on coronal sections which also illustrate the distribution of NE-containing cell bodies, fiber, and terminals. Strong ICSS sites include forebrain structures such as the septum, the diagonal band of Broca, the medial forebrain bundle, and the posterior hypothalamus (Olds & Olds, 1963; see also German & Bowden, 1974, for a review). In the midbrain, the ventral tegmental

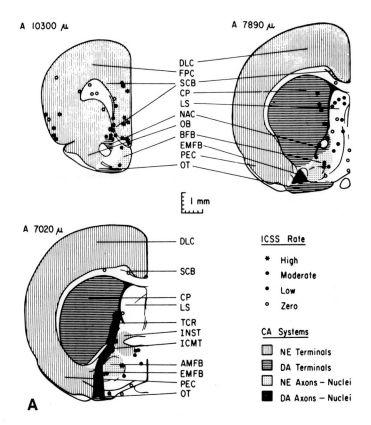

Figure 12-6. Coronal sections mapping (A) telencephalic, (B) diencelphalic, and (C) mesencephalic sites in the rat brain at which ICSS has been explored. The same sections also show the distribution of brain catecholamines. (From German & Bowden, 1974.) Abbreviations: A1, A2, A5, A7: origin of ventral NE system; A6: origin of dorsal NE system (locus coeruleus); A8, A9: origin of nigrostriatal DA systems; A10: origin of mesolimbic DA system; ADNB: anterior dorsal noradrenergic bundle; AMFB: anterior medial forebrain bundle; AMGC: amygdala, n. centralis; AMYG: amygdala, excepting n. centralis; AVNB: anterior ventral noradrenergic bundle; BFB: basal forebrain bundle; CER: cerebellum; CG: central grey; CP: caudate putamen; CVTB: common ventral tegmental bundle; DLC: dorsal and lateral cortex; DNB: dorsal adrenergic bundle; EMFB: external medial forebrain bundle; FPC: frontal pole cortex; HIPP: hippocampus; HT (BL): hypothalamus, basolateral end; HT (PV): hypothalamus, periventricular areas; ICMT: internal capsule, medial tip; INST: interstitial nucleus of stria terminalis; LS: lateral septal area; MGB: medial geniculate body; NAC: nucleus accumbens; NMRF: noradrenergic midbrain reticular formation; OB: olfactory bulb; OT: olfactory tubercle; PC: posterior commissure; PCNB: posterior common noradrenergic bundle; PEC: pyriform and entorhinal cortices and claustrum; PMFB: posterior medial forebrain bundle; PNB: posterior noradrenergic bundle; RN: raphe nuclei; SCB: supracallosal bundle; SCP: superior cerebellar peduncle; ST: stria terminalis; TCR: transcapsular ratiation; VNB: ventral noradrenergic bundle. (From German & Bowden, 1974.)

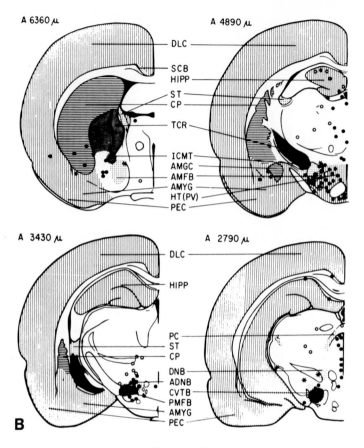

Figure 12-6

area of Tsai, the central grey, and the area just lateral to central grey
support ICSS (Crow, 1972). NE terminals or fibers of passage are found
in all of these sites (see German & Bowden, 1974). Sensitive sites in the
pons include the locus coeruleus (Crow, Spear, & Arbuthnott, 1972;
Farber, Steiner, & Ellman, 1972), the cell bodies of origin of almost
all cortical NE (see Amaral & Sinnamon, 1977, for a review), and the
area around the brachium conjunctivum (Routtenberg & Malsbury,
1969). The medullary area near the nucleus of the solitary tract, which
contains the A_2 noradrenergic cell group (Lindvall & Bjorklund, 1974;
Ungerstedt, 1971), has been shown to support ICSS at high frequencies
of stimulation (Carter & Phillips, 1975).

That ICSS could be obtained from the locus coeruleus (Crow et al.,
1972; Farber et al., 1972) and along the path of its major efferent
projections to the forebrain (Lindvall & Bjorklund, 1974), the dorsal
noradrenergic bundle (Segal & Bloom, 1976), was deemed a strong

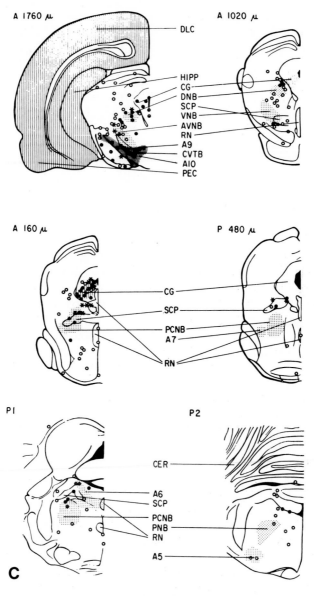

A 1760 μ   A 1020 μ

DLC

HIPP
CG
DNB
SCP
VNB
AVNB
RN
A9
CVTB
A10
PEC

A 160 μ   P 480 μ

CG

SCP

PCNB
A7

RN

P1   P2

CER

A6
SCP

PCNB
PNB
RN

A5

C

Figure 12-6

argument favoring a mediating role of NE in brain-stimulated reward. Further evidence for this hypothesis stemmed from the fact that the medial forebrain bundle, which appears to be the most potent ICSS site (Valenstein, Cox, & Kakolewski, 1970), is the point of convergence of brain NE systems (Lindvall & Bjorklund, 1974; Ungerstedt, 1971). Furthermore, brain stimulation in rewarding sites in the locus coeruleus increased the utilization and turnover of cortical NE (see Arbuthnott, 1976, for a review). Finally, injection of pharmacological agents, such as amphetamine (Stein, 1964) and alpha-methyl-m-tyrosine in conjunction with monoamine oxidase inhibitors (Stein, 1966) that enhance functional brain NE also enhances ICSS; whereas drugs such as 6-hydroxydopamine (6-OHDA) (Breese, Howard, & Leahy, 1971), alpha-methyl-p-tyrosine (Poschel & Ninteman, 1966), and reserpine (Olds, 1959) that decrease functional brain NE inhibit ICSS. (But see Crow's discussion (1976) of the limitations on inferences from these data.)

That the ventral noradrenergic bundle and its cell bodies of origin (A_1, A_2, and A_3) were not originally found to support ICSS was considered a major drawback of the NE hypothesis (Crow, 1976). However, Ritter and Stein (1975) have demonstrated ICSS in the ventral noradrenergic bundle, and the medullary A_2 neurons have been shown to support ICSS at high frequencies (Carter & Phillips, 1975).

A number of investigators (e.g., Corbett & Wise, 1980) noted that in the forebrain and midbrain, the distribution of dopamine (DA) corresponded to sites that supported ICSS. It was shown that pharmacological manipulations favored a mediating role for DA over NE (see Wise, 1978a, for a review). Many of the drug studies that were originally interpreted as implicating a role of NE (e.g., Stein, 1969) were reinterpreted as affecting DA as well (Phillips & Fibiger, 1973; Phillips, Brooke, & Fibiger, 1975). Receptor blocking agents that have a strong affinity specifically for DA receptors, such as spiroperidol and pimozide (Janssen, Niemegeers, Schellekens, Dress, Lenaerts, Pinchard, Schaper, Van Neuten, & Verbruggen, 1968), were found to abolish ICSS (see Wauquier, 1976, for a review). Moreover, the substantia nigra, a site rich in DA-containing cell bodies, was found to support ICSS (Crow, 1972; Phillips, Carter, & Fibiger, 1976). Ritter and Stein (1975) argued that ICSS from electrodes in the region of the A_9 DA-containing neurons was actually mediated by ascending noradrenergic fibers of passage. Stein showed that (a) ICSS could be supported from areas of the ventral noradrenergic bundle that were caudal to any known DA neurons, and (b) 6-OHDA lesions caudal to A_9 resulted in abolition of ICSS from A_9. However, this finding is difficult to interpret because the animals recovered the ICSS response 2 weeks after the lesion.

In an attempt to accommodate the pharmacological data which indicated that the integrity of the DA synapse was critical for the manifestation of ICSS, and the fact that brain-stem sites caudal to any known DA neurons supported ICSS, Crow (1976) and Herberg, Stephens, and Franklin (1976) proposed DA–NE interaction hypotheses. They suggested that DA was necessary for the manifestation of ICSS (and functionally equivalent to incentive), while NE signaled the final attainment of reward (and was functionally equivalent to drive). Antelman and

Caggiula (1977) have suggested that a variety of behaviors (including ICSS) in an aroused animal are facilitated by the suppression of NE and/or the enhancement of DA systems. Although their model uniquely explains reports of enhanced ICSS after locus coeruleus lesions (Farber, Ellman, Mattiace, Holtzman, Ippolito, Halperin, & Steiner, 1976; Koob, Balcom, & Meyerhoff, 1976), it fails to accommodate a large portion of pharmacological data (see above).

In light of the fact that ICSS could be obtained from hindbrain sites, one major problem with the notion of DA-containing neurons and fibers as the sole substrate of brain-stimulation reward is that at those sites there are no DA neurons. Clavier (1976) has refuted the catecholamine (CA) hypotheses and has proposed the existence of a descending noncatecholaminergic ICSS system. Clavier and Routtenberg (1976) showed that bilateral lesions of the locus coeruleus did not abolish ICSS from the dorsal noradrenergic bundle. Farber et al. (1976) also showed that whereas some hypothalamic sites became insensitive to ICSS after lesions of the locus coeruleus, ICSS in medial forebrain bundle (MFB) sites was actually enhanced by these lesions. Moreover, electrolytic (Corbett, Skelton, & Wise, 1977) or 6-OHDA (Clavier, Fibiger, & Phillips, 1976) lesions of the dorsal noradrenergic bundle did not abolish ICSS in the locus coeruleus. These findings refute the notion that a noradrenergic system arising from pontine cell groups provides the neural substrate for ICSS. Moreover, Wise (1978b) has more recently shown, through a series of rate-independent preference tests, that the ICSS response abolition observed after injection of pimozide is, in large part, due to performance-related changes caused by that drug. Furthermore, Clavier and Fibiger (1977) have shown that ICSS from the zona compacta region of the substantia nigra is only transiently affected by 6-OHDA lesions of the nigrostriatal bundle.

The usefulness of inferences based on the correlation of ICSS sites and neurotransmitter distribution in the brain is limited at best. However, that these systems may indeed have an important relationship to ICSS systems is suggested by the pharmacological data and by the findings that animals will self-administer (peripherally or intraventricularly) drugs such as amphetamines (Davis & Smith, 1975) and cocaine (Pickens & Thompson, 1968), which are known to act primarily at CA receptors. It has recently been shown that animals will self-administer amphetamine directly to the nucleus accumbens (Hoebel & Monaco, 1981), a site rich in NE and DA terminals, and NE to the perifornical hypothalamus (Cytawa, Jurkowleniec, & Bialowas, 1980).

More recent investigations suggest that the rewarding effects of opiates may be mediated by positive ICSS sites. This assertion is based in part on the fact that there is a strong correlation between sites that support ICSS and opiate receptor density. ICSS sites in the medial thalamus and the globus pallidus were correctly predicted to exist on the basis of their characterizations as having high opiate receptor density (Stein & Belluzzi, 1979). Many studies have shown that morphine, as well as other agonist injections result in an initial suppression and a subsequent facilitation of ICSS (for a review see Esposito & Kornetsky, 1978). The suppression appears to be attributable to the sedative effects of the drug and exhibits tolerance over repeated drug administrations. The subsequent facilitation appears to be independent of nonspecific performance variables, and does not exhibit tolerance after repeated drug administration (Adams, Lorens, & Mitchell, 1972; Bush, Bush, Miller, & Reid, 1976). Both the suppressive and facilitative effects of morphine on ICSS can be reversed by naloxone (Holtzman, 1976; Nelson, Brutus, Wilson, Farrell, Ocheret, Ellman, & Steiner, 1977). The facilitative effect of morphine on ICSS occurs about 90 minutes after drug injection if rate-free measures (such as threshold) are used (Esposito & Kornetsky, 1977a, 1977b). This corresponds well with the time course of the euphoric effects of morphine in humans. That tolerance does not develop to the facilitative effects of morphine on ICSS has led several investigators to suggest ICSS as a model for drug addiction (see Esposito & Kornetsky, 1978).

While morphine has been shown to facilitate ICSS in the periaqueductal grey, the lateral hypothalamic MFB, the locus coeruleus, the substantia nigra, and the nucleus accumbens, naloxone has been shown to depress ICSS in all of these sites with the exception of the lateral hypothalamic MFB (Stapleton, Merriman, Coogle, Gelbard, & Reid, 1979). Since high levels of catecholamines, as well as opiate receptors, are found at most ICSS sites, the interactive effects of endorphins and catecholamines have been suggested as critical to the mediation of rewarding brain stimulation. Pert and Hulsebus (1975) have shown that the facilitative effects of morphine on ICSS are blocked by prior administration of alpha-methyl-p-tyrosine, a drug that inhibits synthesis of catecholamines. The inferences to be gained on the basis of the correlation of neurochemical substrate and positive ICSS site are limited. However, the rate-free measures provide promising data suggesting that alterations of opiate systems affect the sensitivity of ICSS systems. For example, Esposito, Perry, and Kornetsky (1980) have shown that low doses of naloxone block the threshold-lowering effect of d-amphetamine on ICSS. Further understanding of the mechanism mediating the intracerebral self-administration of morphine may shed further light on the link between opiate systems and brain-stimulation reward.

Relationship of ICSS to Specific Motivational States

It was hypothesized that the neural mechanisms mediating the rewarding effects of brain stimulation also mediate reward during specific motivational states in natural circumstances (Hoebel, 1969). This

notion gained support from the fact that organized patterns of motivated behavior could be elicited in response to hypothalamic brain
stimulation (Caggiula, 1970; MacDonnell & Flynn, 1966; Miller, 1960;
Mogenson, Gentil, & Stevenson, 1971; Vaughan & Fisher, 1962). For
example, lateral hypothalamic brain stimulation elicits a motivated
eating response (Miller, 1960). Brain sites at which this response can be
elicited also always support ICSS (although not all lateral hypothalamic
ICSS sites support eating in response to brain stimulation) (Hoebel &
Teitelbaum, 1962; Margules & Olds, 1962). Similarly, stimulation of
the posterior hypothalamus can result in a copulatory response in male
rats, and those brain sites from which this response is elicited support
ICSS (Caggiula & Hoebel, 1966). In support of the notion that ICSS at
different brain loci is linked to specific motivational states are findings
that the sensitivity of the ICSS response can be altered by physiological
manipulations that alter specific motivated responses. For example,
insulin injection and the presence of food each enhance lateral hypothalamic CSS. ICSS at posterior hypothalamic and septal sites is not influenced by variables affecting feeding (Caggiula, 1967; Hoebel, 1976);
lateral hypothalamic ICSS rates are decreased after a meal, intragastric
infusion of a nutritive stomach load, or glucagon injection (see Figure
12-7). Conversely, castration in male rats depresses ICSS from brain
sites in the posterior hypothalamus but not the lateral hypothalamus.
Testosterone injections reverse the effect of castration on ICSS (see
Figure 12-8) (Caggiula, 1967).

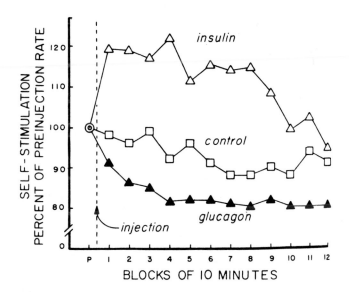

Figure 12-7. Change in the rate of lateral hypothalamic ICSS after injection of
glucagon or insulin. (From Balagura & Hoebel, 1967).

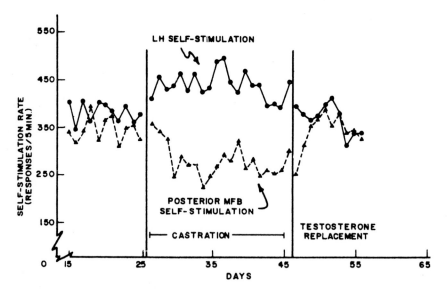

Figure 12-8. Differential effect of castration on rate of ICSS from lateral and posterior hypothalamic sites. Injection of testosterone restores preoperative response rate in rats with electrodes in the posterior hypothalamus. (From Caggiula, 1967.)

    Valenstein, Cox, and Kakolewski (see 1970 for a review) have shown that more than one "motivated" response can be elicited from a single hypothalamic brain site, and this would argue against the idea that these sites are linked to individual motivational states (but see Wise, 1974). Furthermore, peripheral injection of some drugs has been shown to have opposite effects on eating and ICSS elicited from the lateral hypothalamus. For example, amphetamine (a known anorexic agent) enhances ICSS (Stein, 1964) but suppresses eating (Stark & Totty, 1967) in response to brain stimulation. Injection of picrotoxin (a drug known to block receptors for GABA) enhances eating and inhibits ICSS elicited by lateral hypothalamic brain stimulation (Porrino & Coons, 1980). Hoebel maintains, nonetheless, that ICSS is linked to specific motivational functions. Hoebel and co-workers have shown that phenylpropanolamine (an appetite suppressant structurally similar to amphetamine, but without the enhancing effects on activity levels) injected to a lateral hypothalamic site that supports ICSS, eating, and drinking in response to brain stimulation depressed ICSS and elicited eating but had no effect on drinking in response to electrical brain stimulation (Hoebel, Hernandez, & Thompson, 1975; Kornblith & Hoebel, 1976). Experiments along these lines have not, to date, addressed the question of the role of extrahypothalamic brain sites in reward and motivation. The questions arise whether reward at these brain sites represents an independent ICSS system and whether it can be linked to naturally occurring behavior.

Hypothalamic Control of Behavior

It has been well documented, through studies utilizing brain stimulation (see Miller, 1960, 1965), lesion (see Teitelbaum, 1961, for a review), and recording techniques (Oomura, Ooyama, Naka, Yamamoto, Ono, & Kobayashi, 1967), that the hypothalamus plays an important role in controlling certain behaviors. Electrical or chemical stimulation of the hypothalamus can result in the enhancement or attenuation of a variety of behavioral responses. The magnitude and direction of these response alterations are dependent upon the specific stimulation locus within the hypothalamus (e.g., Leibowitz, 1978), the stimulation parameters (e.g., Ball, 1974; Wise, 1968), and the existing physiological and/or environmental conditions (Valenstein et al., 1970).

For example, a variety of hypothalamic manipulations, in addition to electrical stimulation of the lateral hypothalamus, can stimulate feeding in a satiated rat. They include injection of norepinephrine to the anteromedial hypothalamus (Davis & Keesey, 1971; Booth, 1967; Leibowitz, 1978), lesion of the ventromedial hypothalamic area (see Miller, Bailey, & Stevenson, 1950, for a review), and parasagittal hypothalamic knife cut just medial to the fornix (Sclafani, Berner, & Maul, 1973). These stimulated eating responses are characterized by increased taste responsivity (Tenen & Miller, 1964) and are dependent on the integrity of the vagus nerve (see Gold, Sawchenko, De Luca, Alexander, & Eng, 1980; Powley, 1977; Powley, MacFarlane, Markell & Opsahl, 1978; Sawchenko, Leibowitz, & Gold, 1981). Feeding in deprived, but not satiated, rats can be enhanced by injection of dopamine (DA) to the far-lateral hypothalamus (Friedman & Coons, 1979; Leibowitz & Rossakis, 1979).

Conversely, feeding can be inhibited in hungry rats through electrical stimulation of the ventromedial hypothalamic area (Anand & Brobeck, 1951), injection of dopamine or epinephrine to the midlateral (perifornical) hypothalamus (Leibowitz & Rossakis, 1979) or lesion of the lateral hypothalamic area (see Teitelbaum, 1961). Evidence suggests that feeding alterations produced by central drug injection are mediated by postsynaptic receptors in the sensitive hypothalamic sites (see Leibowitz, 1976, for a review). In the case of electrical stimulation and lesion experiments, however, the role of hypothalamic neurons, as opposed to that of extrahypothalamic fibers of passage, has not been specified. Recent studies utilizing injection of kainic acid to the lateral hypothalamus suggest a significant role for hypothalamic neurons in the feeding syndromes seen after electrolytic lesion of that brain region (e.g., Grossman, Dacey, Halares, Collier, & Routtenberg, 1978). Perhaps the most convincing evidence that hypothalamic neurons are part of a homeostatic mechanism controlling feeding comes from the studies of Rolls. He has recorded, in the hypothalamus of monkeys, units that fire selectively to the sight of food, as opposed to other "arousing" stimuli. Furthermore, he has shown that these units fire selectively when the animal is hungry (Rolls, 1976).

Another set of examples comes from reproductive behavior. Cells in and near the ventromedial nucleus of the hypothalmus receive estrogen and facilitate female reproductive behavior (Pfaff, 1980). Preoptic neurons are required for male reproductive behavior (Malsbury & Pfaff, 1974), not only in rats but in a variety of species (Kelley & Pfaff, 1978).

Hypothalamic mechanisms also influence drinking, thermoregulation, aggression, and a variety of species-specific responses in the rat, such as grooming, sniffing, rearing, and locomotion. (For a range of examples see Morgane & Panksepp, 1980.)

Hypothalamic Control of Autonomic Responses

The hypothalamus has been shown to exert an important influence on the viscera through the autonomic nervous system. The original mapping of basal forebrain sites controlling these physiological responses came from the pioneering work of Hess (1954). In his experiments, Hess stimulated thousands of brain sites in hundreds of animals (cats) and measured changes in heart rate, blood pressure, respiration, pupillodilation, micturition, defecation, salivation, eating automatisms such as chewing and licking, sneezing, panting, and defensive movements. Stimulation of the area that Hess designated as the ergotropic sector activates the sympathetic nervous system. The area designated as the trophotropic sector activates the parasympathetic nervous system. The ergotropic (or sympathetic) areas fall mainly in the medial and posterior hypothalamus, including the dorsomedial and ventromedial nuclei, mamillary bodies, and the periventricular system. The trophotropic (or parasympathetic) zone corresponds to the septum, basal forebrain, preoptic area, anterior medial forebrain bundle, and the medial anterior thalamus.

Physiological responses that Hess characterized as "ergotropic," and which we will refer to as "sympathetic," are increased heart rate, respiration, and blood pressure; and pupillodilation. Responses classified as "trophotropic," and which we will refer to as "parasympathetic," include decreased heart rate, respiration, and blood pressure; pupilloconstriction; micturition; defecation; eating automatisms; salivation; and vomiting. Figure 12-9 represents schemata of sagittal sections of the cat brain in which Hess localized control of blood pressure. He constructed comparable maps for all the responses he studied.

Hess' work suggests that autonomic responses compatible with eating are parasympathetic. For example, chewing automatisms, vasoconstriction (in the extremities), and salivation occur during parasympathetic activation. In agreement with this idea, the findings of Beattie and Sheehan (1934) suggest that stimulation of the anterior hypothalamus results in increased gastric pressure (reflecting increased motility). Stimulation of the same site resulted in a drop in blood pressure. Furthermore, stimulation of the vagus nerve resulted in a similar response but of greater magnitude and shorter latency. Vagotomy abolished the hypothalamically stimulated increase in gastric pressure as well as the decrease in blood pressure. Conversely, stimulation of the posterior hypothalamus (which exerts sympathetic control according to the maps of Hess) resulted in decreased gastric pressure and increased blood pressure. Vagotomy had no effect on these responses. Beattie and Sheehan therefore conclude that the hypothalamically stimulated increase in gastric pressure and decrease in blood pressure are vagally mediated parasympathetic responses, while the responses to posterior hypothalamic stimulation are probably mediated by the sympathetic splanchnic nerve.

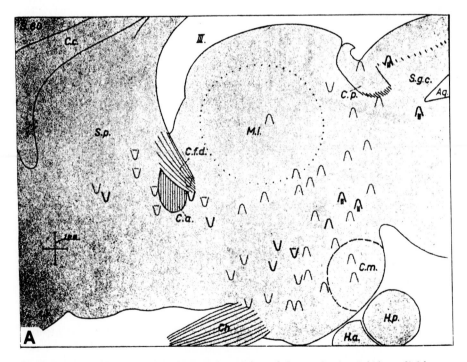

Figure 12-9. Schematic of parasagittal sections of the cat brain at (A) medial hypothalamic, (B) midlateral hypothalamic, and (C) lateral hypothalamic levels. Changes in blood pressure response to electrical stimulation at several loci are indicated. Both keys apply to Figures 12-9A, 12-9B, and 12-9C. (From Hess, 1954.)

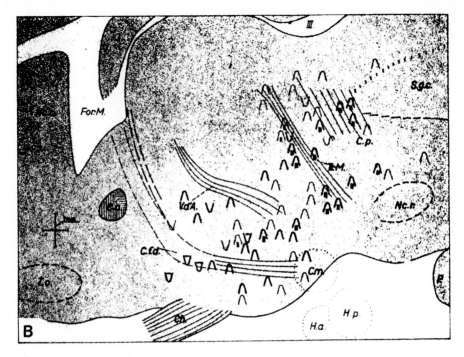

∧ *Blood pressure rise*

∧ *Blood pressure rise with increase in heart rate*

∨ *Blood pressure drop*

Figure 12-9

More recent evidence in agreement with the notion that hypothalamic zones are organized according to a variety of sympathetic and parasympathetic responses comes from the work of Shimazu, Fukada, and Ban (1966). They found that stimulation of the ventromedial hypothalamus resulted in increased blood sugar levels. Subsequent analysis of the liver revealed a concomitant decrease in liver glycogen. This suggests that the hypothalamically stimulated increase in blood sugar can result from glycogenolysis (correlated with sympathetic functions).

More recently, physiologists have tended to restrict each experiment to the study of one or two brain sites, and only a few responses. These experiments provide further information as to the specific autonomic pathways through which the studied responses are mediated. For example, the parasympathetic nervous system generally activated responses that facilitate digestive processes, while sympathetic responses are compatible with a suppression of the digestive process. Misher and Brooks

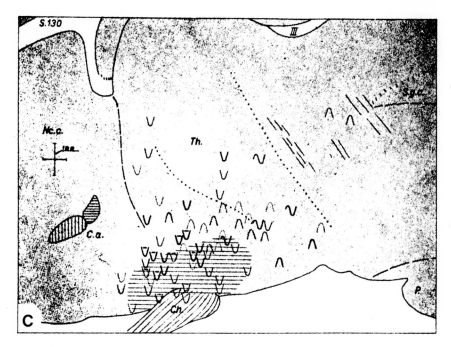

$\bigvee$ Blood pressure drop with decrease in heart rate

$\bigwedge\!\!\bigvee$ Blood pressure drop preceded by pressor wave (diphasic response)

$\bigvee\!\!\bigwedge$ Blood pressure drop with return to normal level before cessation of stimulus

Figure 12-9

(1966) have shown that lateral hypothalamic stimulation (parasympathetic zone) results in increased volume and acidity of gastric secretions. Furthermore, they show that this response is abolished by vagotomy. Shiraishi (1980) has provided electrophysiological evidence that hypothalamically stimulated gastric acid secretion is mediated through the medullary dorsal vagal nucleus.

When a behavioral response and a related autonomic response are stimulated from the same brain site it is tempting to conclude that the behavioral response resulting from the brain stimulation is mediated by the autonomic effects of the stimulation. However, this need not necessarily be the case. An example of how this line of reasoning can be misleading is found in understanding the control, by the supraoptic nucleus, of thirst and ADH release. Increased blood tonicity, stimulation of carotid chemoreceptors, and absence of stimulation of carotid baroreceptors can each result in almost immediate drinking and ADH release. Vasopressin acts on the kidneys to inhibit the release of water in urine. Activation of the osmoreceptors also results in a drinking response. These responses appear to act in parallel. There is no evidence to suggest that vasopressin release causes thirst, or that drinking results from the release of vasopressin (Ramsy, Thrasner, & Keil, 1980).

Autonomic Nervous System Mediation of Hypothalamically Controlled Behavior

Several cases have been shown to exist in which hypothalamic influence on behavior *is* mediated by the autonomic nervous system. Hypothalamically controlled feeding is one such example. Hypothalamic manipulations that result in enhanced feeding have been shown to be prevented by vagotomy. Thus, it appears that these manipulations may enhance feeding by causing an overexpression of parasympathetic activation. The well-known overeating and body weight gain responses that occur after lesions of the ventromedial hypothalamic (VMH) area are accompanied by an increased proportion of body fat, increased release of gastric acid, enlarged size of pancreatic islets, and elevated insulin levels. If animals are placed on restricted feeding schedules (pair-fed to controls), the digestive alterations seen after lesions are somewhat attenuated, but still significantly present (for a review see Powley, 1977; Bray & York, 1979). This suggests that these responses are not secondary results of increased food intake. Vagotomy, however, eliminated overeating totally after VMH lesion. Thus, Powley suggests that lesioning the VMH area (sympathetic zone) results in decreased sympathetic activation and a relatively increased parasympathetic activation, and that these autonomic variables are, in part, responsible for the aberrant behavior following these lesions.

Similarly, both Powley and Opsahl (1976) and Ball (1974) have shown that eating elicited by electrical stimulation of the lateral hypothalamus is attenuated or abolished after vagotomy. Powley and Opsahl have also shown that the effects of vagotomy are behaviorally specific, since stimulation-induced gnawing was unaffected by vagotomy (see Figure 12-10). Furthermore, Gold and co-workers have pointed out that, among the various manipulations that cause obesity in rats, only those achieved through hypothalamic manipulations are reversed by vagotomy (see Table 12-1) (Gold et al., 1980). Obesity resulting from VMH lesion (Powley & Opsahl, 1976), parasagittal knife cut (Gold et al., 1980; Sawchenko, Eng, Gold, & Simson, 1977), hypothalamic norepinephrine injection (Sawchenko et al., 1981), and electrical stimulation of the lateral hypothalamus (Ball, 1974; Powley & Opsahl, 1976) are prevented by vagotomy. Conversely, obesity resulting from access to highly palatable and varied diets (Gold et al., 1980), ovariectomy

AUTONOMIC ASPECTS OF FEEDING

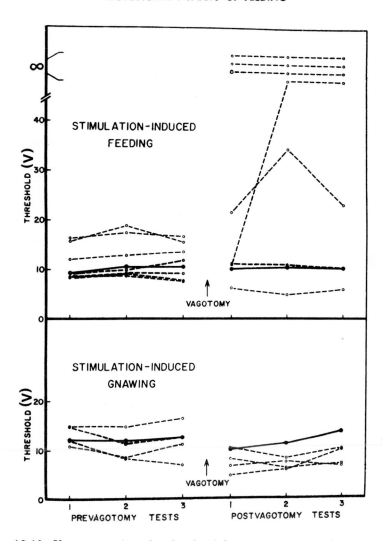

Figure 12-10. Vagotomy raises the threshold for eating, but not for gnawing, induced by hypothalamic brain stimulation. (From Powley & Opsahl, 1976.)

(Eng, Gold, & Wade, 1979), insulin injection (Booth, 1972), and genetic factors (Opsahl & Powley, 1974) is unchanged by vagotomy. Obesity induced by 2-deoxyglucose is attenuated but not abolished by vagotomy (Booth, 1972). Figure 12-11 provides a demonstration of the failure of vagotomy to affect obesity induced by dietary manipulations. Subsequently, these same animals were given hypothalamic knife cuts. The knife cut induced obesity in all but the vagotomized group.

Table 12.1. The Effect of Vagotomy on Obesity Induced by a Variety of Manipulations

Manipulations causing obesity	Obesity prevented by vagotomy	
VMH lesion	yes	Powley & Opsahl, 1976
Parasagittal hypothalamic knife cut	yes	Gold et al., 1980 Sawchenko et al., 1977
Hypothalamic norepinephrine injection	yes	Sawchenko et al., 1981
Electrical stimulation of LH	yes	Ball, 1974 Powley & Opsahl, 1976
2-Deoxyglucose injection	partially	Booth, 1972
Ovariectomy	no	Eng et al., 1979
Supermarket diet	no	Gold et al., 1980
Insulin injection	no	Booth, 1972
Genetic (Zucker) obesity	no	Opsahl & Powley, 1974

Note: LH stands for lateral hypothalamus; VMH, ventromedial hypothalamus.

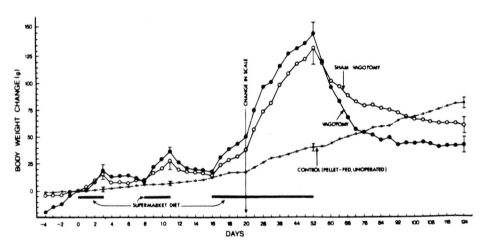

Figure 12-11. Vagotomized and sham-vagotomized rats exhibit dietary obesity compared to pellet-fed controls. A subsequent hypothalamic knife cut induced obesity in sham-vagotomized but not vagotomized animals. (From Gold et al., 1980.)

Correlation of Autonomic Control with Intracranial Self-Stimulation

Hypothesis

In light of the facts that (1) hypothalamic influence on behavior can be mediated partly by the autonomic nervous system and (2) the hypothalamus is a potent brain site for eliciting ICSS, we have posed the following question: Are the positively reinforcing effects of electrical brain stimulation mediated by the autonomic nervous system? In particular, might increases in parasympathetic tone be positively reinforcing, and thereby provide a basis for the ICSS phenomenon?

Three sets of facts triggered this hypothesis. Firstly, the most potent brain site for ICSS lies in the lateral hypothalamic MFB. This site has been mapped as a strong parasympathetic zone by Hess as well as by others. Stimulation in the area of the anterior MFB results in a broad range of parasympathetic responses.

Secondly, hypothalamic areas from which electrical stimulation elicits behavior known to be mediated by the autonomic nervous system are invariably ICSS sites (see above). Furthermore, parasympathetic denervation that abolishes these electrically elicited responses also raises ICSS thresholds elicited from the same hypothalamic site (see Figure 12-12) (Ball, 1974).

Finally, extrahypothalamic sites in the mediobasal forebrain which support high rates of ICSS, such as the septum, diagonal band of Broca, and the medial preoptic area, when stimulated also result in strong parasympathetic responses (see above).

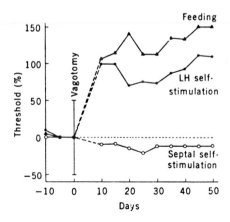

Figure 12-12. Vagotomy raises the threshold for feeding in response to lateral hypothalamic electrical brain stimulation and for ICSS from lateral hypothalamic but not septal sites. (From Ball, 1974.)

Correlation

If our simplest hypothesis is correct, one might expect that all brain sites that support ICSS would also exert excitatory control over the parasympathetic nervous system. Utilizing already existing literature, we have compiled a list of positive ICSS sites at each level of the brain, and have determined, based on what is known through physiological studies of those brain sites, whether they exert either a sympathetic or parasympathetic influence. As can be seen in Table 12-2, the positive ICSS sites in the *forebrain*, which are the basis of our hypothesis, fall in strong parasympathetic zones. However, sites in the *midbrain* that support ICSS (see Figures 12-6C and 12-13A) and which have been linked with autonomic function are in and around the central grey. This area has been shown to be a strong sympathetic zone (Hess, 1954).

At the level of the *pons*, the locus coeruleus, a brain site that supports ICSS (see above and Figure 12-13), is associated with increased heart rate, respiration, and vasodilation, all of which define it as a sympathetic site (although it plays a parasympathetic role with regard to micturition) (see Amarel & Sinnamon, 1977).

The only known ICSS site in the *medulla* is the area of the nucleus of the solitary tract (see Figure 12-14A). That area has been shown to exert a strong parasympathetic influence on heart rate (see Figure 12-14B) (Ciriello & Calaresu, 1980).

Thus, the exploration of ICSS sites and brain sites innervating the parasympathetic nervous system reveals that a one-to-one correspondence between these functions does *not* exist across all levels of the CNS. At forebrain, hypothalamic, and medullary levels, a correspon-

Table 12-2. The Autonomic Effects of Electrical Brain Stimulation at Positive ICSS Brain Sites

	Sympathetic	Parasympathetic
Septum	↓	↑
Diagonal band of Broca		↑
Nucleus accumbens	↓	↑
Medial preoptic area	↓	↑
Lateral preoptic area	↓	↑
Anterior medial forebrain bundle	↓	↑
Anterior hypothalamus	↓	↑
Medial thalamus	↕	↑
Centray grey	↑	
Locus coeruleus	↑	
Nucleus of the solitary tract	↓	↑

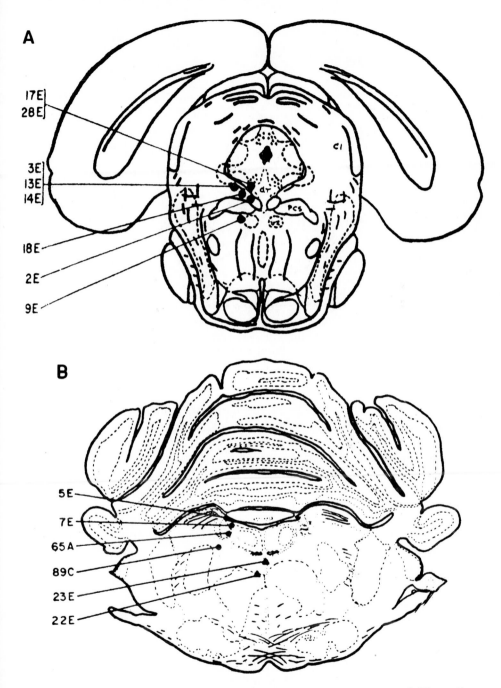

Figure 12-13. ICSS sites in the locus coeruleus at (A) midbrain and (B) pontine levels. Circles indicate positive sites and triangles indicate negative sites. (From Ellman, Ackermann, Bodnor, Jackler, & Steiner, 1975.)

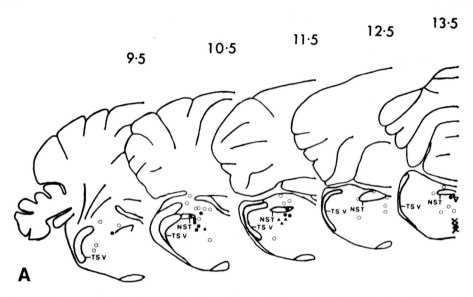

A

Figure 12-14A. Distribution of positive and negative ICSS sites in the medulla oblongata. Open circles denote fewer than 50 responses every 15 minutes; closed circles, 50–200 responses per 15 minutes; triangles, 201–350 per 15 minutes; squares, 351–600 per 15 minutes. Positive sites are restricted to the area of the nucleus of the solitary tract. (From Carter & Phillips, 1975.)

dence occurs in what appears to be a lawful manner; ICSS sites are parasympathetic sites, and few strong parasympathetic sites are not positive ICSS sites. In the midbrain and pons, however, strong sympathetic areas, such as the locus coeruleus and central grey, appear to be associated with sites that support high ICSS rates.

Our prediction, therefore, that brain sites which support ICSS would always facilitate parasympathetic outflow has not been confirmed. This suggests that any simple form of our hypothesis (that increased parasympathetic tone is the substrate of reward during ICSS) may be false. Alternatively, the idea may have merit but the experiments for testing it may be more complicated than envisioned.

Reservations

An implicit assumption among all investigators studying ICSS is that the stimulated systems are also activated during other naturally occurring events. The hypothesis we have put forth represents an attempt to determine whether a known functional system is the mediating mechanism underlying brain-stimulated reward. A more thorough test of this hypothesis would require investigation of the following issues:

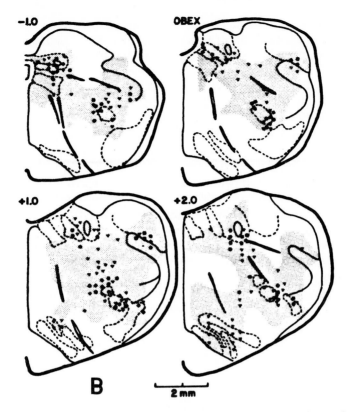

Figure 12-14B. Coronal sections of the medulla from 1 mm caudal to 2 mm rostral to the obex, showing the location of cardioinhibitory sites in the spinal cord. Shaded area indicates region from which cardioinhibition could be elicited by using a stimulation current of 100 μA; closed circles indicate areas where response was elicited by using less than 15 μA; triangles indicate sites at which 15–30 μA elicited the response. (From Ciriello & Calaresu, 1980.)

1. Can ICSS occur in an animal with total denervation of the autonomic nervous system? We were able to find only one study in the literature that addressed this question. Ward and Hester (1969) looked at the combined effect of vagotomy and sympathectomy on ICSS in cats. Several difficulties with this experiment prevent definitive conclusions: (a) the subjects were trained to bar press prior to the lesion by first food depriving them, then conditioning an operant response using food reward, and finally pairing the food with brain stimulation. (b) No sham-lesion control subjects were tested. (c) Only one subject with combined vagotomy and sympathectomy survived the experiment. (d) The authors did not demonstrate that ICSS responses can be acquired in the absence of autonomic influence. We suggest a replication of this study, preferably in rats, where the ICSS response is more stable and robust.

2. That ICSS occurs most effectively at most sites using frequencies of 60–200 Hz raises a question as to whether these systems can be activated at such high frequencies. It is known, for example, that neurons in sympathetic ganglia do not fire in response to stimulation frequencies above 30 per second (Zigmond & Chalazonitis, 1979), and similar frequency limitations may hold for autonomic-related neurons in the hypothalamus (Ellendorff, MacLeod, & Dyer, 1976). If this is true for sympathetic-related neurons, but not parasympathetic-related neurons, then one would imagine high-frequency ICSS in sympathetic sites as blocking activity and actually supporting our original hypothesis. Similarly, it would be of interest to map brain sites supporting ICSS at lower (more physiological) frequencies even though response rates would be significantly depressed.

3. A further question arises as regards our utilization of rate of response (e.g., bar press) as a measure that reflects the magnitude of reward. It has been shown, through the use of a two-choice preference test in which rats are permitted to select ICSS at one of two brain sites, that a slower rate of stimulation at one brain site may be more rewarding than more rapid stimulation at another site (see Hodos & Valenstein, 1962). Since we have utilized an arbitrary minimum response rate for determining whether stimulation at various brain sites is positively reinforcing, we may have omitted sites at which stimulation is rewarding at very low rates. Thus, exploration of sites that support low rates with regard to their reward value as determined by preference tests would be of value.

4. Another source of possible confusion lies in the question whether, when hypothesizing that increased parasympathetic tone is rewarding, it is necessary to take into account the baseline condition of the animal. In other words, could any change in the direction of increased parasympathetic tone be equally rewarding at any point along the "continuum" from sympathetic to parasympathetic tone, or alternatively, are there requirements for the *starting point* on that continuum? Finally, there could be an optimal midpoint on the continuum; in this case, it is conceivable that, under strongly parasympathetic baseline conditions, sympathetic nervous system stimulation would be rewarding. We therefore suggest that selective inactivation of sympathetic and parasympathetic systems (through surgical denervation or pharmacological blockade) be compared to the effect of combined denervation.

5. Our predictions have assumed particular features in the organization of the parasympathetic (and sympathetic) systems across all levels of the brain. For example, stimulation of a parasympathetic zone in the forebrain can activate a wide range of responses including bradycardia, hypotension, stomach motility, salivation, micturition, and pupillary contraction. It is possible, however, that stimulation in

medullary parasympathetic zones activates parasympathetic functions more selectively (e.g., stimulation of the nucleus of the solitary tract causes bradycardia). Thus, if change in a particular parasympathetic function (or large numbers of parasympathetic functions) were required for reward, we would not necessarily expect ICSS sites to correspond as well with parasympathetic zones in the hindbrain. Point-by-point correlations of reward value with effects on a variety of sympathetic and parasympathetic measures in the rat hindbrain would be valuable.

6. Finally, the assumption is implicit in our hypothesis that ICSS at all sites reflects a unitary reward system. There is no firm evidence to support this notion.

References

Adams, W. J., Lorens, S. A., & Mitchell, C. L. Morphine enhances lateral hypothalamic self-stimulation in the rat. *Proc. Soc. Exp. Biol. Med.*, 1972, *140*, 770–771.

Amaral, D. G., & Sinnamon, H. M. The locus coeruleus: Neurobiology of a central noradrenergic nucleus. *Progress in Neurobiology*, 1977, *9*, 147–196.

Anand, B. K., & Brobeck, J. R. Hypothalamic control of food intake in rats and cats. *Yale Journal of Biology and Medicine*, 1951, *24*, 123–140.

Antelman, S. M., & Caggiula, A. R. Norepinephrine-dopamine interactions and behavior. *Science*, 1977, *195*, 646–653.

Arbuthnott, G. W. Further chemical evidence for the involvement of noradrenaline in locus coeruleus self-stimulation. In A. Wauquier & E. T. Rolls (Eds.), *Brain-stimulation reward*. Oxford, England: North-Holland, 1976, pp. 251–260.

Ball, G. G. Vagotomy: Effect on electrically elicited eating and self-stimulation in the lateral hypothalamus. *Science*, 1974, *184*, 484–485.

Beninger, R. J., Bellisle, F., & Milner, P. M. Schedule control of behavior reinforced by electrical stimulation of the brain. *Science*, 1977, *196*, 547–549.

Beattie, J., & Sheehan, D. The effects of hypothalamic stimulation on gastric motility. *Journal of Physiology*, 1934, *81*, 218–227.

Booth, D. A. Localization of the adrenergic feeding system in the rat diencephalon. *Science*, 1967, *158*, 515–517.

Booth, D. A. Modulation of the feeding response to peripheral insulin, 2-deoxyglucose or 3-O-methyl glucose injection. *Physiology and Behavior*, 1972, *8*, 1069–1076.

Brady, J. V. Temporal and emotional effects related to intracranial electrical self-stimulation. In E. R. Ramey & D. S. O'Doherty (Eds.), *Electrical studies on the unanesthetized brain*. New York: Hoeber, 1960.

Bray, G. A., & York, D. A. Hypothalamic and genetic obesity in experimental animals: An autonomic and endocrine hypothesis. *Physiological Reviews*, 1979, *59*, 719–809.

Breese, G. R., Howard, J. L., & Leahy, J. P. Effect of 6-hydroxydopamine on electrical self-stimulation of the brain. *British Journal of Pharmacology*, 1971, *43*, 255–257.

Bush, H. D., Bush, M. A. F., Miller, M. A., & Reid, L. D. Addictive agents and intracranial stimulation: Daily morphine and lateral hypothalamic self-stimulation. *Physiological Psychology*, 1976, *4*, 79–85.

Caggiula, A. R. Specificity of copulation–reward systems in the posterior hypothalamus. *Proceedings of the 75th Annual American Psychological Association Convention*, 1967.

Caggiula, A. R. Analysis of the copulation–reward properties of posterior hypothalamic stimulation in male rats. *Journal of Comparative and Physiological Psychology*, 1970, *70*, 399–412.

Caggiula, A. R., & Hoebel, B. G. "Copulation–reward site" in the posterior hypothalamus. *Science*, 1966, *153*, 1284–1285.

Carter, D. A., & Phillips, A. G. Intracranial self-stimulation at sites in the dorsal medulla oblongata. *Brain Research*, 1975, *94*, 155–160.

Ciriello, J., & Calaresu, F. R. Distribution of vagal cardioinhibitory neurons in medulla of the rat. *American Journal of Physiology*, 1980, *238*, R57–R64.

Clavier, R. M. Brainstem self-stimulation: Catecholamine or non-catecholamine mediation? In A. Wauquier & E. T. Rolls (Eds.), *Brain-stimulation reward*. Oxford, England: North-Holland, 1976, pp. 239–250.

Clavier, R. M., & Fibiger, H. C. On the role of ascending catecholaminergic projections in intracranial self-stimulation of the substantia nigra. *Brain Research*, 1977, *131*, 271–286.

Clavier, R. M., Fibiger, H. C., & Phillips, A. C. Evidence that self-stimulation of the region of the locus coeruleus in rats does not depend upon noradrenergic projections to telencephalon. *Brain Research*, 1976, *113*, 71–81.

Clavier, R. M., & Routtenberg, A. Brain stem self-stimulation attenuated by lesions of medial forebrain bundle but not by lesions of brain stem norepinephrine systems. *Brain Research*, 1976, *101*, 251–271.

Corbett, D., Skelton, R. W., & Wise, R. A. Dorsal bundle lesions fail to disrupt self-stimulation from the region of locus coeruleus. *Brain Research*, 1977, *133*, 37–44.

Corbett, D., & Wise, R. A. Intracranial self-stimulation in relation to the ascending dopaminergic systems of the midbrain: A moveable electrode mapping study. *Brain Research*, 1980, *185*, 1–15.

Crow, T. J. A map of the rat mesencephalon for electrical stimulation. *Brain Research*, 1972, *36*, 265–273.

Crow, T. J. Catecholamine-containing neurones and electrical self-stimulation, 2: A theoretical interpretation and some psychiatric implications. *Psychological Medicine*, 1973, *3*, 66–73.

Crow, T. J. Specific monoamine systems as reward pathways: Evidence for the hypothesis that activation of the ventral mesencephalic dopaminergic neurons and noradrenergic neurones of the locus coeruleus complex will support self-stimulation responding. In A. Wauquier & E. T. Rolls (Eds.), *Brain-stimulation reward*. Oxford, England: North-Holland, 1976, pp. 211–238.

Crow, T. J., Spear, P. J., & Arbuthnott, G. W. Intracranial self-stimulation with electrodes in the region of the locus coeruleus. *Brain Research*, 1972, *36*, 275–287.

Cytawa, J., Jurkowleniec, E., & Bialowas, J. Positive reinforcement produced by noradrenergic stimulation of the hypothalamus in rats. *Physiology and Behavior*, 1980, *25*, 615–619.

Davis, J. R., & Keesey, R. E. Norepinephrine-induced eating: Its hypothalamic locus and an alternate interpretation of action. *Journal of Comparative and Physiological Psychology*, 1971, 77, 394–402.

Davis, W. M., & Smith, S. G. Effect of haloperidol on (+)-amphetamine self-administration. *Journal of Pharmacy and Pharmacology*, 1975, 27, 540–542.

Deutsch, J. A. *The structural bases of behavior*. Chicago: Chicago University Press, 1960.

Deutsch, J. S., & Howarth, C. I. Some tests of a theory of intracranial self-stimulation. *Psychological Review*, 1963, 70, 444–460.

Ellendorff, F., Macleod, N. K., & Dyer, R. G. Bipolar neurones in the rostral hypothalamus. *Brain Research*, 1976, 101, 349–553.

Ellman, S. J., Ackermann, R. F., Bodnar, R. J., Jackler, F., & Steiner, S. S. Comparison of behaviors elicited by electrical brain stimulation in dorsal brainstem and hypothalamus of rats. *Journal of Comparative and Physiological Psychology*, 1975, 88, 816–828.

Eng, R., Gold, R. M., & Wade, G. N. Ovariectomy-induced obesity is not prevented by subdiaphragmatic vagotomy in rats. *Physiology and Behavior*, 1979, 22, 353–356.

Esposito, R. U., & Kornetsky, C. Morphine lowering of self-stimulation thresholds: Lack of tolerance with long-term administration. *Science*, 1977, 195, 189–191. (a)

Esposito, R. U., & Kornetsky, C. Effects of morphine on self-stimulation thresholds to the substantia nigra and the locus coeruleus in the rat. *Soc. Neurosci. Abst.*, 1977, 3, 290. (b)

Esposito, R. U., & Kornetsky, C. Opioids and rewarding brain stimulation. *Neurosci. Biobehav. Rev.*, 1978, 2, 115–122.

Esposito, R. U., Perry, W., & Kornetsky, C. Effects of *d*-amphetamine and naloxone on brain stimulation reward. *Psychopharmacology*, 1980, 69, 187–191.

Falk, J. L. Septal stimulation as a reinforcer of and alternative to consummatory behavior. *Journal of Experimental Analysis of Behavior*, 1961, 4, 213–217.

Farber, J., Ellman, S. J., Mattiace, L. A., Holtzman, A., Ippolito, P. Halperin, R., & Steiner, S. S. Differential effects of unilateral dorsal hindbrain lesions on hypothalamic self-stimulation in the rat. *Brain Research*, 1976, 112, 148–155.

Farber, J., Steiner, S. S., & Ellman, S. J. The pons as an electrical self-stimulation site. *Psychophysiology*, 1972, 9, 105 (abstract).

Friedman, H. R., & Coons, E. E. Dopaminergic modulation of feeding in hungry rats. *Neuroscience Abstracts*, 1979, 5, 217.

Gallistel, C. R. Electrical self-stimulation and its theoretical implications. *Psychological Bulletin*, 1964, 61, 23–34.

Gallistel, C. R. Self-stimulation: The neurophysiology of reward and motivation. In J. A. Deutsch (Ed.), *The physiological basis of memory*. New York: Academic Press, 1973, pp. 175–267.

German, D. C., & Bowden, D. M. Catecholamine systems as the neural substrate for intracranial self-stimulation: A hypothesis. *Brain Research*, 1974, 73, 381–419.

Gibson, W. E., Reid, L. D., Sakai, M., & Porter, P. B. Intracranial reinforcement compared with sugar water reinforcement. *Science*, 1965, 148, 1357–1359.

Gold, R. M., Sawchenko, P. E., De Luca, C., Alexander, J., & Eng, R. Vagal mediation of hypothalamic obesity but not supermarket dietary obesity. *American Journal of Physiology*, 1980, 238(5), R447–R453.

Grossman, S. P., Dacey, D., Halares, A. E., Collier, T., & Routtenberg, A. Aphagia and adipsia after preferential destruction of nerve cell bodies in hypothalamus. *Science*, 1978, *202*, 537-539.

Herberg, L. J. Seminal ejaculation following positively reinforcing electrical stimulation of the rat hypothalamus. *Journal of Comparative and Physiological Psychology*, 1963, *56*, 679-685.

Herberg, L. J., Stephens, D. N., & Franklin, K. B. J. Catecholamines and self-stimulation: Evidence suggesting a reinforcing role for noradrenaline and a motivating role for dopamine. *Physiology and Behavior*, 1976, *4*, 575-582.

Hess, W. R. *Diencephalon: Autonomic and extrapyramidal functions.* New York: Grune & Stratton, 1954.

Hess, W. R. *The functional organization of the diencephalon.* J. R. Hughes (Ed.). New York: Grune & Stratton, 1957.

Hodos, W., & Valenstein, E. S. An evaluation of response rate as a measure of rewarding intracranial stimulation. *Journal of Comparative and Physiological Psychology*, 1962, *55*, 80-84.

Hoebel, B. G. Feeding and self-stimulation. *Annals of the New York Academy of Sciences*, 1969, *157*, 758-778.

Hoebel, B. G. Satiety and the hypothalamus. In D. Noven, W. Wyrwicka, & G. Bray (Eds.), *Hunger: Basic mechanisms and clinical implications.* New York: Raven Press, 1976, pp. 33-50.

Hoebel, B. G., Hernandez, L., & Thompson, R. D. Phenylpropanolamine inhibits feeding, but not drinking, induced by hypothalamic stimulation. *Journal of Comparative and Physiological Psychology*, 1975, *89*, 1046-1052.

Hoebel, B. G., & Monaco, A. T. Self-injection of amphetamine directly into the brain. Presented at *The 52nd Annual Meeting of the Eastern Psychological Association, April, 1981, New York.*

Hoebel, B. G., & Teitelbaum, P. Hypothalamic control of feeding and self-stimulation. *Science*, 1962, *135*, 375-377.

Holtzman, S. G. Comparison of the effect of morphine, pentazocine, cyclazocine on intracranial self-stimulation in the rat. *Psychopharmacologia*, 1976, *46*, 223-227.

Hull, C. L. *Principles of behavior.* New York: Appleton-Century-Crofts, 1943.

Janssen, P. A., Niemegeers, S., Schellekens, K. H. L., Dress, A., Lenaerts, F. M., Pinchard, A., Schaper, W. K. A., Van Nueten, J. M., & Verbruggen, F. J. Pimozide, a chemically novel, highly potent and orally long-acting neuroleptic, Part I: The comparative pharmacology of pimozide, haloperidol and chlorpromazine. *Arzneimittel-Forschung*, 1968, *18*, 261-279.

Kelley, D. B., & Pfaff, D. W. Generalizations from comparative studies on neuroanatomical and endocrine mechanisms of sexual behavior. In J. Hutchison (Ed.), *Biological determinants of sexual behavior.* Chichester, England: Wiley, 1978, pp. 225-254.

Koob, G. F., Balcom, G. J., & Meyerhoff, J. L. Increases in intracranial self-stimulation in the posterior hypothalamus following unilateral lesions in the locus coeruleus. *Brain Research*, 1976, *101*, 554-560.

Kornblith, C., & Hoebel, B. G. Effect of amphetamine, phenylpropanolamine and fenfluramine on feeding, self-stimulation and stimulus-escape. *Pharmacology, Biochemistry and Behavior*, 1976, *5*, 215-218.

Leibowitz, S. F. Brain catecholaminergic mechanisms for control of hunger. In D. Novin, W. Wyrwicka, & G. Bray (Eds.), *Hunger: Basic mechanisms and clinical implications.* New York: Raven Press, 1976, pp. 1-18.

Leibowitz, S. F. Paraventricular nucleus: A primary site mediating adrenergic stimulation of feeding and drinking. *Pharmacology, Biochemistry and Behavior*, 1978, *8*, 163-178.

Leibowitz, S. F., & Rossakis, C. Mapping study of brain dopamine and epinephrine-sensitive sites which cause feeding suppression in the rat. *Brain Research*, 1979, *172*, 101.

Lilly, J. C. Learning motivated by subcortical stimulation: The start and stop patterns of behavior. In H. H. Jasper, L. D. Proctor, R. S. Knighton, W. C. Noshay, & R. T. Costello (Eds.), *The reticular formation of the brain.* Boston: Little, Brown, 1958.

Lindvall, O., & Bjorklund, A. The organization of the ascending catecholamine neuron systems in the rat brain as revealed by the glyoxylic acid fluorescence method. *Acta Physiologica Scandinavica*, Suppl. 412, 1974, 1-48.

MacDonnell, M. F., & Flynn, J. P. Control of sensory fields by stimulation of hypothalamus. *Science*, 1966, *152*, 1406-1408.

Malsbury, C., & Pfaff, D. W. Neural and hormonal determinants of mating behavior in adult male rats: A review. In L. DiCara (Ed.), *Limbic and autonomic nervous systems research.* New York: Plenum Press, 1974.

Margules, D. L., & Olds, J. Identical feeding and rewarding systems in the lateral hypothalamus of rats. *Science*, 1962, *157*, 274-275.

McIntyre, R. W., & Wright, J. E. Parameters related to response rate for septal and medial forebrain bundle stimulation. *Journal of Comparative and Physiological Psychology*, 1965, *59*, 131-134.

Miller, N. E. Analytical studies of drive and reward. *American Psychologist*, 1961, *16*, 739-754.

Miller, N. E. Motivational effects of brain stimulation and drugs. *Federation Proceedings*, 1960, *199*, 846-854.

Miller, N. E. Chemical coding of behavior in the brain. *Science*, 1965, *148*, 328-338.

Miller, N. E., Bailey, C. J., & Stevenson, J. A. F. Decreased "hunger" but increased food intake resulting from hypothalamic lesions. *Science*, 1950, *112*, 256-259.

Misher, A., & Brooks, F. P. Electrical stimulation of hypothalamus and gastric secretion in the albino rat. *American Journal of Physiology*, 1966, *211*, 403-406.

Mogenson, G. J. An attempt to establish secondary reinforcement with rewarding brain stimulation. *Psychological Reports*, 1965, *16*, 163-167.

Mogenson, G. J., Gentil, C. G., & Stevenson, J. A. Feeding and drinking elicited by low and high frequencies of hypothalamic stimulation. *Brain Research*, 1971, *33*, 127-137.

Morgane, P. J., & Panksepp, J. *Handbook of the hypothalamus* (Vol. 3, *Behavioral studies*). New York: Dekker, 1980.

Nelson, W. T., Brutus, M., Wilson, J. E., Jr., Farrell, R. A., Ocheret, D. R., Ellman, S. J., & Steiner, S. S. Effect of morphine on intracrantial self-stimulation in rats. *Soc. Neurosci. Abst.*, 1977, *3*, 298.

Olds, J. Physiological mechanisms of reward. In M. R. Jones (Ed.), *Nebraska Symposium on Motivation.* Lincoln, Nebraska: University of Nebraska Press, 1955.

Olds, J. Adaptive functions of paleocortical and related structures. In H. F. Harlow & C. N. Woolsey (Eds.), *Biological and biochemical bases of behavior.* Madison, Wis.: University of Wisconsin Press, 1958. (a)

Olds, J. Self-stimulation of the brain. *Science*, 1958, *127*, 315-324. (b)

Olds, J. Satiation effects in self-stimulation of the brain. *Journal of Comparative and Physiological Psychology*, 1958, *51*, 675-678. (c)

Olds, J. Studies of neuropharmacologicals by electrical and chemical manipulation of the brain in animals with chronically implanted electrodes. In P. B. Bradley, P. Deniker, & C. Radouco-Thomas (Eds.), *Neuro-Psycho-Pharmacology*. Amsterdam: Elsevier, 1959, pp. 20-32.

Olds, J., & Milner, P. Positive reinforcement produced by electrical stimulation of septal area and other regions of the rat brain. *Journal of Comparative and Physiological Psychology*, 1954, *47*, 419-427.

Olds, J., & Olds, M. E. Drives, rewards, and the brain. In T. M. Newcombe (Ed.), *New directions in psychology* (Vol. 2). New York: Holt, Rinehart & Winston, 1965.

Olds, M. E., & Olds, J. Approach-avoidance analysis of rat diencephalon. *Journal of Comparative and Physiological Psychology*, 1963, *120*, 259-295.

Oomura, Y., Ooyama, H., Naka, P., Yamamoto, T., Ono, T., & Kobayashi, N. Some stochastical patterns of single unit discharges in the cat hypothalamus under chronic conditions. *Annals of the New York Academy of Sciences*, 1967, *157*, 666-689.

Opsahl, C. A., & Powley, T. L. Failure of vagotomy to reverse obesity in the genetically obese Zucker rat. *American Journal of Physiology*, 1974, *226*, 34-37.

Pert, A., & Hulsebus, R. Effect of morphine on intracranial self-stimulation behavior following brain amine depletion. *Life Sciences*, 1975, *17*, 19-20.

Pfaff, D. W. *Estrogens and brain function: Neural analysis of a hormone-controlled mammalian reproductive behavior.* New York: Springer-Verlag, 1980.

Phillips, A. G., Brooke, S. M., & Fibiger, H. C. Effects of amphetamine isomers and neuroleptics on self-stimulation from the nucleus accumbens and dorsal noradrenergic bundle. *Brain Research*, 1975, *85*, 13-22.

Phillips, A. G., Carter, D. A., & Fibiger, H. C. Dopaminergic substrates of intracranial self-stimulation in the caudate nucleus. *Brain Research*, 1976, *104*, 221-232.

Phillips, A. G., & Fibiger, H. C. Dopaminergic and noradrenergic substrates of positive reinforcement: Differential effects of D- and L-amphetamine. *Science*, 1973, *179*, 575-577.

Pickens, R., & Thompson, T. Cocaine-reinforced behavior in rats: Effects of reinforcement magnitude and fixed-ratio size. *Journal of Pharmacology and Experimental Therapeutics*, 1968, *161*, 122-129.

Pliskoff, S. S., Wright, J. E., & Hawkins, T. D. Brain stimulation as a reinforcer: Intermittent schedules. *Journal of the Experimental Analysis of Behavior*, 1965, *8*, 75-88.

Porrino, L. J., & Coons, E. E. Effects of GABA receptor blockade on stimulation-induced feeding and self-stimulation. *Pharmacology, Biochemistry and Behavior*, 1980, *12*, 125-130.

Poschel, B. P. H., & Ninteman, F. W. Norepinephrine: A possible excitatory neurohormone of the reward system. *Life Sciences*, 1963, *10*, 782-788.

Poschel, B. P. H., & Ninteman, F. W. Hypothalamic self-stimulation: Its suppression by blockade of norepinephrine synthesis and reinstatement by methamphetamine. *Life Sciences*, 1966, *5*, 11-16.

Powley, T. L. The ventromedial hypothalamic syndrome, satiety, and a cephalic phase hypothesis. *Psychological Review*, 1977, *84*, 89-126.

Powley, T. L., & Opsahl, C. A. Autonomic changes of the hypothalamic feeding syndrome. In D. Novin, W. Wyrwicka, & G. Bray (Eds.), *Hunger: Basic mechanisms and clinical implications.* New York: Raven Press, 1976.

Powley, T. L., MacFarlane, B. A., Markell, M. S., & Opsahl, C. A. Different effects of vagotomy and atropine on hypothalamis stimulation-induced feeding. *Behavioral Biology*, 1978, *23*, 306–325.

Ramsay, D. J., Thrasher, T. N., & Keil, L. C. Stimulation and inhibition of drinking and vasopressin secretion in dogs. In S. Yoshida, L. Share, & K. Yagi (Eds.), *Antidiuretic hormone.* Tokyo: Japan Scientific Societies Press, and Baltimore: University Park Press, 1980, pp. 97–113.

Ritter, S., & Stein, L. Self-stimulation in the mesencephalic trajectory of the ventral noradrenergic bundle. *Brain Research*, 1975, *81*, 145–157.

Rolls, E. T. The neurophysiological basis of brain-stimulation reward. In A. Wauquier & E. T. Rolls (Eds.), *Brain-stimulation reward.* Oxford, England: North-Holland, 1976, pp. 65–88.

Routtenberg, A., & Malsbury, C. Brain stem pathways of reward. *Journal of Comparative and Physiological Psychology*, 1969, *68*, 22–30.

Sawchenko, P. E., Eng, R., Gold, R. M., & Simson, E. L. Effects of selective subdiaphragmatic vagotomies on knife cut induced hypothalamic hyperphagia. *International Conference on the Regulation of Food and Fluid Intake, 6th, Paris, 1977.*

Sawchenko, P. E., Leibowitz, S. F., & Gold, R. M. Evidence for vagal involvement in eating elicited by adrenergic stimulation of the paraventricular nucleus. *Brain Research*, 1981, *225*, 249–269.

Sclafani, A., Berner, C. N., & Maul, G. Feeding and drinking pathways between the medial and lateral hypothalamus in the rat. *Journal of Comparative and Physiological Psychology*, 1973, *85*, 20–51.

Segal, M., & Bloom, F. E. The action of norepinephrine in the rat hippocampus, III: Hippocampal cellular responses to locus coeruleus stimulation in the awake rat. *Brain Research*, 1976, *107*, 499–511.

Seward, J. P., Uyeda, A. A., & Olds, J. Resistance to extinction following cranial self-stimulation. *Journal of Comparative and Physiological Psychology*, 1959, *52*, 294–299.

Shimazu, T., Fukuda, A., & Ban, T. Reciprocal influences of the ventro-medial and lateral hypothalamic nuclei on blood glucose level and liver glycogen content. *Nature*, 1966, *210*, 1178–1179.

Shiraishi, T. Effects of lateral hypothalamic stimulation on medulla oblongata and gastric vagal neural responses. *Brain Research Bulletin*, 1980, *5*, 45–250.

Sidman, M., Brady, J. V., Conrad, D. G., & Schulman, A. Reward schedules and behavior maintained by intracranial self-stimulation. *Science*, 1955, *122*, 830–831.

Skinner, B. F. *The behavior of organisms.* New York: Appleton-Century-Crofts, 1938.

Smith, N. S., & Coons, E. E. Temporal summation and refractoriness in hypothalamic reward neurons as measured by self-stimulation behavior. *Science*, 1970, *169*, 782–784.

Spies, G. Food versus intracranial self-stimulation reinforcement in food deprived rats. *Journal of Comparative and Physiological Psychology*, 1965, *60*, 153–157.

Stapleton, J. M., Merriman, V. J., Coogle, C. L., Gelbard, S. O., & Reid, L. D. Naloxone reduces pressing or intracranial stimulation of sites in the periadueductal gray area, accumbens nucleus, substantia nigra, and lateral hypothalamus. *Physiological Psychology*, 1979, *7*, 427–436.

Stark, P., & Totty, C. W. Effects of amphetamines on eating elicited by hypothalamic stimulation. *Journal of Pharmacology and Experimental Therapeutics*, 1967, *158*, 272–278.

Stein, L. Secondary reinforcement established with subcortical stimulation. *Science*, 1958, *127*, 466–467.

Stein, L. Self-stimulation of the brain and the central stimulant action of amphetamine. *Federation Proceedings*, 1964, *23*, 836–841.

Stein, L. Psychopharmacological aspects of mental depression. *Canadian Psychiatric Association Journal*, 1966, *11*, 34–49.

Stein, L. Chemistry of purposive behavior. In J. T. Tapp (Ed.), *Reinforcement and behavior*. New York: Academic Press, 1969.

Stein, L., & Belluzi, J. D. Brain endorphins: Possible role in reward and memory formation. *Federation Proceedings*, 1979, *38*, 2468–2472.

Szabo, I. Path neuron system of medial forebrain bundle as a possible substrate for hypothalamic self-stimulation. *Physiology and Behavior*, 1973, *10*, 315–328.

Szabo, I., Lenard, L., & Kosaras, B. Drive decay theory of self-stimulation: Refractory periods and axon diameters in hypothalamic reward loci. *Physiology and Behavior*, 1974, *12*, 329–343.

Teitelbaum, P. Disturbances in feeding and drinking behavior after hypothalamic lesions. In M. A. Jones (Ed.), *Nebraska Symposium on Motivation*. Lincoln, Nebraska: University of Nebraska Press, 1961.

Tenen, S. S., & Miller, N. E. Strength of electrical stimulation of the lateral hypothalamus, food deprivation, and tolerance for quinine in food. *Journal of Comparative and Physiological Psychology*, 1964, *58*, 55–62.

Terman, M., & Kling, J. W. Discrimination of brightness differences by rats with food or brain stimulation reinforcement. *Journal Exp. Anal. Behavior*, 1968, *11*, 29–37.

Thorndike, E. L. *Animal intelligence*. New York: Macmillan, 1911.

Trowill, J. A., Panksepp, J., & Gandelman, R. An incentive model of rewarding brain stimulation. *Psychological Review*, 1969, *76*, 264–281.

Ungerstedt, U. Stereotaxic mapping of the monoamine pathways in the rat brain. *Acta Physiologica Scandinavica*, 1971, *Suppl. 367*, 1–48.

Valenstein, E. S., Cox, V. C., & Kakolewski, J. W. Reexamination of the role of the hypothalamus in motivation. *Psychological Review*, 1970, *77*, 16–31.

Vaughan, E., & Fisher, A. E. Male sexual behavior induced by intracranial electrical stimulation. *Science*, 1962, *137*, 758–760.

Ward, J. W., & Hester, R. W. Intracranial self-stimulation in cats surgically deprived of autonomic outflow. *Journal of Comparative and Physiological Psychology*, 1969, *67*, 336–343.

Wauquier, A. The influence of psychoactive drugs on brain self-stimulation in rats: A review. In A. Wauquier & E. T. Rolls (Eds.), *Brain-stimulation reward*. Oxford, England: North-Holland, 1976, pp. 123–170.

Wise, R. A. Hypothalamic motivational systems: Fixed or plastic neural circuits? *Science*, 1968, *162*, 377–379.

Wise, R. A. Lateral hypothalamic electrical stimulation: Does it make animals "hungry"? *Brain Research*, 1974, *67*, 187–209.

Wise, R. A. Catecholamine theories of reward: A critical review. *Brain Research*, 1978, *152*, 215–247. (a)

Wise, R. A. Neuroleptic attenuation of intracranial self-stimulation: Reward or performance deficits. *Life Sciences*, 1978, *22*, 535–542. (b)

Zigmond, R. E., & Chalazonitis, A. Long-term effects of preganglionic nerve stimulation on tyrosine hydroxylase activity in the rat superior cervical ganglion. *Brain Research*, 1979, *164*, 137–152.

Chapter 13

Brain Mechanisms in Hedonic Processes

ELIOT STELLAR

Introduction

From the start of physiological psychology in Wilhelm Wundt's laboratory in 1879, there has been a concern with the biological basis of
sensation, including feeling or feeling tone. In 1894, William James
offered a theory, later known as the James–Lange theory, of how our
feelings of emotion such as fear arose. He knew about the cardiovascular and visceral reflexes that occurred in emotion and theorized that it
was the sensation of those changes that led to the experience of fear.
In a similar vein, Cannon (1934) directed our attention to the sensations of hunger and thirst, arising as his experiments indicated from
local changes in the stomach and throat. These theories put the emphasis on the role of peripheral factors and concerned themselves with the
sensations or feelings that could be reported by humans. Bard (1928)
and Lashley (1938), in contrast, emphasized the central nervous system's role in emotion and motivation and studied animal behavior
rather than human experience. The so-called Cannon–Bard theory
(Cannon, 1927), in contradistinction to the James–Lange theory, thus
assumed a central hypothalamic mechanism that gave rise to the peripheral cardiovascular and visceral changes in emotion, and through direct
cortical influences produced the experience of emotion. In a separate
development, Richter (1942-1943) and Adolph (1943) turned our
attention toward physiological regulations and the role that motivated
behavior played. Thus, through a coalescence of these historic trends
were born our modern behavioristic concepts of the physiology of

motivation. But it is well to remember that it was not long ago that we did not talk about motivated behavior but rather focused on the sensations associated with emotion, hunger, thirst, and so forth, and their peripheral biological basis. It is less than 50 years that we have had any conception of the role of the central nervous system in motivated behavior, and we have learned much detail during this period. Armed with these advances in knowledge, it is time that we again address questions of sensation, feeling, and affect in humans, and animals as well, and ask about the biological basis of hedonic experience.

Physiology of Motivation

Back in 1954, when I first published my thoughts about the physiology of motivation, my emphasis was on animal behavior, particularly consummatory behavior such as eating, drinking, copulation, and attack (Stellar, 1954). In this chapter, I want to address a range of hedonic processes involved in motivation as well: appetitive or approach behavior, reward and reinforcement, and hedonic experience, the feelings of pleasantness and unpleasantness that humans can report. In 1954, motivation was defined as increased activity that was goal oriented if the appropriate goal object, such as a female rat in heat, was present. One of the major points I tried to convey was that motivated behavior was under multifactor control (Figure 13-1), so that in hunger, for example, stimuli arising in the mouth and in the gut would contribute in an additive way to the final common neural pathway to behavior. Also contributing, often in essential ways, were changes in the internal environment such as increases or decreases in blood temperature, osmotic pressure, or circulating hormones. Furthermore, it was argued that learning played an important role, particularly in the ability of sensory stimuli to arouse the animal to motivated behavior, but possibly also in changes in the internal environment.

One of the strengths of the theory was that it postulated the same multifactor mechanisms in the satiation of motivated behavior as in its arousal. In fact, it went so far as to postulate dual central neural mechanisms, one for arousal or excitation and one for satiation or inhibition. Since the literature at that time showed that significant increases and decreases in eating, drinking, sexual behavior, sleep, and emotional behavior could be produced by hypothalamic lesions, it was postulated that the hypothalamus might contain the control mechanisms that integrated sensory and humoral influences as well as past experience into the expression of motivated behavior.

Given this central role ascribed to the hypothalamus, it was nonetheless recognized that the hypothalamus was just part of a larger limbic system operating in motivated behavior (Figure 13-2). In addition to

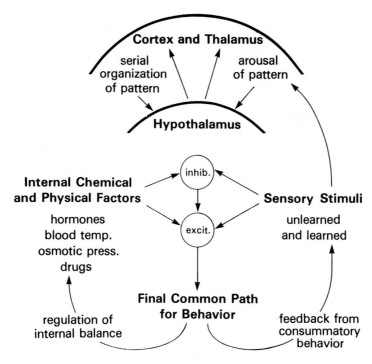

Figure 13-1. Multifactor control of motivated behavior through hypothalamic mechanisms, envisaged in 1954.

efferent output of the hypothalamus directed to the rostral forebrain and to the response mechanisms of the brain stem and spinal cord, it was clear that the hypothalamus had extensive afferent input from the cortex, amygdala, septal nuclei, olfactory bulb, and reticular formation to say the least. In addition, since the hypothalamus lined the third ventricle and was highly vascularized, it was thought likely that it would contain receptor regions for hormones and other changes in the internal environment important in motivated behavior. We also knew at that time of the neurosecretory role of hypothalamic neurons and their effects on the anterior and posterior pituitary, but we did not know how extensive this control system was or that hypothalamic neurosecretions might be released into the ventricles and into the substance of the brain itself. The complexity and the richness of these mechanisms have been demonstrated many times in the intervening years, but nowhere more clearly than in Pfaff's (1980) study of the brain mechanisms involved in reproductive behavior.

In addition, we now know that there is a whole new chemical world of neurotransmitters and neuromodulators that is clearly involved in the physiology of motivation. A literal highway of long neural path-

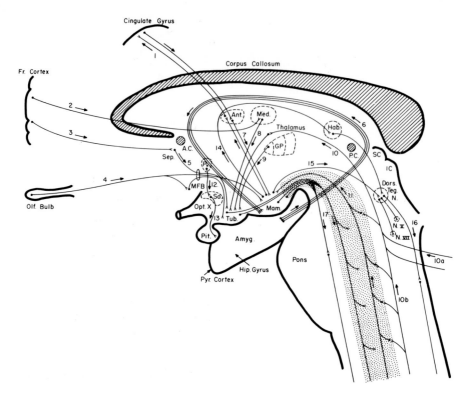

Figure 13-2. Major afferent and efferent connections of the hypothalamus as they were known in 1954.

ways runs from cell bodies in the brain stem to the hypothalamus and through it on their way to rostral forebrain structures (Figure 13-3). These systems, particularly those involving the catecholamines, have to be part of the mechanism we were trying to envisage in 1954. Quite clearly, many neruopeptides are also involved through either their central neural or peripheral action or both. The endogenous opiates, for example, have been implicated in appetite and are important in pain and mood as well. Cholecystokinin (CCK), a gut and brain peptide, appears to be a satiety factor, as Smith (Gibbs, Young, & Smith, 1973) and his colleagues have shown, depressing the amount of food an animal will ingest in a meal. Some of the exogenously administered CCK's effects must be peripheral, for they can be blocked by vagotomy in the rat. But some must be central, for Della-Fera and Baile (1979) have shown that intraventricular injection of cholecystokinin/octapeptide (CCK-8) in the sheep blocks food intake. Even more striking, Della-Fera and her colleagues (Della-Fera, Baile, Schneider, & Grinker, 1981) went on to show that intraventricular administration of an antibody to CCK increases food intake in their sheep. Similar satiety effects have now been obtained by Kissileff and his colleagues (Kissileff, Pi-Sunyer, Thornton, & Smith, 1981) by intravenous administration of CCK-8 to humans who not only reduce food intake, but also report feelings of satiety.

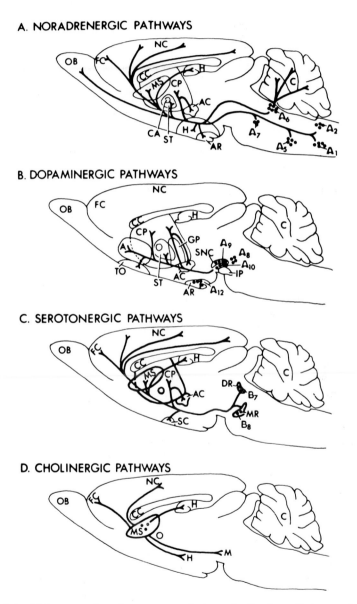

Figure 13-3. Major neural pathways to and through the hypothalamus, involving different neurotransmitters (Harvey, 1973).

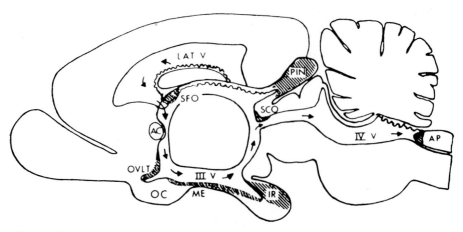

Figure 13-4. Seven circumventricular organs of the rat's brain that lie outside the blood–brain barrier. SFO, subfornical organ; OVLT, organum vasculosum of the lamina terminalis; ME, median eminence; IR, infundibular recess; SCO, subcommissureal organ; PIN, pineal; AP, area postrema (Phillips, 1978).

One of the big questions in all of these experiments with peripherally administered peptides has been whether they can cross the blood–brain barrier, but we now know that one way they may influence the brain is through the circumventricular organs that lie outside the blood–brain barrier (Figure 13-4). This possibility is clearly shown by Epstein (1978) in his work with the potent dipsogen, angiotensin. This peptide, made in the brain as well as the periphery, is believed to exert its effects on the subfornical organ (SFO) of the rat. Femtomole amounts of angiotensin, for example, administered directly to the SFO, result in very significant water intake. Furthermore, presumably through a similar mechanism, steady infusion of angiotensin into the ventricle not only causes rats to drink as much as their body weight in water overnight, but also to drink enormous quantities of 3% NaCl solutions that they normally avoid. Detailed analysis of the anatomical pathways involved in these mechanisms (Figure 13-5) may now be possible with the newer anatomical tracing methods, as studies of the connections of the SFO are now revealing (Miselis, in press).

Figure 13-5. Detailed anatomical connections of the subfornical organ, determined ▶ by an anterograde tracing method in which labeled amino acid is injected among the cell bodies in the SFO. Then with autoradiographic methods the pathways (left) and terminal fields (right) of the SFO are determined. NM, n. medianus of medial preoptic area; OVLT, see Figure 13-4; SONa, Supraoptic n. anterior; SONt, Supraoptic n. tuberal; PVN, paraventricular; NC, n. circularis; PeV, periventricular area; Pfd, dorsal perifornical area; LH, lateral hypothalamus; fx, fornix; sm, stria medullaris; ac, anterior commissure; oc, optic chiasm; ot, optic tract. (Adapted from Miselis.)

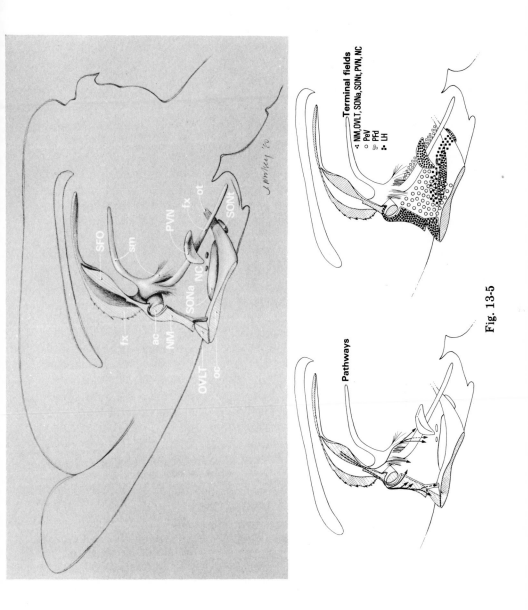

Fig. 13-5

Terminal fields
∴ NM, OVLT, SONa, SONt, PVN, NC
○ PeV
ᵍᵖ PFd
♣ LH

Pathways

Motivation and Hedonic Processes

As these examples illustrate, most of our emphasis in the study of the physiology of motivation has been on consummatory behavior where we really did not have to address the basic questions of motivation, for we could talk about feeding behavior, drinking, copulation, maternal behavior, attack, or thermoregulatory behavior. Neal Miller was one of the few people who kept drawing our attention to appetitive and operant measures of motivation (1956). The classic Miller, Bailey, and Stevenson paper (1950) concluded that hyperphagic rats with VMH lesions had "decreased hunger but increased food intake" because they would not work for food (operant measure) or eat if the food was adulterated with quinine (appetitive measure). Most of us dismissed this phenomenon as a "finickiness" in consummatory behavior of the sort that Teitelbaum (1955) described. But Teitelbaum himself went on to point out that the best test of whether behavior was motivated was whether an animal would learn an arbitrary operant to achieve the appropriate goal of the motivated behavior (1966).

Another major challenge to our preoccupation with consummatory behavior came with Olds and Milner's discovery of self-stimulation in 1954. Here were reward and reinforcement functions of the limbic system. To some degree they were related to the mechanisms of consummatory behavior, for the same parameters that increased and decreased sexual behavior and food intake increased or decreased self-stimulation, as the experiments of Margules and Olds (1962) and Hoebel and Teitelbaum (1962) showed. But very early, in 1956, Olds postulated "pleasure centers in the brain" and thus added another possible limbic system function. He envisaged two systems: (1) a lateral system, mainly the medial forebrain bundle and its rostral and caudal connections, that is hedonically positive in that the rat will work very hard to turn on electrical stimulation there; and (2) a medial, periventricular system in the hypothalamus and midbrain that is hedonically negative in that the rat will work very hard to turn off electrical stimulation there when it is initiated by the experimenter.

Others have also raised the question of hedonic process and its neural basis. Certainly Pfaffmann (1960) does in his discussion of the "pleasures of sensation" resulting from afferent gustatory stimulation. Earlier, P. T. Young (1959) looked at food preference behavior as a measure of hedonic process. He trained rats to choose repeatedly between minute tastes of solutions (1 or 2 drops), so that postingestional factors were not of consequence. Thus, for example, he found that rats preferred the highest concentrations of sucrose solutions (40–50%) rather than concentrations near isotonic levels (5–10%) that were preferred in preference tests utilizing ingestion. So the appetitive and consummatory measures do not always agree, depending, as Mook (1963) showed in the rat with an esophogeal fistula, on the postingestional consequences of consummation. If postingestional consequences are minimized by putting water into the stomach as the fistulated rat drinks glucose and sucrose solutions, the preference functions (Figure 13-6) faithfully follow the intensity of afferent gustatory nerve impulses (Figure 13-7) shown by Hagstrom and Pfaffmann (1959). So sensory input itself can be hedonic. However, lest we think only of taste, it is well to remember Harry Harlow's concept of "tactile comfort" (Harlow & Zimmermann, 1959), so important in the normal affective development of the rhesus monkeys and the rest of us I am sure. Perhaps one even better example of the hedonic aspect of somesthetic stimulation is the effect of thermal stimulation and thermal comfort and discomfort. We'll talk about that shortly.

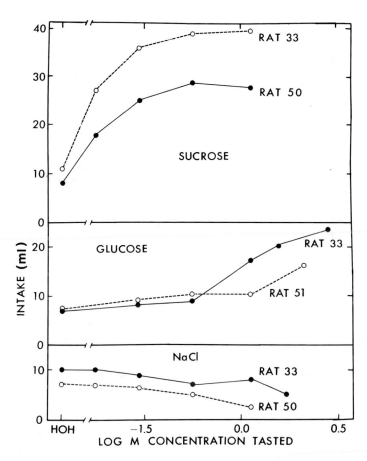

Figure 13-6. Preference curves for sucrose, glucose, and NaCl in fistulated rat where only water reaches the stomach (Mook, 1963). Compare with Figure 13-7.

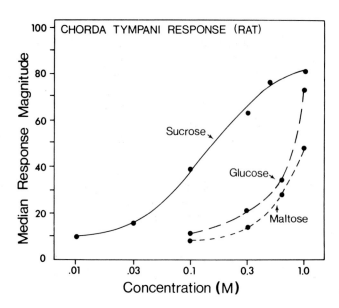

Figure 13-7. Electrophysiological response of the chorda tympani to sucrose and glucose solutions (Hagstrom & Pfaffmann, 1959).

The question of hedonic process comes up quite directly in our studies of motivated behavior in human subjects where we not only measure food intake or thermoregulatory response, but also obtain verbal reports of hedonic experience or ratings on a hedonic scale. Although we do not usually directly study the neural mechanisms at work in human motivation, doing human experiments that parallel animal studies can be most instructive, as you will see.

Evolution of Hedonic Processes

However, before we look at some of our human studies and see how they relate to parallel animal studies, we should recognize that we are dealing with a continuum of functions of the limbic system. At the simplest level are the *physiological regulations.* Next are the two aspects of motivated behavior: *consummatory behavior,* which may serve those regulations; and *appetitive behavior,* which may be an unlearned approach or withdrawal or may be the performance of an arbitrary operant. *Reward and reinforcement* are also involved, for they are important in teaching an animal to perform an operant and the stimuli associated with these processes can be said to have incentive value or hedonic value. In the case of humans, we also deal with *hedonic experience*, pleasantness and unpleasantness, pleasure and pain.

The continuum we are talking about, in fact, should be even broader than the limbic system and the vertebrates that possess it, as Epstein has pointed out (Chapter 2, this volume). He quite properly includes the invertebrates in his continuum and argues that, in the absence of affective expression, their eating, drinking, mating, and similar behaviors should be classified as instinctive rather than motivated. This evolutionary perspective is important, for behavior has developed over the long reaches of phylogeny and new properties emerged, gradually or abruptly, as new properties of the nervous system developed. Thus, we should expect that examination of existing representatives of phylogeny should show emergence of motivated behavior from instinctive behavior, the emergence of reward processes that reinforce new operant behavior, and the emergence of hedonic experience. Theoretically, there should be precursors of each emergence, showing up in incomplete or weak form, so that we should expect to see some aspects of motivational and reward processes in the invertebrates and some aspects of hedonic experience in infrahuman mammals. In all cases, we are dealing with constructs that we infer, not only from the behavior of individual species that we study, but from seeing that species in evolutionary perspective.

Thermoregulatory Processes

Some of these issues are illustrated when we compare experiments on temperature regulation in animals and humans. We know that thermoregulatory responses can be elicited in warm-blooded animals not only by extremes of ambient temperature, but also by heating or cooling the anterior hypothalamus and preoptic area (Satinoff, 1964). Dogs, for example, will shiver and vasoconstrict, or pant and vasodilate, when this region of the brain is cooled or heated, even when ambient temperature is neutral (Fusco, Hardy, & Hammel, 1961). Normally temperature receptors in the skin serve to signal the hypothalamic mechanisms at the same time that core temperature may be decreased or increased, directly signaling the hypothalamus with cooler or warmer blood. In addition to such physiological responses, animals also use thermoregulatory behavior to conserve or lose heat. Quite simply, they will move from a cold to a warmer part of the environment or from a hot to a cooler region. Even poikilothermic animals such as lizards and other reptiles will thermoregulate behaviorally when they cannot regulate physiologically. Satinoff has shown that physiological and behavioral thermoregulation may be separated in animals like the rat, for anterior hypothalamic and preoptic lesions will impair physiological temperature regulation, but will not interfere with behavioral thermoregulation (Satinoff & Rutstein, 1970). Similarly, lesions in the lateral hypothalamus will impair behavioral thermoregulation without much damage to physiological regulation (Satinoff & Shan, 1971).

The easiest way to test behavioral thermoregulation in the laboratory rat is to allow it to press a lever to turn on heat or cold in the face of the opposite ambient temperature. Originally this work was done in one direction with a cold box and a heat lamp, but a more elegant setup was devised by my colleague and former student, John Corbit (1969, 1973). He used the system shown in Figure 13-8. Hot or cold air was flowed at a very high rate over the rat in a small chamber. Physiological regulation was overwhelmed by the large airflows, but the animal could respond behaviorally. A press of the lever would switch the flow from hot to

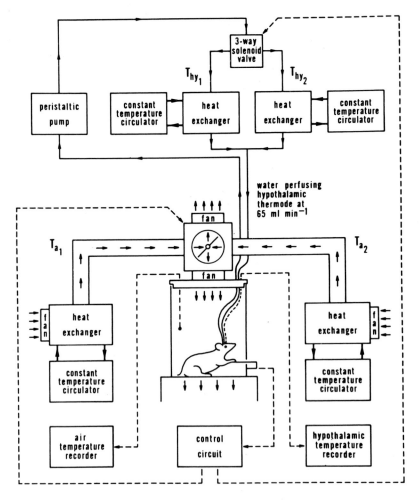

Figure 13-8. Experimental setup for operant control of peripheral temperature and anterior hypothalamic temperature (Corbit, 1973).

cold or cold to hot for a 15-sec period. The setup also allowed the experimenter to flow cold or hot water through U-shaped steel tubes implanted as thermodes in the anterior hypothalamus. Again the rat could press a lever to get a 15-sec flow of hot water when the brain was being cooled by a steady flow of cold water and vice versa.

Quite clearly, the rat performed adaptive thermoregulatory responses in both ambient temperature and brain temperature experiments, showing that both skin temperature change and brain temperature change can be both motivating and rewarding. How rapidly the animal pressed the lever was a function of the extreme of temperature. For example, when the brain was heated, the higher the temperature, the more rapidly the rat pressed for a brief shot of cold water (Figure 13-9). In many ways, this is an example of thermal self-stimulation of the brain to parallel electrical self-stimulation of the brain, so we are talking about CNS mechanisms of thermal reinforcement.

Perhaps even more interesting was the fact that the rat would heat its skin when its brain was cooled and vice versa. It would also heat its brain when its skin was cooled and vice versa. Quite clearly, information from temperature receptors in the skin and temperature of the brain is integrated in the anterior hypothalamic-preoptic area. This phenomenon is illustrated in Figure 13-10, where the rat's rate of responding to cool its brain is shown as a function of different skin temperatures over a range of low to high brain temperatures.

At the same time, Corbit was able to show that the animal knew where its problem was, for if its brain was cooled and it had a choice of warming its skin or warming its brain, it behaved appropriately and warmed its brain (Corbit & Ernits, 1974). Similarly, it behaved appropriately when its skin was cooled and preferred to warm its skin over warming its brain when given a choice.

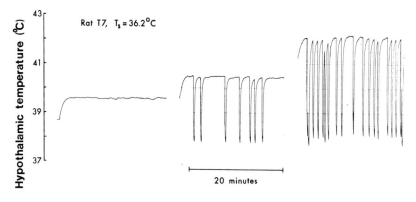

Figure 13-9. Increase in operant responding for 15 sec of anterior hypothalamic cooling as a function of increasing hypothalamic temperature (Corbit, 1973).

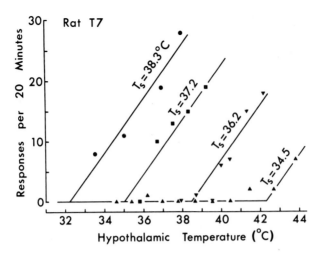

Figure 13-10. Rate of operant responding in order to cool hypothalamic temperature as a function of different skin temperatures over a range of brain temperatures (Corbit, 1973).

So the animal experiments show that body temperature can be regulated physiologically through temperature-sensitive neural mechanisms in the anterior hypothalamus and preoptic area. Given appropriate operant responses, body temperature can also be regulated by behavior that meets the major criterion of motivated behavior in that the responses vary in vigor as a function of the degree of temperature extreme the animal faces, either on its skin or in its brain. Under these conditions an operantly produced change in temperature on the skin or in the brain is a highly rewarding hedonic process.

What we don't know directly, of course, is whether the animal has a hedonic experience as it indulges in its vigorous hedonic behavior. Parallel experiments, done noninvasively, on humans, make their hedonic experience as well as their hedonic behavior clear. In his doctoral dissertation, my former graduate student, Raymond Hawkins, immersed human subjects in constant-temperature hot or cold baths up to their necks (1975). Then he had them stand up out of the water and take a shower that started at tub temperature, but that could be made hotter or colder with the turn of a dial. Their instructions were to find the most pleasant shower temperature. If the subject was kept in the tub a short time, there was no change in rectal temperature, so only skin temperature was increased or decreased. At longer exposures, however, rectal temperature changed about .5°C, and as Figure 13-11 shows, it made quite a difference. As quickly as possible, subjects with elevated rectal temperatures turned the shower down to very cold; those with lowered internal temperatures took long hot showers.

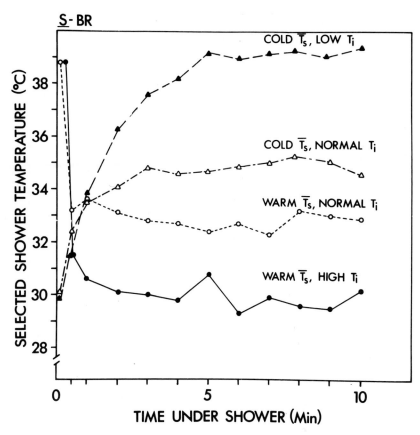

Figure 13-11. Shower temperature selected as most pleasant by a human subject after skin temperature (T_s) was raised or lowered and after core temperature (T_i) was also raised or lowered (Hawkins, 1975).

Subjectively, the subjects reported the hot and cold tubs as very unpleasant, especially after their core temperature changed. The showers, on the other hand, were extremely pleasant, in fact hedonically sensational. If only skin temperature was changed in the tub and rectal temperature remained normal, then the shower temperature was less extreme (Figure 13-11) and the hedonic experience was modest.

Hawkins also had his subjects replicate the procedure of Cabanac (1971) in which, while immersed in different tub temperatures, they dipped their hands in buckets of water of different temperature and rated them on a hedonic scale. As Figure 13-12 shows, when body temperature was raised or lowered, the most pleasant hand temperatures were close to the opposite extremes, even temperatures the subjects called "biting cold" and "burning hot." Thus, the hedonic quality of an

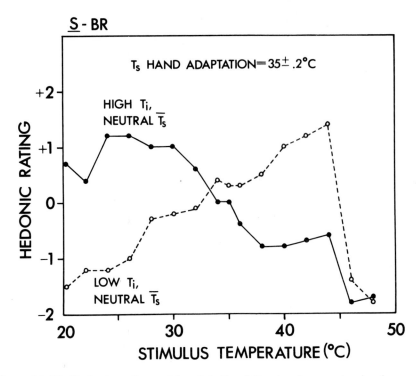

Figure 13-12. Hedonic rating of hand baths (stimulus temperature) when core temperature (T_i) was raised or lowered by whole-body immersion in a constant-temperature bath (Hawkins, 1975).

external stimulus depends heavily on the state of the internal environment (core temperature).

Quite clearly, then, human subjects behave like rats, and in addition, report intense hedonic experiences as their body temperatures are raised or lowered (very unpleasant) and they are given the opportunity to make ratings of different hand temperatures or take showers at temperatures of their own choice (the opposite extreme is most pleasant).

Taken together, these findings suggest that there is a temperature-sensitive limbic mechanism, centered in the anterior hypothalamus and preoptic area, that is responsive to afferent impulses from skin temperature receptors and to core temperature in an additive way. This mechanism generates physiological responses that work to defend and restore body temperature. Working through the lateral hypothalamus, they also generate intense thermoregulatory motivated behavior and make temperature change of the skin or brain highly rewarding. Assuming there is a similar neural process in humans, it also generates intense hedonic experiences of discomfort and comfort, unpleasantness and pleasantness.

Hedonic Processes in Taste and Hunger

Similar analyses and comparisons of humans and animals are also possible in the study of hunger and thirst motivation, in sexual behavior,
aggression, maternal behavior, and so forth, but none are as well worked
out as the case of thermoregulatory behavior. I'll mention two efforts
briefly. One is Cabanac's study (1971) of the pleasantness and unpleasantness of glucose solutions as a function of the ingestion of glucose.
He had subjects taste and swallow 50-ml mouthfuls of 20% glucose
solutions once every 3 minutes and judge both their sweetness and their
hedonic qualities. Sweetness ratings did not change, but within 10 trials
(500 ml in 30 minutes), ratings of pleasantness turned to unpleasantness (Figure 13-13). However, if the solutions were not swallowed, but
merely tasted and spit out, there was no change in pleasantness ratings.
Preloads of 500 ml of 20% glucose produced ratings of unpleasantness
even when the test glucose mouthfuls were not swallowed, but intravenous glucose injections did not. We were able to replicate some of
these findings in trained subjects some years ago, but drew the tentative
conclusion that the change in hedonic ratings was produced by gastric
distension, slight nausea, and the consequent reluctance to ingest more

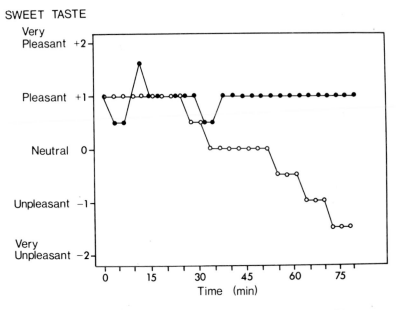

Figure 13-13. Change in the rating of the pleasantness of 50-ml 20% sucrose solution, depending on whether the solution was swallowed (open circles) or spit out
(closed circles) (Cabanac, 1971).

glucose solution, for 500-ml preloads of water and 10% glucose produced the same effect as 20% glucose preloads.

The second study is our effort to compare direct intragastric eating by stomach tube in humans and animals (Stellar, 1967). You will recall that animals eventually regulate their intake when they eat via stomach tube (Epstein & Teitelbaum, 1962). In order to train them to press the lever that activates the pump that delivers the food to the stomach, it is necessary to give them a tiny oral reward for each press. We did not have to do that when we instructed our human subjects to feed themselves by stomach tube. They regulated their intake as well as they did when eating orally, as you can see in Figure 13-14. However, intragastric feeding was not as satisfying as oral feeding, as the hunger ratings in Figure 13-15 show. Just as in the case of animals, the oral factors are contributing something to the hedonic process over and above the regulation of food intake. In the animal studies, we call it "reward"; in the human studies, we call it "hedonic experience." The question is, how different are they?

Drive and Reward Processes

Self-Stimulation

At this point, I'd like to shift back to animal experiments and focus on some studies that attempt to separate the drive and reward components of motivation and hedonic process. My starting point is the work of Gallistel and his students (1973), who followed up on Deutsch's division of self-stimulation into a drive function and reward function (Deutsch & Howarth, 1963). Using running speed in an alleyway for self-stimulation in the goal box, this approach was able to show that rats ran faster for a given level of reward if they received a "free" brain stimulation as a priming (drive) stimulation just before they were allowed to run. The more intense the priming, the faster running. With priming held constant, increasing the intensity of stimulation in the goal box (reward) also increased running speed. The effect of rewarding stimulation lasted a long time, so that animals running slowly for weak reward stimulations run slowly when first tested the next day. If reward stimulation intensity was increased, running speed gradually increased over 6–10 trials and reached a new higher asymptote of running speed. Tested 24 hours later, the animals began running at the high speed, indicating a memory for the previous intensity of rewarding stimulation.

It was very different for the priming stimulation. As soon as it was increased in intensity, running speed increased. Then if priming was decreased, running speed on that trial decreased. Furthermore, the effects of priming, unlike those of rewarding stimulation, decayed rapidly. So, for example, if the rat was made to wait 20 or 30 sec after

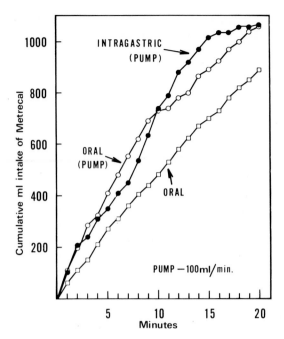

Figure 13-14. Comparison of voluntary intragastric intake of a liquid diet by stomach tube (intragastric pump) with intake by mouth (oral pump).

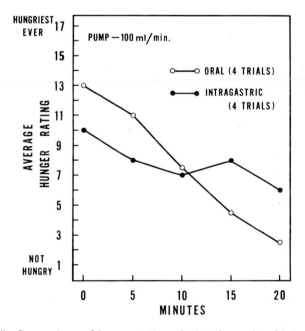

Figure 13-15. Comparison of hunger ratings during the oral and intragastric intake shown in Figure 13-14.

intense priming, it ran much more slowly than if it ran immediately after priming; after 60–90 sec, the decay was almost complete. So if priming represents the drive component of self-stimulation, it is a transient function that decays very rapidly compared to the reward function, which seems to involve memory.

Approach and Withdrawal

An important analysis of what such electrical stimulation of the brain means in terms of hedonic processes outside the runway was carried out by J. R. Stellar in Gallistel's laboratory (Stellar, Brooks, & Mills, 1979). He dealt with the two systems described by Olds and prepared rats with electrodes in the positively reinforcing lateral system, in the medial forebrain bundle of the lateral hypothalamus, and rats with electrodes in the negative medial, periventricular system of the hypothalamus. Rats with lateral placements self-stimulated; rats with medial placements worked to turn stimulation off as soon as it came on. He then explored the animals' response to a variety of stimuli that naturally evoked either approach or withdrawal behavior and he compared the effect of these stimuli with and without simultaneous brain stimulation.

When the animals were tested under lateral hypothalamic stimulation, responses to aversive external stimuli were reduced and responses to positive external stimuli were increased. Thus, for example, the rats did not show escape or avoidance response to shock from a grid floor during lateral hypothalamic stimulation, although they did show flexor reflexes and prancing on the grid at the intensities of foot-shock used; they responded positively to a tactile probe around the mouth and chewed on it and pursued it during lateral hypothalamic stimulation; they did not withdraw from a cotton swab containing a strong ammonia solution that was previously avoided, and in fact, approached it (one rat took it in its mouth); they did not show startle responses to intense sounds; they responded as positively to weak sugar solutions that they had previously ignored as they had to strong sugar solutions without lateral hypothalamic stimulation.

Medial hypothalamic stimulation increased the vigor of withdrawal from aversive stimuli and attenuated the response to positive stimuli. For example, it took increasing sugar concentration by a factor of 10 in order to elicit a positive response under medial hypothalamic stimulation. With the same tests, bilateral lateral hypothalamic lesions greatly reduced approach responses and increased withdrawal or avoidance responses.

Thus there is evidence for an approach system and a withdrawal system within the brain that can be activated by electrical stimulation that itself is either rewarding or aversive. When the reward system is activated, responses to external stimuli are biased in the direction of approach so that response to negative stimulation is blocked or attenuated and response to positive stimulation is increased. When the aversive system is stimulated, the reverse is true and response to positive stimulation is greatly attenuated or blocked. Presumably there is normally a hedonic balance between the approach and withdrawal systems until some internal change in brain state biases responding to external stimuli in the positive or negative hedonic direction.

Drive and Reward in Food Motivation

Quite clearly, both drive state and reward determine hedonic behavior, whether it be in self-stimulation or approach and withdrawal behavior. In an effort to explore drive and reward processes in food-motivated behavior, I decided to adopt Gallistel's runway and use running speed as a measure of motivated behavior as the degree of food deprivation and the intensity of food reward were varied. Given the ability to separate drive and reward functions, the next question was, where in the sequence of motivated behavior does the satiety factor, CCK, act? On the drive function? On the reward function? How much of CCK's satiety effect is on rewarding properties of taste stimuli and incentives, how much on the postingestional effects of food and fluid intake? I've made a start and would like to report my preliminary results here and tell you something of my plans to probe the neural mechanisms further.

The basic runway procedure is to train a hungry rat to run from start box to goal box for a small food reward (.3 gram of wet mash or 2 drops of fluid food). The distance is 1 meter and performance is expressed as running speed in centimeters per second, the reciprocal of running time from start to goal. The clock is started when the start-box door goes up and is stopped when the rat puts its head into the food compartment. For convenience, the goal box then becomes the start box and the animal shuttles back to food at the opposite end. When the animal is highly motivated, it takes its stance at the door like a track star, bolts out as the door opens, runs directly to the goal box, puts its head in the food compartment, and eats.

When the animal's motivation is low, it may hesitate before leaving the start box and watch the door go up, it may stop in the runway and groom or sniff, it may retrace its steps back into the start box, it may stop and rear, exploring the wire mesh roof of the runway, it may hesitate before entering the goal box or putting its head in the food compartment; but according to the rules of the procedure, the parameters must be such that it always ingests the reward. Quite clearly the running speed measure reflects the competition among drives to explore, groom, and approach food and eat, as well as how fast the animal runs.

A testing session consists of 11 trials and the median running speed is taken as the measure of performance for that session.

The first exploration of the running speed measure compares running speed in the runway to amount ingested in 1-hour meal as a function of hours of deprivation (Figure 13-16A, B vs. Figure 13-16C) and also as a function of concentration of sucrose solution (Figure 13-16D vs. E).

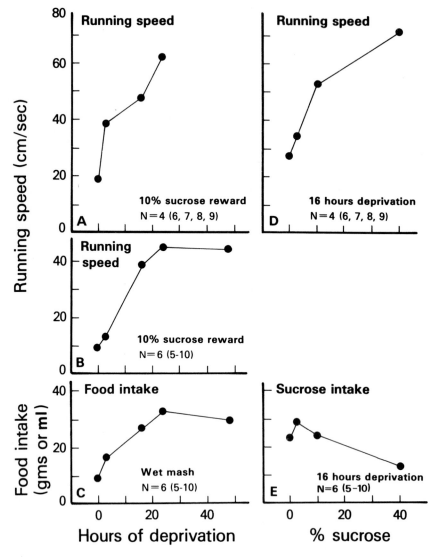

Figure 13-16. Effects of varying food deprivation on food intake (C) and running speed (A, B) compared to the effects of varying the concentration of sucrose on intake (E) and running speed (D).

Quite clearly running speed increases as a function of deprivation up to
24 hours, but there is no further increase at 48 hours. The food intake
measure shows the same function. It is quite different with the sucrose
concentration function. Running speed increases monotonically up to
the highest concentration tested (40%), but ingestion shows a peak at
10% and a sharp drop at 40%, presumably the result of negative postingestional feedback.

The Effects of CCK

The next step was to look at the effects of CCK-8 injected intraperitoneally. The basic procedure in these tests was to habituate the animals to intraperitoneal (i.p.) saline injections 15 minutes before the
meal or the runway test. Then a 2-day crossover design was used in
which half the animals received CCK on the first day and saline on the
second day and the other half were tested in the reverse order. The results show than an i.p. dose of 2 μg/kg of CCK-8 (roughly equivalent
to 40 Ivy dog units) depressed food intake (wet mash), as previously
shown in the literature, particularly in the first 30 minutes (Figure
13-17). A similar depression was produced in running speed for wet
mash in three repetitions of the 11-trial test 15, 60, and 105 minutes
after CCK (Figure 13-17).

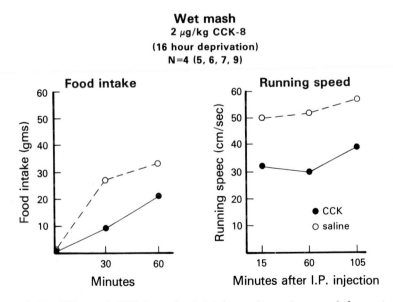

Figure 13-17. Effect of CCK-8 on food intake and running speed for wet mash
reward.

The lawful nature of CCK's effect on running speed is indicated in Figure 13-18, where a dose response function (1.0, 1.5, and 2.0 μg/kg of CCK-8) shows that with increasing doses the initial depression of running speed becomes greater and lasts longer across the three test sessions. A similar finding with food intake is shown in Figure 13-19.

In order to compare the relative effect of CCK on taste alone with taste plus nutritive and osmotic postingestional effects, saccharin and sucrose were selected for study. The initial exploration was to see the effect of CCK-8 on the ingestion of a preferred saccharin solution (.13%) under 24-hour food deprivation conditions and of a preferred sucrose solution (10%) under conditions of food satiation. These results are shown in Figure 13-20. In addition, a mixture of 3% glucose and .13% saccharin was studied because rats ingest twice as much of this solution in a 1-hour test as they do of 10% sucrose when satiated, and by this measure the mixture is highly palatable.

When our explorations are complete, we will have a parametric study of the effects of CCK-8 on ingestion and running speed, using a range of concentrations of sucrose and saccharin and the glucose–saccharin mixture. This procedure will allow us to explore the effects of CCK on the reward function, and with a suitable range of deprivations, on the drive functions. Only a start in these parametric studies has been made, looking at the effect of CCK-8 on running speed to 40% sucrose under supersatiation conditions in which the animals have pellets all the time and are fed a wet mash meal just before the runway test so that they have full stomachs. The results (Figure 13-21) show that 2 μg/kg of

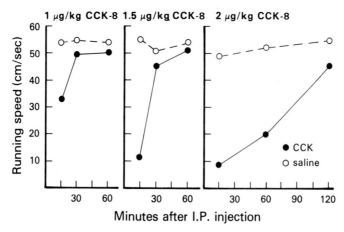

Figure 13-18. Increasing depression of running speed with increasing dose of CCK-8.

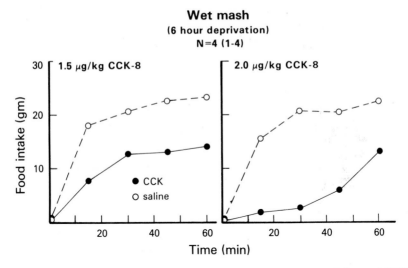

Figure 13-19. Increasing depression of food intake with increased dose of CCK-8.

CCK-8 has a minimal effect on this highly rewarding stimulus. Finally, a control was done with thirsty rats running to water reward and it was shown that there is no CCK effect here (Figure 13-21).

Quite clearly CCK has a satiety effect on the appetitive response to food, where postingestional effects are minimal. It also has a satiety effect on the ingestion of sucrose and saccharin, for it depresses the intake of both. The saccharin effect is interesting, for its ingestion does not have any postingestional nutritive or osmotic effects, and thus the

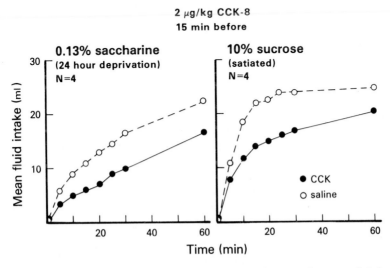

Figure 13-20. Effects of CCK-8 in depressing saccharin and sucrose intake.

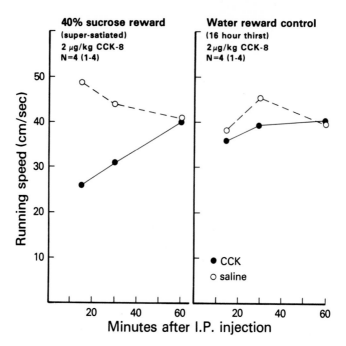

Figure 13-21. Effect of CCK-8 on running speed of the "supersatiated" rat to 40% sucrose reward (left). Control test, showing no effect of CCK-8 on running speed of thirsty rats for water reward (right).

consummatory response is controlled only by taste. Comparing saccharin and sucrose in the runway will be most interesting and instructive, as will further investigation of the "highly palatable glucose–saccharin mixture." Preliminary results show that CCK-8 had hardly any effect on either the ingestion of the glucose–saccharin mixture or running speed to it in the runway.

As we look to future experiments, it will be most interesting to examine intraventricular administration of CCK-8 in the rat. So far there have not been consistent reports of a satiety effect with central CCK in the rat, but very clear results have been obtained in sheep. Our hope is that the runway measure will be very sensitive to central CCK and that we will be able to study CCK's central neural effects. Also in the immediate future are collaborative experiments on thirst with Alan Epstein in which we plan to assess the effect of intraventricular angiotensin on running speed for water and NaCl solutions.

My hope is that studying the appetitive side of motivation in the runway will bring us closer to a method of investigating the hedonic processes in animals. In these first experiments, it should allow us to ask new questions about the satiety effects of CCK and where in the motivational sequence it acts. It is to be hoped that it will lead us rather directly to the brain mechanisms involved.

Discussion

Taken together, the experimental findings and theoretical considerations put forward in this chapter lead to a number of conclusions and speculations.

1. The limbic system of the vertebrate brain mediates a wide variety of motivated behaviors, some of which contribute to physiological regulations and the adaptation of the organism (e.g., drinking, eating, thermoregulatory behavior) and some of which are not involved in physiological regulation or the survival of the individual (e.g., sexual behavior, maternal behavior). All are under multifactor control and are dependent on some combination of external stimuli and internal states.

2. The limbic system may contain dual mechanisms, responsible for arousal and satiation, approach and withdrawal, and positive and negative reinforcement. It is possible these are the excitatory and inhibitory mechanisms suggested in 1954, but that is still not proven as a general case. In the cycles of behavior, the balance between these two systems swings from one to the other, probably not frequently to the extremes and rarely for long at the point of neutrality. Might we speculate that these two systems are the substrates for Solomon's opponent processes (Solomon & Corbit, 1974)?

3. While it is clear that there are specific mechanisms for each kind of behavior, we are not certain how the specificity, expressed through the final common pathway to behavior, comes about. Some of it is due to the guiding and directing action of stimuli and stimulus patterns (e.g., sweet or salty taste, lordosis); some is due to specific internal environment conditions, acting on central neural receptor mechanisms (e.g., thermal sensitivity of the anterior hypothalamus); some of it may be due to highly specific integrative mechanisms for each major kind of behavior. We just don't know.

4. Despite the specificity of motivated behaviors, all involve the same hedonic processes: approach or withdrawal, reinforcement, hedonic experience. Is there a final common hedonic pathway, as Olds implied in the concept of "pleasure center"? Or are the hedonic mechanisms themselves specific? Or is there some other mechanism by which the common hedonic properties of motivated behavior are generated?

5. Sensory stimuli are arousing and motivating and may depend on the state of the internal environment for their potency, but not always. Theoretically, they should also be satiating (full gut?). They also, of course, can be reinforcing, both rewarding and punishing, leading to approach and withdrawal, thus acting as incentives.

6. As Kety (1970) has pointed out, the catecholamines may be ideally suited to broadcast significant biological events and thus serve as the

basis of the reinforcement of learning. There is evidence for their roles in both motivated behavior and reinforcement, but it is not specific or definitive as yet.

7. The peptides are involved in both arousal (angiotensin) and satiation (CCK), and given what we are learning of their central neural effects and the diverse neurosecretory functions of the brain, they should play a central role in hedonic processes.

8. Drive and reward functions may be experimentally separable in food motivation as well as in self-stimulation and we may be able to identify separate neural mechanisms involved. Presumably such agents as angiotensin and CCK have different effects on drive functions (arousal and satiation) and on reward (reinforcement) and incentive (learned arousal) functions, but this remains to be determined experimentally.

9. Finally, can we speculate about hedonic experience? Taken in evolutionary perspective, what we identify as hedonic experience in man emerges over phylogeny in a wide range of behavioral precursors. In the simplest of organisms, taxes, reflexes, and instinctive behaviors serve ingestive behavior, defense, and reproduction. These behaviors may not qualify as motivated behavior, for they may not be influenced by the internal state of the organism, there may be no affective display (Epstein), and the animal may not be able to learn to perform an arbitrary operant to achieve its goal (Teitelbaum). Yet the animal may become hyperactive when deprived, it may show strong approach and withdrawal behavior, it may show food preferences, for example, and these may be thought of as the precursors of motivated behavior. The blowfly is a good example because it eats in response to the intensity of the taste stimuli, is not responsive to its internal nutritive state, and stops eating in response to the stimulation of the full foregut. Yet it becomes hyperactive when deprived, accepts and rejects, and has food preferences (Dethier, 1964).

In the vertebrates, motivated behavior clearly emerges in that the animal may show the behavior only under certain states of the internal environment, clearly performs arbitrary operant responses to obtain its goals, and thus is responsive to reward and reinforcement. Many of the reflexes and other physiological responses remain, as is obvious in the case of temperature regulation. Some of the precursors of hedonic experience may occur in infrahumans, as judged primarily by approach and withdrawal behavior, affective expression, and the potent effects of reinforcement. These can only be inferred, but should not be ignored. We used the example of thermoregulatory behavior in rats; Olds inferred pleasure in self-stimulation; Harlow talked about tactile comfort in monkeys; Pfaffmann described the pleasures of taste sensation; Bard (1940) vividly described the affective display of the female cat in heat before and after mating, but stopped short of inferring orgasm.

In humans, we have the reflexes and physiological regulations that automatically adapt the organism, we have approach and withdrawal, appetitive and consummatory motivated behavior, reward and reinforcement of learning, affective display, and hedonic experience. As in other vertebrates, the limbic system seems clearly involved in all of these hedonic processes, one would think all the more extensively for the more complex and highly evolved of them.

Acknowledgments. This research was supported by USPHS MH15767 and a grant from the Grant Foundation.

References

Adolph, E. F. *Physiological regulations.* Lancaster, Pa.: Jacques Cattell, 1943.

Bard, P. A diencephalic mechanism for the expression of rage with special reference to the sympathetic nervous system. *American Journal of Physiology*, 1928, *84*, 490-515.

Bard, P. The hypothalamus and sexual behavior. *Research Publication of the Association for Research in Nervous and Mental Disease*, 1940, *20*, 551-579.

Cabanac, M. Physiological role of pleasure. *Science*, 1971, *173*, 1103-1107.

Cannon, W. B. The James–Lange theory of emotions: A critical examination and an alternative theory. *American Journal of Psychology*, 1927, *39*, 106-124.

Cannon, W. B. Hunger and thirst. In C. Murchison (Ed.), *A handbook of general experimental psychology.* Worcester, Mass.: Clark University Press, 1934.

Corbit, J. D. Behavioral regulation of hypothalamic temperature. *Science*, 1969, *166*, 256-258.

Corbit, J. D. Voluntary control of hypothalamic temperature. *Journal of Comparative and Physiological Psychology*, 1973, *83*, 394-411.

Corbit, J. D., & Ernits, T. Specific preference for hypothalamic cooling. *Journal of Comparative and Physiological Psychology*, 1974, *86*, 24-27.

Della-Fera, M. A., & Baile, C. A. Cholecystokinin octapeptide: Continuous picomole injections into the cerebral ventricles of sheep suppress feeding. *Science*, 1979, *206*, 471-473.

Della-Fera, M. A., Baile, C. A., Schneider, B. S., & Grinker, J. A. Cholecystokinin antibody injected in cerebral ventricles stimulates feeding in sheep. *Science*, 1981, *212*, 687-689.

Dethier, V. G. Microscopic brains. *Science*, 1964, *143*, 1138-1145.

Deutsch, J. A., & Howarth, C. I. Some tests of a theory of intracranial self-stimulation. *Psychological Review*, 1963, *70*, 444-460.

Epstein, A. N. The neuroendocrinology of thirst and salt appetite. In W. F. Ganong & L. Martini (Eds.), *Frontiers in neuroendocrinology.* New York: Raven Press, 1978, pp. 101-134.

Epstein, A. N., & Teitelbaum, P. Regulation of food intake in the absence of taste, smell, and other oropharyngeal sensations. *Journal of Comparative and Physiological Psychology*, 1962, *55*, 753-759.

Fusco, M. M., Hardy, J. D., & Hammel, H. T. Interaction of central and peripheral factors in physiological temperature regulation. *American Journal of Physiology*, 1961, *200*, 572-580.

Gallistel, C. R. Self-stimulation: The neurophysiology of reward and motivation. In J. A. Deutsch (Ed.), *The physiological basis of memory*. New York: Academic Press, 1973.

Gibbs, J., Young, R. C., & Smith, G. P. Cholecystokinin decreases food intake in rats. *Journal of Comparative and Physiological Psychology*, 1973, *84*, 488-495.

Hagstrom, E. C., & Pfaffmann, C. The relative taste effectiveness of different sugars for the rat. *Journal of Comparative and Physiological Psychology*, 1959, *52*, 259-262.

Harlow, H. F., & Zimmermann, R. R. Affectional responses in the infant monkey. *Science*, 1959, *130*, 421-432.

Harvey, J. A. Discussion: Use of the ablation method in the pharmacological analysis of thirst. In A. N. Epstein, H. R. Kissileff, & E. Stellar (Eds.), *The neuropsychology of thirst*. Washington, D. C.: V. H. Winston & Sons, 1973, pp. 293-306.

Hawkins, R. C. *Human temperature regulation and the perception of thermal comfort*. PhD thesis, University of Pennsylvania, 1975.

Hoebel, B. G., & Teitelbaum, P. Hypothalamic control of feeding and self-stimulation. *Science*, 1962, *135*, 375-377.

James, W. The physical basis of the emotions. *Psychological Review*, 1894, *1*, 516-529.

Kety, S. S. The biogenic amines in the central nervous system: Their possible roles in arousal, emotion, and learning. In F. O. Schmitt (Ed.), *The neurosciences second study program*. New York: Rockefeller University Press, 1970, pp. 324-336.

Kissileff, H. R., Pi-Sunyer, F. X., Thornton, J., & Smith, G. P. C-terminal octapeptide of cholecystokinin decreases food intake in man. *American Journal of Clinical Nutrition*, 1981, *34*, 154-160.

Lashley, K. S. An experimental analysis of instinctive behavior. *Psychological Review*, 1938, *45*, 445-471.

Margules, D. L., & Olds, J. Identical "feeding" and "rewarding" systems in the lateral hypothalamus of rats. *Science*, 1962, *135*, 374-375.

Miller, N. E. Effects of drugs on motivation: The value of using a variety of measures. *Annals of the New York Academy of Sciences*, 1956, *65*, 318-333.

Miller, N. E., Bailey, C. J., & Stevenson, J. A. F. Decreased "hunger" but increased food intake resulting from hypothalamic lesions. *Science*, 1950, *112*, 256-259.

Miselis, R. R. The efferent projections of the subfornical organ: A circumventricular organ within a neural network subserving water balance. *Brain Research*, in press.

Mook, D. G. Oral and postingestional determinants of the intake of various solutions in rats with esophageal fistulas. *Journal of Comparative and Physiological Psychology*, 1963, *56*, 645-659.

Olds, J. Pleasure centers in the brain. *Scientific American*, 1956, *193*, 105-116.

Olds, J., & Milner, P. Positive reinforcement produced by electrical stimulation of septal area and other regions of rat brain. *Journal of Comparative and Physiological Psychology*, 1954, *47*, 419-427.

Pfaff, D. W. *Estrogens and brain function*. New York: Springer-Verlag, 1980.

Pfaffmann, C. The pleasures of sensation. *Psychological Review*, 1960, *67*, 253-268.

Phillips, M. I. Angiotensin in the brain. *Neuroendocrinology*, 1978, *25*, 354-377.

Richter, C. P. Total self-regulatory functions in animals and human beings. *Harvey Lectures*, 1942-1943, *38*, 63-103.

Satinoff, E. Behavioral thermoregulation in response to local cooling of the rat brain. *American Journal of Physiology*, 1964, *206*, 1389-1394.

Satinoff, E., & Rutstein, J. Behavioral thermoregulation in rats with anterior hypothalamic lesions. *Journal of Comparative and Physiological Psychology*, 1970, *71*, 77-82.

Satinoff, E., & Shan, S. Loss of behavioral thermoregulation after lateral hypothalamic lesions in rats. *Journal of Comparative and Physiological Psychology*, 1971, *77*, 302-312.

Solomon, R. L., & Corbit, J. D. An opponent-process theory of motivation, I: Temporal dynamics of affect. *Psychological Review*, 1974, *81*, 119-145.

Stellar, E. The physiology of motivation. *Psychological Review*, 1954, *61*, 5-22.

Stellar, E. Hunger in man: Comparative and physiological studies. *American Psychologist*, 1967, *22*, 105-117.

Stellar, J. R., Brooks, F. H., & Mills, L. E. Approach and withdrawal analysis of the effects of hypothalamic stimulation and lesions in rats. *Journal of Comparative and Physiological Psychology*, 1979, *83*, 446-466.

Teitelbaum, P. Sensory control of hypothalamic hyperphagia. *Journal of Comparative and Physiological Psychology*, 1955, *48*, 156-163.

Teitelbaum, P. The use of operant methods in the assessment and control of motivational states. In W. K. Honig (Ed.), *Operant behavior: Areas of research and application.* Englewood Cliffs, N.J.: Prentice-Hall, 1966.

Young, P. T. The role of affective processes in learning and motivation. *Psychological Review*, 1959, *66*, 104-125.

Chapter 14

Motivation and Psychological Stress

Neal E. Miller

Motivation, Learning, and Performance

Some conditions are much more effective in producing learning and performance than are others. For example, if one wants to train a rat to run from the starting box at one end of a long narrow alley to a goal box containing food at the other end, the learning and performance, if any, will be exceedingly poor if the animal has just been completely satiated on that type of food and will be vastly better if the animal is 15% underweight and has also been deprived of food for 23 hours. Similarly, with water in the goal box, there will be little learning and performance if the rat has just been satiated on water and much better learning and performance if the rat has been water-deprived. It is convenient to refer to the functionally similar effects of these different deprivations as "drives."

In the absence of food for the food-deprived rat or water for the water-deprived one, the learning and performance of running also are either poor or absent. It is convenient to refer to the food and water as "rewards" or "reinforcements." The joint effects of an appropriate drive and an appropriate reward are often referred to as "motivation."

Another convenient way of producing learning and performance is to use an alley, the floor of which is a grid through which an electric shock is administered to the feet of the rat. Under these conditions, the rat will quickly learn to run from the grid to an insulated platform where he escapes from the electric shock. So it becomes convenient to refer to the electric shocks as a drive and escape from shocks as a reward.[1]

Furthermore, the hunger–food, thirst–water, shock–escape from shock that are effective in causing the animal to learn to run faster down the alley are also effective in producing a stronger strength of pull if the animal has been habituated to wear a little harness, like that illustrated in Figure 14-1, and is temporarily restrained on the way to the goal. With mammals, the same operations that are effective in producing learning in the alley are effective also in producing other types of learning, such as pressing a bar. Thus, one finds that one is describing a certain amount of orderliness in nature.

Motivation in Conflict Behavior

The role of motivation is brought out especially clearly in the study of approach–avoidance conflict (Miller, 1959, 1980a). If, after an animal has been trained to run down an alley to secure food as a reward, he is given a brief electric shock at the goal, whether or not he will continue to run to the goal is a function of the amount of food deprivation as measured in hours and weight loss and the strength of electric shock as measured in milliamperes (mA). The same thing is true of a water-deprived rat running to the goal of water. With suitably designed experiments, the points where the strengths of approach and avoidance are equal when measured by conflict are quite comparable to those where they are equal as measured by strength of pull.

Design for Testing the Utility of an Intervening Variable

We have found it useful to use words like drive, reinforcement, and motivation to describe certain common effects of a number of different manipulations. Now let us discuss the problem at a more rigorous level. If one is dealing with the effects of a single manipulation, amount of water given to a deprived animal immediately before testing, upon a single measure, the amount of water consumed, as Figure 14-2 shows, there is no point in using an intervening variable such as thirst; it merely complicates the description.

The situation is different if one is dealing with the effects on a deprived animal of three manipulations—14 ml of water given to a

---

[1] The foregoing effects are vividly illustrated in a 16 mm motion picture film (also available as a videotape) entitled "Motivation and Reward in Learning" distributed by McGraw-Hill, New York. For a more thorough discussion of functional definitions of drive and reward, see Miller (1959).

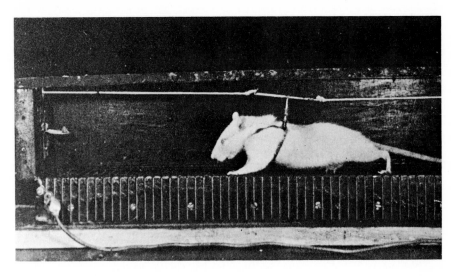

Figure 14-1. Rat temporarily restrained partway to the goal in order to record strength of pull as a measure of performance.

deprived animal by mouth versus 14 ml of water injected directly into the stomach via a chronic fistula versus no preloading—and is using two measures of the effect—the amount of water subsequently drunk and the effect on the rate of performance of bar pressing reinforced on a variable-interval schedule. Then, as Figure 14-3A shows, describing all of the direct relationships is rather complex and, as Figure 14-3B shows, using thirst as an intervening variable becomes more economical. But for such a description to be legitimate, any two manipulations that produce an equal effect on thirst as determined by one of the measures must produce an equal effect on the same thirst as indicated by the other measure. In other words, there must be a perfect correlation between the measures, since they all presume to indicate the same thing, namely, thirst. Figure 14-4 shows the results of an experiment designed

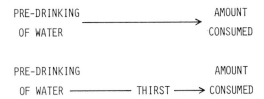

Figure 14-2. When only one treatment and one measure of its effects are involved, it is simpler to represent the direct relationship between them than to insert an intervening variable such as thirst.

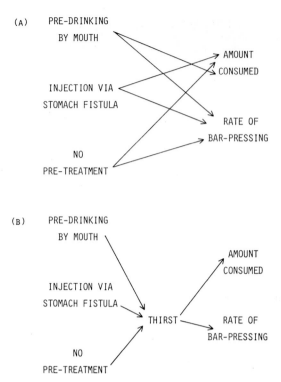

Figure 14-3. When the effects of three treatments on two measures are involved, it can be simpler to use an intervening variable, such as thirst, than to state each of the direct relationships separately.

to test this prediction. It can be seen that the results are what would be expected if we were dealing with only a single intervening variable. Unfortunately, the design necessary to test for the justification of using a single intervening variable, comparing the effects of two or more manipulations on two or more measures, is seldom used. This problem has been discussed and illustrated in more detail elsewhere (Miller, 1959, 1967).

The concepts of physical science are so useful and convincing because their functional unity and generality are confirmed by tests of the foregoing design. Electricity generated in different ways—by chemical reaction in a battery, by an electrostatic machine, or by wires cutting lines of magnetic force—has the same effect on a variety of measures, such as repulsion of like charges on an electrometer, deposition of silver in an electroplating bath, or production of a magnetic field that deflects the needle on a meter. Carrying the matter still further, we note that electrons produced in a variety of ways all have the same charge, and a number of different ways of measuring this charge all agree. In biologi-

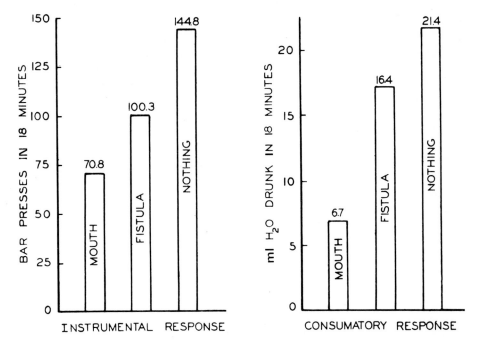

Figure 14-4. Effects of three treatments given to water-deprived rats on two measures of performance. The treatments were 14 ml of water drunk normally by mouth immediately before, 14 ml of water administered via a chronic stomach fistula, and no prewatering. The measures were bar presses reinforced on a variable-interval schedule and milliliters drunk in separate 18-minute tests. (Data from Miller, Sampliner, & Woodrow, 1957.)

cal science, tests of this kind often tell us that our simple initial conceptualization is inadequate. Instead of selecting on the basis of parsimony, evolution often selects on the basis of redundance.

Osmolarity Is Not Enough

The value of experiments designed to compare the effects of two or more treatments on two or more measures is illustrated by the studies of some of the students in my laboratory. In a series of separate tests, Novin (1962) studied the effect of a number of experimental operations—hours of water deprivation, injection of saline intravenously by chronic fistula, feeding dry food to hungry rats, drinking water—on two measures. One of these was volume of water consumed; the other was conductance of the brain tissue as an index of electrolyte content and hence of effective osmolarity of body fluid. He found that each of the experimental operations affected both the measures in the direction that would be expected if thirst were regulated only by osmoreceptors. But then he designed an experiment to compare the effects of the first two of these treatments on both of the measures. The results are presented in Figure 14-5. You can see that the injection of hypertonic saline produced a larger change in conductivity than did the period of water deprivation, but the comparison was in the opposite direction for the amount of water drunk. This is a negative correlation instead of the kind of perfect positive correlation that would be expected if only one factor were involved. Clearly, the amount drunk must be determined by something besides electrolyte concentration, a conclusion that was not apparent from the separate studies. Novin surmised that this something might be extracellular volume. Later, Stricker (1966) performed a series of experiments confirming that something more than effective osmotic pressure is involved and showing that the additional factor is extracellular volume.

Learning that there are at least two different factors involved in thirst is a definite advance in understanding its mechanism. But for many purposes thirst may behave as a relatively unitary variable; it may not always be necessary to speak of different kinds of thirst any more than it usually is necessary to differentiate among the various isotopes of lead.

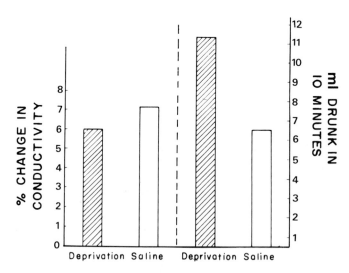

Figure 14-5. Injection of hypertonic saline produces a greater increase in conductivity than does a period of water deprivation, but elicits less drinking than does the deprivation. Therefore, a single intervening variable cannot account for the results. (From Novin, 1962.)

Some General Effects of Psychological Stress

As has been pointed out elsewhere (Miller, 1980b, c, 1981), a large number of clinical observations, epidemiological studies, and studies of the effects of drastic life changes show that conditions that may loosely be described as stressful have a tendency to produce an increased incidence of undesirable mental and physical effects. Some of the stressors that have been studied are bombing raids, combat, immigration to a radically different social environment, rapid drastic changes in the same environment, disasters, social disorganization, crowding, lack of control, loud noise, loss of social support, and loss of loved ones. Some of the effects produced are the entire range of neurotic and even psychotic symptoms, gastrointestinal disturbances and ulcers, sudden cardiac death, hypertension, strokes, cardiac arrhythmias, increased susceptibility to a wide variety of diseases, and increased incidence of cancer. Although many of these studies have used clever controls, it is extremely difficult to rule out confounding factors such as sanitation, pollution, and such dietary factors as saturated fats, fiber, and salt. However, mechanisms of the brain and its neurohumoral systems are being discovered that could account for many of the foregoing effects. But the exact roles of specific mechanisms linking the effects of specific stressors to specific symptoms remain to be worked out. Furthermore, experimental studies in which confounding factors can be rigorously controlled are confirming a number of the physical effects of a number of behavioral stressors. I shall summarize a few of these, concentrating on one uniquely psychological stress that may be described as fear.

Effects of Discrimination and Coping on Stomach Lesions and Other Physical Consequences of Chronic Fear

From the point of view of analytical design, a series of experiments performed by Dr. Jay Weiss and his associates in his section of my laboratory are especially illuminating. In one type of experiment, male albino rats weighing approximately 200 grams were tested in groups of three. Each rat was semirestrained in a separate soundproof compartment and had fixed electrodes attached to its tail. Electrodes on the first two rats were wired in series so that the animals received exactly the same strength of electric shocks. For the first rat, a distinctive tone preceded the occurrence of the shock so that the rat could learn the discrimination of when it was dangerous and when it was safe. For the second rat, the same tone sounded the same number of times but its occurrence was not correlated with the shocks so that there was no way for that rat to learn the discrimination. The third rat was a control for the effects of confinement and food deprivation. He received the same tones but no electric shocks (Weiss, 1970).

Figure 14-6 shows the stomachs of three such rats. The stomach of the control rat shows virtually no lesions, while the stomach of the rat receiving the unsignaled, and hence unpredictable, shocks shows a large number of lesions. The stomach of the rat receiving shocks that were signaled by a tone, and hence predictable, shows far fewer lesions; it is quite similar to that of the nonshocked control rat. That these striking results are indeed typical is shown by Figure 14-7, which presents the average length of lesions in the groups receiving these three types of treatment. You can see that the purely psychological variable of being able to learn the discrimination between when it is dangerous and when it is safe produced a striking reduction in the amount of damage to the stomach.

Figure 14-8 illustrates the apparatus used in the next experiment. Again, the electrodes on the tails of the first two rats are wired in series so that they receive exactly the same electric shocks. The only difference between these two rats is the fact that the first, or avoidance-learning, rat can turn off the shocks for himself and his partner by

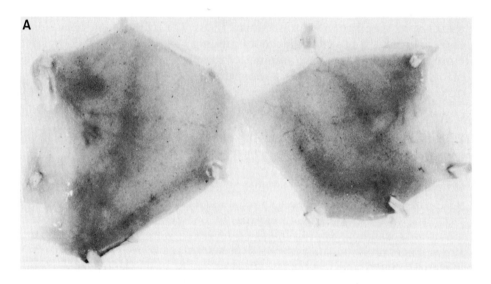

Figure 14-6. Effects of a purely psychological variable, having the opportunity to learn a discrimination, on stomach lesions. (A) Stomach of a control rat, exposed to the same restraint and food deprivation but no electric shocks. (B) Stomach from a rat that received unsignaled shocks and hence was unable to learn a discrimination. Extensive lesions show up as black spots. (C) Stomach of a rat that received exactly the same shocks, but they were preceded by a tone so that he could learn to discriminate when it was dangerous and when it was safe. (From photographs by Jay Weiss.)

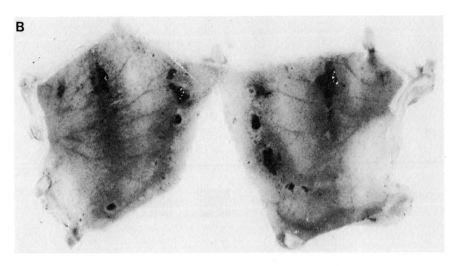

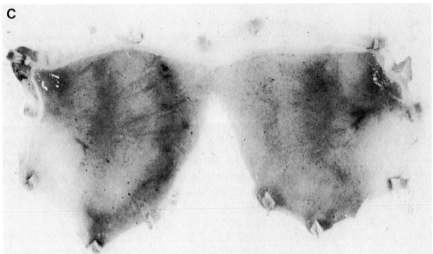

Fig. 14-6

rotating the little wheel. The tone signals the imminence of shock for both rats. If the first one turns the wheel quickly enough, he avoids the shock; if he fails to do this, he turns off the shock by rotating the wheel. The second rat is exposed to the same wheel but it is not connected to the shock-control apparatus; he is dependent on the responses of his partner. The third rat is the control receiving no electric shocks. The left side of Figure 14-9 shows the results of an experiment of this kind. It can be seen that the purely psychological variable of being able to control the shocks by performing a simple coping response of rotat-

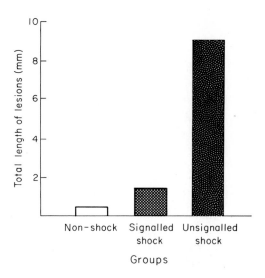

Figure 14-7. The average amount of gastric lesions in groups of control rats receiving no shock and of experimental rats receiving signaled shocks or unsignaled shocks of equal physical intensity. (From Miller, 1972, based on data by Weiss, 1970.)

ing the wheel produces a great reduction in the number of stomach lesions induced (Weiss, 1968, 1971a).

But if the conditions are made slightly different, so that every time the experimental rat turns the wheel he gives himself a shock and his partner a shock via the electrodes on the tail so that he has to take a shock in order to turn off the longer train of shocks, or in other words, is in an avoidance–avoidance conflict, the results are dramatically different (Weiss, 1971b). In this case, as the right side of Figure 14-9 shows, the difference between the groups is exactly reversed—the rat that has to perform the coping response has far more lesions than his yoked control. Both rats receive exactly the same number of shocks, so again the only difference between the two groups is a purely psychological variable. The opposite results of the two experiments also involve a purely psychological variable—whether the coping response is a simple one or whether it involves conflict. That the same variable, being able to perform the coping response, can have opposite results under different conditions shows the need for caution in generalizing from the results of a single experiment. Attempts at practical applications must be checked by carefully evaluated pilot experiments.

In these and other experiments, Weiss and his associates studied the effects of discrimination and coping on other measures in addition to stomach lesions. They found that the treatments that produced increased stomach lesions also produced higher levels of plasma corticosterone (Weiss, 1971a), depleted brain norepinephrine (Weiss, Stone

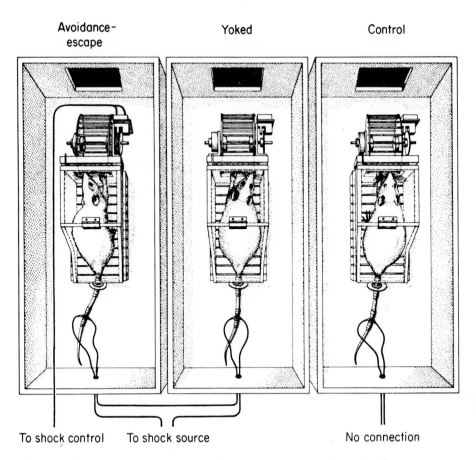

Figure 14-8. Apparatus for studying the effects of the ability to perform a simple coping response on gastric lesions. The avoidance–escape rat can control the shock by rotating the little wheel. Since fixed electrodes on the tails are wired in series, the yoked rat receives exactly the same shocks but his wheel is not connected to shock control. The control rat receives no shocks, but the same confinement and food deprivation. (Adapted from Weiss, 1972.)

& Harrell, 1970; Weiss, Glazer, & Pohorecky, 1976), more inhibition of eating when food was presented in the experimental situation [a test called the *conditioned emotional response* (CER) that has been used as a measure of fear] (Weiss, 1968), and an aftereffect of behavioral depression that interfered with the subsequent learning of a shuttle-avoidance response in a different experimental situation (Weiss, Glazer, Pohorecky, Bailey, & Schneider, 1979; Weiss, Goodman, Losito, Corrigan, Charry, & Bailey, 1981).

Because of the direction and consistency of the foregoing results, it is reasonable to conceptualize them in the way that is depicted in

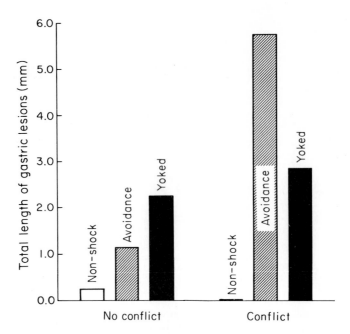

Figure 14-9. Being able to perform a simple coping response to avoid the shocks reduces the stomach lesions for the avoidance rat even though his yoked control receives exactly the same shocks. The relationship is reversed, however, in a conflict situation in which the avoidance rat must give himself and his partner a brief shock in order to avoid a longer train of shocks. (From Miller, 1972, based on data by Weiss, 1971b.)

Figure 14-10. Each of the treatments presented on the left side can be considered to increase fear, which has the indicated effect on each of the measures represented on the right side. The 17 effects predicted from this diagram that have been tested yielded the expected results. Three of them have not yet been tested: the effect of unpredictable versus predictable shock on the depletion of norepinephrine, and the effects of a conflict-inducing coping response on the depletion of nor-epinephrine and on the inhibition of eating in the CER test. Experiments determining whether or not each of these predicted results will come out in the correct direction provide further possibilities for testing the correctness and parsimony of the conceptualization represented in Figure 14-10.

The fact that a single intervening variable appears to account for these results is of course more significant than the exact name attached to that variable. As far as these particular results are concerned, instead of fear it could be called a conditioned emotional response, a condi-

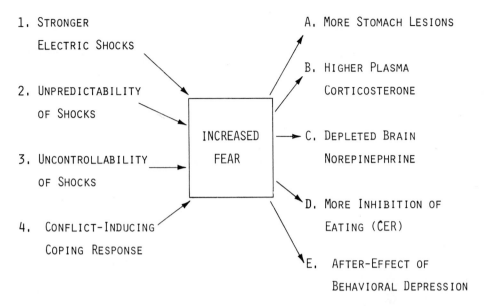

1. STRONGER ELECTRIC SHOCKS

2. UNPREDICTABILITY OF SHOCKS

3. UNCONTROLLABILITY OF SHOCKS

4. CONFLICT-INDUCING COPING RESPONSE

INCREASED FEAR

A. MORE STOMACH LESIONS

B. HIGHER PLASMA CORTICOSTERONE

C. DEPLETED BRAIN NOREPINEPHRINE

D. MORE INHIBITION OF EATING (CER)

E. AFTER-EFFECT OF BEHAVIORAL DEPRESSION

Figure 14-10. How the effects of the four treatments (at the left) in a series of experiments by Jay Weiss on the five measures he studied (at the right) can be summarized in terms of a single intervening variable, such as increased fear.

tioned aversive state, stress, learned high arousal, or the fight–flight response.

If the internal response involved in this experiment is indeed fear, we should predict that it will serve as a drive and that escape from fear will serve as a new reward to reinforce the learning of a new response (Miller, 1948). Thus, if a rat that had been subjected to this type of experiment were repeatedly placed in the apparatus without any further electric shocks and were given an opportunity to perform a specific response, such as pressing a lever, that would release him from the apparatus, we would expect him to learn the response that allows him to escape. Then variables 1–4 will be expected to increase the performance of that escape response. We should also predict that each of the variables 1–4 will produce increased levels of plasma epinephrine.

Conner, Vernikos-Danellis, and Levine (1971) found that rats given unpredictable, uncontrollable shocks to their tails had less elevation of plasma corticosterone if they had the opportunity to attack each other than if they did not. On the basis of this observation, Weiss, Pohorecky, Salman, and Gruenthal (1976) tested the effects on stomach lesions of being able to attack, and found that this opportunity also reduced them. From this, one would predict that it would reduce measures C, D, and E.

Possible Shortcomings of Simple Formulation in Terms of Fear

With the investigation of more experimental manipulations, one might eventually expect to find exceptions to this rule that whatever treatment changes one of the measures on the right side will produce the same change in the other measures. Such an exception will mean that there are other ways, in addition to fear, of affecting some of these measures. To take an extreme example, either adrenalectomy or a pharmacological block will reduce the elevation of plasma corticosterone, but it might not necessarily reduce stomach lesions, the depletion of brain norepinephrine, the inhibition of eating, or the aftereffect of behavioral depression. It should be worthwhile to perform at least some of these tests.

In an experiment following up on Weiss's study of the effects of a coping response on stomach lesions, Tsuda and Hirai (1975) found that, compared with helpless yoked control rats, those that could escape the electric shock by a single bar press had fewer stomach lesions, but those that had to press the bar 10 times in order to escape had more lesions. From this, the formulation represented in Figure 14-10 would have to predict that the latter group would show more fear than their yoked controls by all of the other measures, including the CER and learning and performing a response to escape from the apparatus. If they did not do this, and it seems intuitively plausible that they might not, one would have to conclude that some factor other than fear is involved in the stomach lesions.

In considering the possible shortcomings of the formulation represented in Figure 14-10, one must bear in mind two lessons from the history of science. First, a theory may be instrumental in advancing science because it stimulates the experiments that show the need for a better one (Smyth, 1947). Second, a theory that accounts for a number of facts usually is not overthrown by contradictory facts but only by a better theory (Conant, 1947).

Are There Qualitatively Different Types of Stress?

Bailey and Weiss (unpublished results) find that the unpredictability of electric shocks produces not only an increase in stomach lesions, but also an increase in cardiac lesions. Will variables 1, 3, and 4 also produce such increases? It is conceivable that 3, uncontrollability of shocks, could decrease them. In other words, rats that learn to perform a simple coping response of rotating a wheel might possibly have more cardiac lesions than their yoked partners who do not learn and perform any active response.

The foregoing type of analysis poses an important problem: Are there qualitative differences in "stresses" so that one kind of stress predisposes to one kind of physical symptom and another kind predisposes to a different type? In attacking this problem, one will have to distinguish it from two different but also significant problems, namely, do different strengths or durations of the same stress predispose to different symptoms, and does the same episode of stress produce different symptoms at different times after it is over? At present, aside from some challenging experiments by Mason, Maher, Hartley, Mougey, Perlow, and Jones (1976), there is little evidence on the possible qualitatively different physical effects of qualitatively different stressors. This is because most investigators, with the exception of Mason's group, have confined themselves to studying the effects of a number of different treatments on a single measure or the effects of a single treatment on a number of different measures. They have not used the design that we have been illustrating: studying the effects of a number of different treatments on a number of different measures.

Two Responses to Fear

A dangerous situation frequently elicits one of two contrasting patterns of response (Miller, 1951). One of these involves heightened activity, running, screaming, and displaying warning signals such as the white underside of the raised tail of a deer. If the animal is cornered, it may also involve fighting. Cannon (1953) has characterized this as the fight–flight response. The other pattern is that of crouching and freezing, remaining motionless and mute but alert. Death-feigning may be an extreme form of this pattern, or may conceivably be a different one. In response to a predator, the first pattern is functionally useful in escape or defense, the second one in remaining concealed. An animal may shift rapidly from one to the other, as when a pheasant remains crouched motionless until almost stepped on and then suddenly flies away to alight at a distance, again to remain motionless and concealed.

These different patterns of overt skeletal activity appear to have different physiological components. For example, Corson and Corson (1975) found that in a situation where electric shocks were administered, there tended to be two types of dogs, one that responded with the flight–fight pattern of sympathetic arousal, tachycardia, salivation, panting, and increased secretion of ADH; and another one that did not. Williams (1975) describes two patterns of response that produce increases in blood pressure. One is analogous to Cannon's flight–fight response in which there is an increase in cardiac output produced by an increase in heart rate and stroke volume, the peripheral resistance of the large muscles decreases, and that of the viscera increases, with the total resistance remaining relatively the same. The second pattern is characterized by an increased peripheral resistance without an increase in cardiac output; in fact, there often is a reduced heart rate. He believes this second pattern is one of vigilance. Hypertension tends to evolve from the first to the second.

Anderson and Tosheff (1973) and Anderson (1981) found that if dogs are trained in an avoidance response at the same time of day for many days, their response during the avoidance training involves increased blood pressure produced primarily via increased heart rate and cardiac output, but that after considerable training, before the onset of trials each day a response of anticipatory hypertension begins to appear, characterized primarily by increased peripheral resistance, decreased kidney perfusion, and lowered heart rate. Anderson (personal communication) also has found that if the dogs are salt-loaded via large infusions of isotonic saline, which in themselves will not produce hypertension, the combination of such salt-loading and the avoidance training causes a chronic blood pressure elevation of the second type. Anderson refers to the anticipatory hypertension as part of an orienting response; I would tentatively consider it to be a response to fear and thus predict that an animal showing it would, if given an opportunity, learn to escape from the apparatus.

At present, I tend to believe that it is most useful to consider these two contrasting patterns of response to a dangerous situation as two different innate response patterns to fear, but it is conceivable that adtional research will show that it is useful to deal with these two patterns directly without any reference to fear.

Additional Cardiovascular Consequences of Fear

Lown and Wolf (1971) found that in dogs with experimental infarcts produced by tying off a coronary artery, increased activity of the sympathetic nervous system produced by stimulation of the stellate ganglion caused cardiac arrhythmias that progressed to fibrillation and sudden death. In another experiment, Lown, Verrier, and Corbalan (1973) used electrical stimulation via a chronic electrode in the ventricle to produce a preventricular contraction (PVC) like the ones that often occur in a damaged heart. Gradually increasing the strength of current, they found that the stage just short of fatal fibrillation was the one in which a single stimulation elicited a series of PVCs. Then they found that if dogs were tested without any electric shocks to their feet in a room where they had previously received such shocks, the threshold for the stage just short of sudden death was much lower than it was when they were tested in a room where they had previously been petted and fed. Since no electric shocks were delivered during the test, the difference must have been produced by having learned to fear the one room.

In experiments on pigs with an experimentally induced infarct, Skinner, Lie, and Entman (1975) found that when these pigs were not adapted to the laboratory or were tested by unfamiliar experimenters, a lethal arrhythmia was produced. The foregoing observations are in line with Järvinen's (1955) finding that patients with myocardial infarction are five times as likely to undergo sudden death when unfamiliar staff are making ward rounds than they are in any other comparable time.

If indeed fear is the intervening variable, as represented in Figure 14-10, we would expect that suitable experiments would show that the incidence of fatal fibrillation could be increased by unpredictability of electric shock, uncontrollability of shocks, and a conflict-inducing response.

Friedman and Dahl (1975) trained rats to press a bar for food and then induced an approach–avoidance conflict by having the depression of the bar administer shock through the grid on which the rats stood. They found that extensive treatment of this kind induced hypertension in a strain of rats selected for susceptibility to hypertension induced by a high-salt diet, but did not in a strain selected for resistance to salt-induced hypertension. They also found that separate exposures to equal amounts of hunger and electric shock produced less hypertension than the procedure involving approach–avoidance conflict. If we extend our fear model to this situation, we will have to predict that the approach–avoidance conflict will produce an increase in all of the measures on the right side of Figure 14-10. In fact, a similar experiment by Sawrey, Conger, and Turrell (1956) has shown that rats exposed to such a conflict have more stomach lesions than those exposed to the separate elements of food deprivation and electric shock. Both the latter experiment and the one by Friedman and Dahl were marred by the fact that, instead of being administered by fixed electrodes, the shocks were administered via a grid floor that might conceivably have allowed the experimental and yoked control animals to have performed different responses which caused the shocks to be received in a less painful way by one of the groups (Miller, 1963).

Immune Responses

Anything that affects immune responses obviously will have wide significance for medicine. Psychological stress is known to increase the level of corticosteroids in the blood, which are known to suppress a number of aspects of the immune system. This could be one explanation of the already mentioned epidemiological, clinical, and life-change data showing that conditions that might loosely be described as stressful increase the incidence of a wide range of diseases and even malignancies. Other mechanisms, such as the catecholamines, growth hormone, and direct innervation of lymph nodes and other tissues involved in immune reactions, could also be involved. On the other hand, a number of confounding factors, such as the neglect of hygienic behavior, could also be involved in the epidemiological, clinical, and life-change data. But the case is made much stronger by a number of carefully controlled experiments demonstrating effects of stress on the immune system.

A considerable number of the just-mentioned experiments subjected animals such as mice, rats, monkeys, and chimpanzees to the stressor of avoidance conditioning, a procedure that certainly induces fear. A number of other procedures have been used, such as housing animals in isolation or rotating the home cage on a phonograph turntable. Some experiments have subjected human subjects to conditions such as sleep deprivation and loud noises. Most of these experiments have used indirect measures of effects on the immune system such as increased susceptibility to experimentally induced bacterial and viral infections and to implanted tumors. A few experiments have used direct measures of the immune system such as the level of interferon, the ability of macrophages to ingest bacteria, the ability of natural killer cells to disrupt labeled tumor cells, or the number of lymphocytes and their responsiveness to stimulation via a mitogen (Ader, 1981; Miller, 1980b; Riley, 1981a, b; Stein, Schiavi, & Camerino, 1976).

Although most of the foregoing experiments found that the stressors reduced the effectiveness of the immune system, a number of equally good studies have failed to produce any effect or have produced reliable effects in the opposite direction. These conflicting results indicate that the problem is complex and far from being completely understood. Most of the studies have involved the comparison of only two groups—a presumably normal group compared with a group submitted to additional stressors. But as Vernon Riley (1981b) has beautifully demonstrated, the conditions in the average animal room are well above true baseline levels so that the so-called normal control group may actually be subjected to considerable variable unknown levels of stress. Thus, it is entirely possible that some of the conflicting results are produced by something as simple as the two points being measured by different studies being on different parts of a nonmonotonic (e.g., inverted U-shaped) curve for the effect of the intensity, the duration, or the rebound aftereffects of stress. We need systematic studies aimed at determining a number of points on the foregoing curve for effects of stressors on direct measures of different aspects of the immune system (Miller, 1980b). A first simple step in this direction is a study showing that four levels of increasing stress produce increasing suppression of the reaction of T cells to a mitogenic stimulus (Keller, Weiss, Schleiffer, Miller, & Stein, 1981). We also need to investigate the detailed neurohumoral mechanisms involved.

Neurohumoral Mechanisms

In his pioneering investigations of the flight–fight response, Cannon (1953) emphasized the role of the sympathetic nervous system and of the catecholamines epinephrine and norepinephrine, while in his pioneering investigations, Selye (1956) emphasized the role of ACTH and the corticosteroids. Unfortunately, many subsequent investigators have studied one or the other of these two systems, but very few have studied both. The advent of powerful new techniques is opening up increasing opportunities for studying the effects of these and other neurohumoral mechanisms involved in the physiological effects of psychological stress.

In addition to studying effects on corticosteroids and catecholamines, Mason et al. (1976) have studied effects on growth hormone, thyroxine, sex hormones, vasopressin, oxytocin, and insulin. They have shown that effects of a given situation, for example, the chronic confinement of a monkey in a restraining chair, rise and fall at different rates. In studying the reactions of paratroop recruits to a series of training jumps, Ursin, Baade, and Levine (1978) have observed similar phenomena of different time courses for different physiological responses. To the extent that these hormones and physiological responses are involved in the medically significant effects of psychological stress, we will not expect all of these effects to be explained in terms of one single intervening variable. At present, it is probably wisest to consider stress as an area of research rather than as a unitary phenomenon (Miller, 1980b).

Questions About Aversive Motivation and Stress

This chapter has illustrated many examples of physical effects of a psychological stress that might be referred to as fear. But fear can also be considered as a drive, and escape from fear as a reward. Therefore, in each of these examples it is highly probable that the stressful situation would motivate the learning and performance of an escape response. In other words, in many of these situations there is a close and conceivably identical relationship between stress and motivation. Will all situations that have been described as stressful function also as aversive motivation? Certainly it seems highly plausible that given the opportunity, the subjects would learn a response to escape from the treatments that have been involved in many experiments on stress: very loud sounds, sleep deprivation, difficult tasks, crowding on commuter trains, rapidly paced dangerous work in sawmills, and so on. A number of experiments have shown functional similarities between fear and an aversive motivation elicited by frustration (Barry, Wagner, & Miller, 1962).

Conversely, are all aversive motivations stressful in that they will produce medically adverse physical effects of the type that we have described? This, too, seems plausible but should be critically investigated experimentally. At least, a certain level of strength or duration may be required. Another significant question is, do different types of aversive motivation produce different physically adverse effects?

Joyful Levels of Arousal

The medically significant effects of positive emotions and motivations have received vastly less investigation than have those of the negative or aversive ones. There are two opposing possibilities, neither of which may turn out to be a generally applicable answer. One is that any strong arousal, be it in a happy or an aversive situation, functions as a stress that can produce adverse physical consequences; the other is that the arousal of strong happy emotions powerfully counteracts the adverse effects of stressors and has a generally favorable effect on health. Frankenhaeuser (1976) and her students have elegantly demonstrated that aversive situations such as threats, crowding, lack of control, understimulation, and overstimulation increase urinary levels of catecholamines and their metabolites. Then she investigated the effects of a pleasantly exciting situation, a bingo game rigged so that everyone was winning. The subjects were happily excited and indubitably would have learned a response to get into the situation rather than to avoid it. But to her surprise, the subjects had just as high levels of catecholamines and their metabolites as subjects previously studied in extremely aversive situations. Therefore, she advanced the hypothesis that catecholamines vary with arousal while corticosteroids, which she is just beginning to investigate, vary with aversiveness.

Seymour Levine has long maintained that levels of corticosteroids are subject to behavioral modification in either direction. For example, Goldman, Coover, and Levine (1973) found that opposite shifts in schedules of reinforcement can change levels of plasma corticosterone in opposite directions: Shifts to schedules of reinforcement that deliver fewer or no rewards produce elevations, while those to markedly improved schedules produce reductions. But are these effects and those of other consummatory responses that the authors have described potent and general ones, or are they merely reducing toward normal an increased level of corticosteroids induced by the frustration of a strongly motivated subject who is responding to signals associated with the availability of food pellets or other goal objects but not receiving them rapidly enough?

Pavlov (1927) describes the counterconditioning that occurs when a painful stimulus is made the signal for the delivery of food to a hungry dog:

> Subjected to the very closest scrutiny, not even the tiniest and most subtle objective phenomenon usually exhibited by animals under the influence of strong injurious stimuli can be observed in these dogs. No appreciable changes in the pulse or in the respiration occur in these animals, whereas such changes are always most prominent when the nocuous stimulus has not been converted into an alimentary-conditioned stimulus.

Suggestively similar effects have been reported by Beecher (1956), who has observed that when soldiers have been subjected to extremely harrowing and hazardous conditions of combat, a severe wound that means they will escape further combat by being sent home often does not evoke the reactions of severe pain. Nor do these soldiers request the morphine that would be required after a comparably severe injury that did not have good connotations.

This phenomenon of counterconditioning deserves more detailed study with the much more powerful modern techniques for investigating physiological and hormonal effects. Will counterconditioning reduce the level of catecholamines and corticosteroids, and reverse other hormonal effects of fear and pain? Twenty years ago I showed that animals can be trained to resist the behavioral effects of pain and fear, and raised the question whether such effects were achieved at the expense of increased physiological costs or had the opposite effect of reducing physiological costs (Feirstein & Miller, 1963; Miller, 1960). Now powerful techniques are much more readily available for answering such questions. In order to avoid confounding by effects of food deprivation, it would be interesting to determine what effects could be produced in satiated animals by a highly preferred sweet solution.

More extensive and analytical research on the effects of joyful emotions (Cousins, 1979), of a sense of humor, of tender loving care, of the laying on of hands, of social supports, and of placebo effects will have, in my opinion, considerable prospects of yielding medically significant results.

References

Ader, R. Behavioral influences on immune responses. In S. M. Weiss, J. A. Herd, & B. H. Fox (Eds.), *Perspectives on behavioral medicine.* New York: Academic Press, 1981, pp. 163–182.

Anderson, D. E. Inhibitory behavioral stress effects upon blood pressure regulation. In S. M. Weiss, J. A. Herd, & B. H. Fox (Eds.), *Perspectives on behavioral medicine.* New York: Academic Press, 1981, pp. 307–319.

Anderson, D. E., & Toshoff, J. G. Cardiac output and total peripheral resistance changes during preavoidance periods in the dog. *Journal of Applied Physiology*, 1973, *34*, 650-654.

Barry, H., III, Wagner, A. R., & Miller, N. E. Effects of alcohol and amobarbital on performance inhibited by experimental extinction. *Journal of Comparative and Physiological Psychology*, 1962, *55*, 464-468.

Beecher, H. K. Relationship of significance of wound to pain experienced. *Journal of American Medical Association*, 1956, *61*, 1609-1613.

Cannon, W. B. *Bodily changes in pain, hunger, fear and rage* (2nd ed.). Boston: C. T. Branford, 1953.

Conant, J. B. *On understanding science.* New Haven: Yale University Press, 1947.

Conner, R. L., Vernikos-Danellis, J., & Levine, S. Stress, fighting and neuroendocrine function. *Nature*, 1971, *234*, 564-566.

Corson, S. A., & Corson, E. O'L. Constitutional differences in physiologic adaptation to stress and disease. In G. Serban (Ed.), *Psychopathology of human adaptation.* New York: Plenum Press, 1976, pp. 77-94.

Cousins, N. *Anatomy of an illness.* New York: Norton, 1979.

Feirstein, A. R., & Miller, N. E. Learning to resist pain and fear: Effects of electric shock before versus after reaching goal. *Journal of Comparative and Physiological Psychology*, 1963, *56*, 797-800.

Frankenhaeuser, M. The role of peripheral catecholamines in adaptation to understimulation and overstimulation. In G. Serban (Ed.), *Psychopathology of human adaptation.* New York: Plenum Press, 1976, pp. 173-191.

Friedman, R., & Dahl, K. The effect of chronic conflict on the blood pressure of rats with a genetic susceptibility to experimental hypertension. *Psychosomatic Medicine*, 1975, *37*, 402-416.

Goldman, L., Coover, G. D., & Levine, S. Bidirectional effects of reinforcement shifts on pituitary-adrenal activity. *Physiology and Behavior*, 1973, *10*, 209-214.

Järvinen, K. A. J. Can ward rounds be a danger to patients with myocardial infarction? *British Medical Journal*, 1955, *1*, 318-320.

Keller, S. E., Weiss, J. M., Schleifer, S. J., Miller, N. E., & Stein, M. Suppression of immunity by stress: Effect of a graded series of stressors on lymphocyte stimulation in the rat. *Science*, 1981, *213*, 1397-1399.

Lown, B., Verrier, R., & Corbalan, R. Psychologic stress and threshold for repetitive ventricular response. *Science*, 1973, *182*, 834-836.

Lown, B., & Wolf, M. Approaches to sudden death from coronary heart disease. *Circulation*, 1971, *44*, 130-132.

Mason, J. W., Maher, J. T., Hartley, L. H., Mougey, E. H., Perlow, M. J., & Jones, L. G. Selectivity of corticosteroid and catecholamine responses to various natural stimuli. In G. Serban (Ed.), *Psychopathology of human adaptation.* New York: Plenum Press, 1976, pp. 147-171.

Miller, N. E. Studies of fear as an acquirable drive, I: Fear as motivation and fear reduction as reinforcement in the learning of new responses. *Journal of Experimental Psychology*, 1948, *38*, 89-101.

Miller, N. E. Learnable drives and rewards. In S. S. Stevens (Ed.), *Handbook of experimental psychology.* New York: Wiley, 1951, pp. 435-472.

Miller, N. E. Liberalization of basic S-R concepts: Extensions to conflict behavior, motivation and social learning. In S. Koch (Ed.), *Psychology: A study of a science* (Study 1, Vol. 2). New York: McGraw-Hill, 1959, pp. 196-292.

Miller, N. E. Learning resistance to pain and fear: Effects of overlearning, exposure and rewarded exposure in context. *Journal of Experimental Psychology*, 1960, *60*, 137-145.

Miller, N. E. Animal experiments on emotionally-induced ulcers. *Proceedings of the world congress on psychiatry*, June 4-10, 1961, Montreal (Vol. 3). Toronto: University of Toronto Press, 1963, pp. 213-219.

Miller, N. E. Behavioral and physiological techniques: Rationale and experimental designs for combining their use. In C. F. Code & W. Heidel (Eds.), *Handbook of physiology*, Section 6: *Alimentary canal* (Vol. 1, *Food and water intake*). Washington, D. C.: American Physiological Society, 1967, pp. 51-61.

Miller, N. E. Interactions between learned and physical factors in mental illness. *Seminars in Psychiatry*, 1972, *4*, 239-254.

Miller, N. E. Applications of learning and biofeedback to psychiatry and medicine. In H. I. Kaplan, A. M. Freedman, & B. J. Sadock (Eds.), *Comprehensive textbook of psychiatry* (3rd ed.). Baltimore: Williams & Wilkins, 1980, pp. 468-484. (a)

Miller, N. E. A perspective on the effects of stress and coping on disease and health. In S. Levine & H. Ursin (Eds.), *Coping and health* (NATO Conference Series). New York: Plenum Press, 1980, pp. 323-353. (b)

Miller, N. E. Effects of learning on physical symptoms produced by psychological stress. In H. Selye (Ed.), *Selye's guide to stress research.* New York: Van Nostrand Reinhold, 1980, pp. 131-167. (c)

Miller, N. E. An overview of behavioral medicine: Opportunities and dangers. In S. M. Weiss, J. A. Herd, & B. H. Fox (Eds.), *Perspectives on behavioral medicine.* New York: Academic Press, 1981, pp. 3-22.

Miller, N. E., Sampliner, R. I., & Woodrow, P. Thirst-reducing effects of water by stomach fistula vs. water by mouth measured by both a consummatory and an instrumental response. *Journal of Comparative and Physiological Psychology*, 1957, *50*, 1-5.

Novin, D. The relation between electrical conductivity of brain tissue and thirst in the rat. *Journal of Comparative and Physiological Psychology*, 1962, *55*, 145-154.

Pavlov, I. P. *Conditioned reflexes* (G. V. Anrep, trans.). London: Oxford University Press, 1927.

Riley, V. Biobehavioral factors in animal work on tumorigenesis. In S. M. Weiss, J. A. Herd, & B. H. Fox (Eds.), *Perspectives on behavioral medicine.* New York: Academic Press, 1981, pp. 183-214. (a)

Riley, V. Psychoneuroendocrine influences on immunocompetence and neoplasia. *Science*, 1981, *212*, 1100-1109. (b)

Sawrey, W. L., Conger, J. J., & Turrell, E. S. An experimental investigation of the role of psychological factors in the production of gastric ulcers in rats. *Journal of Comparative and Physiological Psychology*, 1956, *49*, 457-461.

Selye, H. *Stress and disease.* New York: McGraw-Hill, 1956.

Skinner, J. E., Lie, J. T., & Entman, M. L. Modification of ventricular fibrillation latency following coronary artery occlusion in the conscious pig: The effects of psychologic stress and beta-adrenergic blockade. *Circulation*, 1975, *51*, 656-667.

Smyth, H. D. From X-rays to nuclear fission. *American Scientist*, 1947, *35*, 485-501.

Stein, M., Schiavi, R. C., & Camerino, M. Influence of brain and behavior on the immune system. *Science*, 1976, *191*, 435-440.

Stricker, E. M. Extracellular fluid volume and thirst. *American Journal of Physiology*, 1966, *211*, 232-238.

Tsuda, A., & Hirai, H. Effects of the amount of required coping response tasks in gastrointestinal lesions in rats. *Japanese Psychology Research*, 1975, *17*, 119-132.

Ursin, H., Baade, E., & Levine, S. (Eds.). *Psychobiology of stress: A study of coping men.* New York: Academic Press, 1978.

Weiss, J. M. Effects of coping responses on stress. *Journal of Comparative and Physiological Psychology*, 1968, *65*, 251-260.

Weiss, J. M. Somatic effects of predictable and unpredictable shock. *Psychosomatic Medicine*, 1970, *32*, 397-408.

Weiss, J. M. Effects of coping behavior in different warning signal conditions on stress pathology in rats. *Journal of Comparative and Physiological Psychology*, 1971, 77, 1-13. (a)

Weiss, J. M. Effects of punishing the coping response (conflict) on stress pathology in rats. *Journal of Comparative and Physiological Psychology*, 1971, 77, 14-21. (b)

Weiss, J. M. Psychological factors in stress and disease. *Scientific American*, 1972, *226* (No. 6), 104-113.

Weiss, J. M., Glazer, H. I., & Pohorecky, L. A. Coping behavior and neurochemical changes: An alternative explanation for the original "learned helplessness" experiments. In G. Serban & A. Kling (Eds.), *Animal models in human psychobiology.* New York: Plenum Press, 1976, pp. 141-173.

Weiss, J. M., Glazer, H. I., Pohorecky, L. A., Bailey, W. H., & Schneider, L. H. Coping behavior and stress-induced behavioral depression: Studies of the role of brain catecholamines. In R. Depue (Ed.), *The psychobiology of the depressive diosorders: Implications for the effects of stress.* New York: Academic Press, 1979, pp. 125-160.

Weiss, J. M., Goodman, P. A., Losito, B. G., Corrigan, S., Charry, J. M., & Bailey, W. H. Behavioral depression produced by an uncontrollable stressor: Relationship to norepinephrine, dopamine, and serotonin levels in various regions of rat brain. *Brain Research Reviews*, 1981, *3*, 167-205.

Weiss, J. M., Pohorecky, L. A., Salman, S., & Gruenthal, M. Attenuation of gastric lesions by psychological aspects of aggression in rats. *Journal of Comparative and Physiological Psychology*, 1976, *90*, 252-259.

Weiss, J. M., Stone, E. A., & Harrell, N. Coping behavior and brain norepinephrine level in rats. *Journal of Comparative and Physiological Psychology*, 1970, 72, 153-160.

Williams, R. B. Physiologic mechanisms underlying the association between psychosocial factors and coronary heart disease. In W. D. Gentry & R. B. Williams (Eds.), *Psychosocial aspects of myocardial infarction and coronary care.* St. Louis: C. V. Mosby, 1975, pp. 37-50.

Chapter 15

A Physiological and Psychological Analysis of Pain: A Potential Model of Motivation

DAVID J. MAYER and DONALD D. PRICE

Stimuli that give rise to the perception of pain are powerful motivating forces throughout the animal kingdom. Thus, pain shares with the more traditionally studied motivational systems an interspecies generality that presumably has evolved because of its critical survival value. However, the study of pain as an instigator of behavior offers a number of unique advantages that could allow more rapid and detailed understanding of the physiological and psychological mechanisms of motivational states.

Probably the most important advantage in this regard is the ease with which stimuli giving rise to pain can be quantified and manipulated. Unlike the stimuli giving rise to thirst and hunger (hours of deprivation) stimuli producing pain (e.g., heating of the skin) directly and reliably activate known receptors. In addition, such stimuli can be quite brief in duration (milliseconds) and can be repeated at short intervals. Such attributes make feasible the utilization of electrophysiological techniques such as evoked potentials and poststimulus spike histograms. These techniques are not feasible with the more extended events initiating other motivational states. Thus, the events leading to behavior elicited by noxious stimuli offer the potential of being traced through the nervous system.

Another advantage for pain as a motivational model is that pain, as best such things can be known, is organized and perceived similarly among a wide range of mammalian species including man. Behaviors associated with noxious stimuli ranging from simple flexion reflexes to organized escape and avoidance responses appear to be very similar in rats, cats, monkeys, and man. For example, both flexion reflexes and avoidance responses will occur in all of these species when the skin is heated to approximately 45°C, and this is the temperature at which humans first report pain. In addition, at least at the levels so far examined, the anatomical organization and physiological responses of the neural elements appear to be quite similar among studied species. Thus, it appears likely that knowledge of pain gleaned from animal studies has wide applicability to other species including man.

Finally, in this regard, it should be pointed out that a great deal is already known about the neurobiology and psychology of pain, and it is an area of intense current interest. This probably results from the immense magnitude of clinical problems associated with pain. Regardless of the reasons for this interest, it is a distinct advantage to study a topic of broad interest, since interdisciplinary approaches often provide information and insights not as easily accessible in areas of narrower and less intense interest.

A Short Historical Perspective

It seems reasonable to suppose, at least in higher organisms, that without affect there can be no motivation. Behavior appears to be an attempt by organisms to alter their affective state. Curiously, a historical examination of the study of pain reveals that the affective and thus motivational aspects of pain have often been ignored. Although early thinkers, most explicitly Aristotle, considered pain as pure affect, the opposite of pleasure, the advent of post-Renaissance scientific thinking has tended to obscure this point of view. Beginning with Descartes and continuing until quite recently, a mechanistic approach toward the analysis of pain has prevailed. Although there have been dissenters along the way, the advent of physiology and classical psychophysics, with their expertises lying in the analysis of sensation, has resulted in the analysis of pain being subsumed within the framework of sensory systems.

The stage was set for this approach with Müller's "doctrine of specific nerve energies." Müller (1842) stated explicitly that sensation resulted from the activity of peripheral nerves impinging on the brain. Pain was not recognized as a separate sensation but was included in the sensation of touch. Thus, pain was officially relegated to the sensorial world. Von Frey and others further developed Müller's doctrine with the notion that pain sensation occupies separate sensory channels from other somatic sensations. Such an approach culminated in the search for specific pain receptors, channels, and centers in the brain.

There can be little doubt that a sensorial analysis of pain has contributed a great deal to our understanding of the neurobiology of pain, and the school of thought is prevalent to the present day (Perl, 1980). Dissenting voices, however, sporadically interjected that this approach failed to account for a great deal of clinical and behavioral data. This dissention culminated in the work of Melzack and Wall (1965) and its extension by Melzack and Casey (1968). They recognized and expanded the notion that the pain experience includes more than sensory dimensions. This approach has become known as the *gate control* theory of pain.

Although a detailed description of this theory is not possible here, we will summarize several relevant aspects. The theory indicates that, first of all, there are at least three dimensions to the pain experience:

1. A *sensory-discriminative* component, which functions to analyze the sensory information in a somatic input such as location, rate of onset, and intensity;
2. an *affective-motivational* component, which drives the organism to take action with regard to input; and
3. a *cognitive-evaluative* component, which allows comparison of the present input with past experience.

Melzack and Casey (1968) and Melzack (1973) made explicit suggestions about neural structures and systems that were associated with these various dimensions of the pain experience. The sensory-discriminative component was associated with the neospinothalamic system including the ventrobasal complex of the thalamus and somatosensory cortex. The motivational-affective dimension was related to a paramedial ascending system ascending in the spinal cord to the reticular formation and having rich interconnections with the limbic system. As would be expected, the higher order processing of the cognitive-evaluative dimension was associated, at least in part, with the cerebral cortex. One goal of this chapter will be to examine these proposed subdivisions of the pain experience and their associated neural structures in the light of current knowledge.

The original description of the gate control theory (Melzack & Wall, 1965) focused a great deal of attention on the physiological mechanism of pain transmission at the level of the spinal cord and dorsal horn. It was proposed that complex interactions between various inputs occur even at this initial processing stage. We will review the considerable new information about neural processing of noxious stimuli at this level of the nervous system.

A final aspect of the pain experience that was explicitly recognized by the gate control theory was that pain can often show great variability in relation to the actual magnitude of the sensory stimulus. It was proposed that the neural processing of pain is modulated by centrifugal control systems at every stage of afferent processing. At the time the theory was proposed, little specific information was available about this aspect of pain physiology. However, a great deal has been learned about these systems in the past 10 years, and we will review this work here.

Psychophysical and Psychological Aspects of Pain

Although pain is conceptualized by some as a sensation and by others as an emotional feeling, the phenomenon is best considered as an experience that contains at least both elements. Thus, if we are to understand the phenomenon of pain as it occurs in our experience, we need to ask how sensory and affective components of pain are constituted in our experience as well as how these components are interrelated. This inquiry into experience is necessary before one can even begin to distinguish neurophysiological mechanisms that are relatable to each component. However, once the different aspects of pain are sufficiently understood, we can outline a strategy for identifical of their neural substrates.

The neurophysiological study of pain offers the unique opportunity to administer controlled nociceptive stimuli and to compare neural responses to these stimuli with sensory and affective responses to similar controlled stimuli. This approach could allow us to determine which neural structures and mechanisms are involved in different aspects of pain. The more general implication of this approach is that it could provide knowledge about neural mechanisms of sensation, arousal, and affect per se. The following discussion will first review the phenomenology and psychophysics of different dimensions of pain experience and then focus on a strategy whereby psychophysics and neurophysiology can be combined to identify the neural substrates for these different dimensions.

The Sensory Aspects of Pain

The sensory–discriminative dimension of pain refers to the experience of the intensity, duration, location, and unique quality (e.g., burning, aching, sharp, dull) of sensations normally reported as unpleasant. As has been done for other somatosensory modalities, a number of stimulus–response relationships have been determined for painful sensations. The most precise relationships have been established with the use of radiant heat or contact heat. Heat-induced pain can be controlled, quantitatively administered, and produced in such a manner as to produce little or no tissue damage. The following discussion will emphasize the major findings derived from studies of heat-induced pain.

The threshold for thermally evoked pricking pain occurs at skin temperatures of 44–45°C, regardless of the rate of temperature increase used to arrive at these temperatures (Hardy, 1953). This independence between threshold intensity and rate differs markedly from the sense of warmth, the perceived intensity of which is very much dependent on the rate of temperature increase. Moreover, the threshold intensity required for heat-induced pain exhibits much less spatial summation than that observed for warmth. The constancy of heat-induced pain raises the question whether the thresholds for reflex avoidance responses to pain are similar. Hardy (1953) has shown that the threshold for the heat-induced flexion reflex in spinal man averages $44.1 \pm 0.75°$C, and this end point, like that for pain, is independent of the rate of temperature increase. The similar parametric requirements for heat-induced pain and flexion reflex support the hypothesis that both are subserved at least in part by common neural mechanisms. The stability of these thresholds under specific experimental contexts should not be misconstrued as indicating that they are unmodifiable. The threshold of heat-induced pain is influenced by the immediate past history of thermal stimulation and includes such factors as the number, duration, and intensities of previous stimuli. For example, long duration, low intensity noxious heat stimuli can evoke primary hyperalgesia, which is accompanied by a lowering of pain threshold and an augmentation of the intensity of suprathreshold pain (Beitel & Dubner, 1976; Hardy, Wolff, & Goodell, 1952).

As with other sensory modalities, the magnitude of painful sensation intensity increases as a direct function of stimulus intensity (Adair, Stevens, & Marks, 1968; Price, Barrell, & Gracely, 1980). In fact, a rather precise relationship has been established between skin temperatures in the noxious range (i.e., 45–51°C) and perceived magnitudes of painful sensation (Price et al., 1980). This relationship is best described as a power function whose exponent is 2.3 (see Figure 15-1). As can be seen from Figure 15-1, the relationship is linear when plotted in log–log coordinates and has a slope of 2.3.

Beyond these similarities to other sensory modalities, there are stimulus–response features that are uniquely characteristic of pain. These characteristics may be termed *radiation, slow temporal summation,* and *afterresponses.* They have been described for pathological types of pain and for certain types of experimental pain (Noordenbos, 1959).

Radiation is often a distinct characteristic of suprathreshold pain. At the threshold for heat-induced pain, the sensation is often that of a pricking sensation that is confined within the area of stimulation (Hardy et al., 1952). However, higher suprathreshold temperatures evoke painful sensations that are perceived as spreading to surrounding skin areas. Yet these areas are not in contact with the thermode and their temperatures are not elevated from normal levels (Price et al., 1978). Similarly, many chronic pains and pathological pains

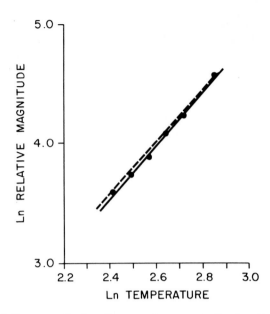

Figure 15-1. Relative magnitudes of neuronal responses (broken line) and sensation intensities (solid line) resulting from different levels of noxious heat applied to the skin. The log relative magnitudes are plotted against log temperature. Temperature was calculated in terms of the difference between the applied noxious temperature and baseline temperature $(T_1 - T_0)$. Both psychophysical and neuronal responses appear to be power functions with exponents of 2.2–2.3. The psychophysical and neuronal data are based on Price et al. (1980) and Price, Hayes, Ruda, & Dubner (1978), respectively.

radiate or trigger pains in body sites distant from the original stimulus (Noordenbos, 1959; Melzack, 1973).

Another aspect of some types of pain is that they increase in intensity with repeated stimulation, that is, they exhibit *slow temporal summation*. One experimental form of this phenomenon is second pain. When a brief noxious stimulus is applied to the distal part of an extremity, an initial sharp well-localized pain is followed about 1 sec later by a burning or throbbing pain. The second pain is less well localized and often outlasts both the stimulus and the arrival of the primary afferent impulses that evoke it. If only one stimulus is given, the second pain may be difficult to detect and masked to an extent by the first pain (Price, 1972; Price, Hu, Dubner, & Gracely, 1977). However, if the stimulus evoking it is repeated at a frequency of once every 3 sec or less, second pain clearly becomes more intense with each successive stimulus (Price et al., 1977). Moreover, once summated, this type of pain outlasts the train of stimuli that evoked it. Similarly, postherpetic neuralgia pain exhibits the same characteristics of diffuse localization, slow temporal summation, and afterresponse (Noordenbos, 1959). The similarities between experimentally induced second pain and certain forms of pathological pain indicate that the latter reflect an exacerbation of existing physiological mechanisms.

Another aspect of the sensory–discriminative component of pain is the "quality" of sensation. The sensory qualities of pain are unique and are described by words such as aching, burning, dull, and wrenching. These qualities are dependent to an extent on the kind of body tissue that is being stimulated. They are not simply the experience of "overstimulation." For example, when one gradually increases a squeeze applied to a fold of skin, the sensation of pressure changes to that of a sharply penetrating well-localized sensation. This sensation is not perceived as simply a continuation of the feeling of pressure. An experimentally more familiar example is the transition between heat-induced warmth and pain. As skin temperatures increase, the perception of warmth (between 35 and 42°C) changes to that of a "burning" or "pricking" pain (Hardy et al., 1952). This transition is perceived clearly as a change in quality of sensation and not merely as a change in intensity along the same continuum. Quality appears to be a critical characteristic that distinguishes painful sensations from other types of skin sensations. Although painful sensations are often perceived as more intense than other types of sensations, occasional subtle aches or soreness sensations can be only slightly detectable, yet painful.

Both the unique qualities of painful sensations and their unique spatial and temporal characteristics support the idea that pain is, at least in part, a sensory modality. This idea is consistent with the fact that there are several types of receptors that are specialized to respond to one or more forms of noxious stimulation.

Arousal

The arousal dimension of pain refers to the extent to which painful sensations dominate experience and occupy ongoing thoughts and intentions. To put it another way, it is the magnitude of attention directed toward the painful experience. Arousal may be experienced as an abrupt interruption, as in the case of an unexpected intense noxious stimulus, or it may be experienced as more or less continuous.

Cognitive–Evaluative Aspects

A person often experiences pain in terms of meanings. As others (Bakan, 1968; Buytendyck, 1961) have pointed out, these include one or more of the following possibilities: (a) the experience of being interrupted (i.e., having one's thoughts, projects, or goals interrupted); (b) the experience of having to endure a difficult or intense burden over time; and (c) the experience of being concerned about one's future health or well-being. All three meanings can coexist in the same person; they are not mutually exclusive. The type of painful sensation interacts with perceived situational factors to constitute these meanings. For example, a person who associates mild abdominal pain with indigestion is responding to a radically different context than is a person who associates abdominal pain with cancer. The intensities of sensation for both pains may be similar, but the cancer patient is likely to have a higher level of concern for future well-being. The person with indigestion is more likely to feel inconvenienced or interrupted. The unique manner in which a person gives meanings to painful sensations and the particular way these meanings are constituted make up the cognitive–evaluative dimension of pain (Melzack & Casey, 1968; Melzack, 1973). Both sudden acute pain and chronic pain are experienced in terms of meanings. A person who unexpectedly stubs his toe may experience an abrupt interruption of his immediate intentions and may be suddenly concerned about the future implications of this event. The chronic-pain patient simply has a much longer period of time in which to reflect on the meanings of his or her painful situations.

Affective Components

The cognitive–evaluative aspects of pain are intimately related to affective aspects of pain. Indeed, they often are the antecedents of affective responses. For example, a patient who is starting to have pain from cancer may experience the pain as mild in terms of sensation intensity. However, its presence reminds the patient of impending deterioration and it is experienced as a serious threat to future health. Anxiety and/or fear would be the likely emotional response of this patient. On the other hand, a low-back-pain patient's life activities may be seriously curtailed as a result of pain. Pain may be experienced as a constant interruption. A patient who usually leads an active life is likely to experience frustration or despair (Buytendyck, 1961). Depression sets in when one feels that there is little or no hope of living a normal active life. The depressed chronic-pain patient often views his or her pain as an inevitable burden. Thus, the affective dimension of pain is based on meanings that one gives to the painful sensations *and* to the painful situation. These meanings are associated with goals, desires, and expectations that are interrelated with the life context of the patient.

This explanation fits well with Schacter and Singers' (1962) "cognitive theory of emotional reaction." This theory contends, with experimental evidence, that the physiological arousal pattern is similar for a variety of emotions, both positive and negative. They suggest that distinctions between "affective" states are largely the result of *situational* cues that are *cognitively* processed. For pain, these cognitive factors are likely to include one's ongoing goals, desires, and expectations. As Buytendyck (1961) has pointed out, an adequate explanation of pain depends on an adequate theory of human emotion. Both pain theory and emotion theory must take into account the role of arousal, meanings, cognition, and the interrelationships among all these factors.

That different and unique cognitive factors influence the affective dimension of pain indicates that there is no unique and invariant emotion that is associated with pain. The affective dimension of pain can be manifested as anxiety, frustration, depression, or anger, depending on how the sensation and situation are appraised. Although the context is often simpler than and usually dissimilar to ordinary life situations, experimental pain can be felt in terms of different emotional feelings. For example, investigators often include a distress scale in assessment of ischemic pain or cold pressor pain (Johnson, 1973). Distress is a natural, though by no means invariant, reaction to the *situation* of ischemic pain. Ischemic pain slowly mounts over time and the sensations are of a distinctly "unnatural" character. The ambiguity inherent in this experimental paradigm facilitates anxiety rather than other types of emotional reactions. On the other hand, more abrupt noxious stimuli, such as electrical shocks to the skin or teeth, more often evoke annoyance or feelings of frustration.

Several experimental studies have shown how cognitive factors influence and sometimes radically alter affective responses to experimentally controlled noxious stimuli. Johnson's (1973) study of pain evoked by forearm ischemia revealed that subjects who received a description of the sensations produced by ischemia had lowered levels of distress as compared to subjects who only received a description of the procedure. Sensation intensities were unaffected by this difference in description. Diazepam, a common tranquilizer, also has been shown to reduce perceived unpleasantness but not sensation intensities associated with pains evoked by tooth shock (Gracely, McGrath, & Dubner, 1976a).

In an attempt to integrate assessment of psychological context in experimental studies of pain, Price et al. (1980) used psychophysical methods to analyze experiential factors that selectively influence one or the other dimension of pain. In one study, subjects made cross-modality matching responses to several dimensions of their experience, including sensory intensity and unpleasantness. Nonnoxious (35–42°C) and noxious (45–51°C) skin temperature stimuli were randomly interspersed during each experimental session. Changes in expectation were induced by preceding one half of the noxious stimuli with a warning signal. As shown in Figure 15-2A, the average responses of these subjects indicated that 45–51°C noxious temperatures were felt as less

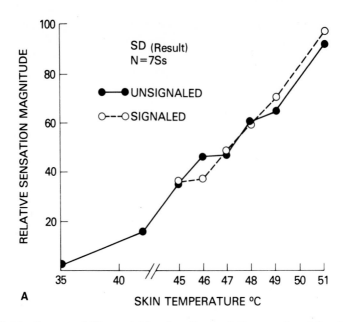

Figure 15-2A. Cross-modality matching functions relating produced line lengths to sensation intensities evoked by increases in skin temperature. Line lengths are transformed into numbers along a 0–100 continuum after the maximum response of each subject is set to 100. The filled and open circles represent responses during unsignaled and signaled trials, respectively. (From Price et al., 1980.)

unpleasant when preceded by a warning signal. In contrast, sensation magnitudes evoked by these same skin temperatures were unaffected by the warning signal (see Figure 15-2B). Thus, only the magnitudes of unpleasant feelings are lowered by decreasing one's expectation of avoiding pain. Part of what is aversive about some experimental pains is one's lack of certainty about what sensations to expect or when to expect them.

Another aspect of this same study was that subjects were instructed to arrive at their affective judgments in two ways. In one session, they compared the outcome of each stimulation with what they wanted to happen (*affect–result* responses). In the other session, they simply focused on the pleasantness or unpleasantness of each sensation as it was experienced (*affect–process* responses). All subjects' affect–result responses were more positive (or less unpleasant) than affect–process responses. These results underscore the critical influence of expectation and the manner in which one evaluates sensations on affective responses to noxious stimulation. These experiential factors can be measured and taken into account during experimental studies of pain.

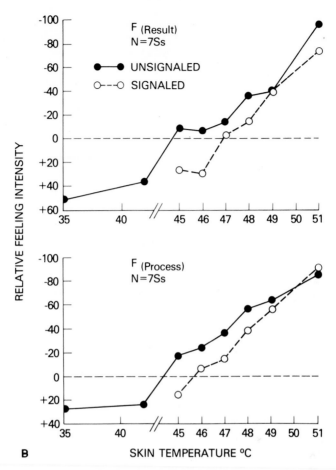

Figure 15-2B. Cross-modality matching functions relating produced line lengths of perceived magnitudes of positive or negative feelings evoked by increases in skin temperature. As in Figure 15-2A, maximum responses are set to 100 for each subject. The ordinates are divided into positive and negative scales corresponding to positive and negative feeling intensity, respectively. The upper (result) and lower (process) graphs are based on two different ways of judging unpleasantness. (From Price et al., 1980.)

A Strategy for Studying Neural Mechanisms of Pain

Psychophysical studies of pain have provided invaluable information about how different dimensions of pain experience are related to stimulus parameters and to situational factors. If different components of pain bear different relationships to these parameters, then one should be able to use this information to help identify neurons and neural mechanisms related to these components. Such a strategy has been useful in identifying neurons that subserve the sensory–discriminative aspects of pain (Price & Dubner, 1977). In brief, four distinct lines of evidence used to identify sensory–discriminative nociceptive neurons are as follows: (1) selective stimulation of the candidate neuron(s) gives rise to a painful sensation that has sensory characteristics normally associated with pain; (2) responses of the candidate neuron to controlled nociceptive stimulation show parallels to human psychophysical responses to similar stimulation; (3) reduction or abolition of the neuron's responses to nociceptive stimulation results in a decrease in sensory–discriminative responses to nociceptive stimulation; (4) the neurons have anatomical connections consistent with a role in sensory–discriminative aspects of pain.

These criteria can be extended to identify neurons that are involved in the various components of pain. At early stages of nociceptive information processing, such as at the level of primary afferents, selective stimulation of nociceptive neurons normally gives rise to all dimensions of pain. At some level of the neuraxis, we might expect that application of the foregoing criteria would reveal nociceptive neurons that are more involved in affect than in sensory discrimination. For example, selective stimulation of such central neurons (criterion 1) would evoke affective components of pain with few or no sensory–discriminative components. Furthermore, as would be predicted by psychophysical experiments described above, neurons participating exclusively in affective responses would respond to graded heat stimuli less intensely when such stimuli are preceded by a warning signal. Similarly, the tranquilizer Diazepam, which is known to reduce affective but not sensory responses to noxious stimuli, would reduce responses of "affective" neurons to similar stimuli.

In the following section we will review current knowledge about neurons and neural mechanisms involved in the various components of pain. In the context of this review, we will consider the level of the neuraxis at which the various components of pain are likely to become differentiated, keeping in mind the criteria discussed above. It is hoped that this approach will illuminate a means whereby the neural basis of the interrelationships between pain sensation, affect, and motivation can be understood.

Primary Cutaneous Afferents

The receptors that signal impending tissue damage are not uniformly sensitive. They fall into several categories, depending on their responses to mechanical, thermal, and chemical stimulation and on the conduction velocities of the axons that supply them (Price & Dubner, 1977).

Although nociceptive afferents have been shown to innervate several types of tissue, those innervating the skin have been most extensively studied and are strongly implicated in pain mechanisms. Their essential characteristics are summarized below.

Aδ high-threshold mechanoreceptive (Aδ HTM) afferents that respond only to intense mechanical stimuli and conduct between 4 and 40 m/sec have been described in the skin of the cat and in monkey extremities. Many respond only to stimulus intensities that produce overt tissue damage, others give threshold responses to nondamaging pressure applied to the skin (>1 g/mm^2). Most important, all such HTM primary afferents respond to noxious or potentially damaging skin stimuli with the highest impulse frequency. They are particularly sensitive to excitation by sharp objects but are relatively insensitive to heat. Therefore, they seem well adapted for transmitting information that is related to the localized pricking pain produced by mechanical stimuli. So far, primary afferents of this type have not been identified in human nerves.

Aδ heat-nociceptive afferents conducting between 3 and 20 m/sec have recently been identified in the limb and facial skin of monkeys. Like Aδ HTM afferents, these afferents respond to intense mechanical stimulation. However, unlike the Aδ HTM afferents, Aδ heat-nociceptive afferents respond monotonically to increases in receptive-field skin temperature. These responses positively accelerate, the steep portion of the curve occurring in the 45–53°C range. Threshold temperatures for these afferents are usually below noxious or painful levels (40–44°C), but highly noxious skin temperatures (>50°C) evoke maximum responses. The role of these neurons in signaling pain is clearly established. They are the only myelinated primary afferents innervating the skin of the extremities that can be reliably activated by noxious heat. Thus, heat-induced first pain, the latency of which corresponds to the activity in the small myelinated Aδ fibers, must be initiated by impulses in the Aδ heat afferents. Neither this first pain nor the responses of the Aδ heat afferents outlast the duration of the heat stimulus. Both the intensity of the first pain in man and the responses of the Aδ heat afferents in monkeys are progressively reduced during brief repeated application of heat stimuli to the same spot on the hand. Thus, the characteristics of heat-induced first pain can be largely accounted for by the response characteristics of Aδ heat-nociceptive afferents. Recently it has been shown that these afferents excite neurons of origin of the spinothalamic tract of monkeys (Price et al., 1978). Therefore, Aδ heat-nociceptive afferents have central connections consistent with a role in pain. However, direct confirmation of their functional role in man awaits their identification and analysis in human nerves.

C-fiber polymodal nociceptive afferents form an extremely important group of peripheral fibers, since they constitute 80–90% or more of the C-fiber population of primates. They innervate the skin of the monkey (Beitel & Dubner, 1976) and man (Torebjork, 1974) and are characterized by their responses to noxious mechanical, noxious heat, and chemical irritant stimuli. Some also respond to intense cold (less than 10°C). These polymodal nociceptive afferents have several important properties such as sensitization to repeated applications of low-intensity noxious stimuli and response suppression by high-intensity noxious stimuli. They respond with their highest frequency to two or more forms of intense cutaneous stimuli, but also respond weakly to mechanical (1–10 g) and thermal (38–43°C) stimuli that are clearly not painful to human observers. They may, therefore, provide some information about nonpainful sensations.

There is little doubt that C-fiber polymodal nociceptive afferents signal tissue damage and contribute directly to pain sensations in man. Brief heat pulses evoke distinct first and second pain (Price et al., 1977). Except for the very small population of C warm afferents that respond to noxious heat, polymodal nociceptive afferents are the predominant C afferent group activated by this stimulus in primates and are the peripheral population that is most likely accountable for heat-induced second pain.

Like the responses of Aδ heat-nociceptive afferents, those of C-fiber polymodal afferents became progressively reduced in monkeys during a train of 3-sec interpulse interval heat pulses. When an identical train of heat pulses was applied to the hands of human observers, second pain increased in intensity. Thus, second pain summation occurs when the afferents evoking it are partially suppressed and must be critically dependent on prolonged summation in the central nervous system. This explanation is supported by the observation that second pain is increased to an even greater extent when the location of the probe on the skin changes between successive heat pulses so that different receptors are activated with each stimulus. These observations are consistent with a study by Collins, Nulsen, and Randt (1960) in which the exposed sural nerve was electrically stimulated in awake humans. They found that a single volley in C afferents (Aδ were blocked by cold) did not evoke any sensation, but that repetitive stimulation at 3 per second evoked mounting, burning pain.

C-fiber polymodal nociceptive afferents excite many of the same spinothalamic tract neurons that are activated by Aδ heat-nociceptive afferents (Price et al., 1978). Therefore, they have central synpatic connections adapted to play a role in pain mechanisms.

There is little doubt that all of the major classes of primary nociceptive afferents activate all dimensions of pain. The different types of pain evoked by selective stimulation of each class result in sensations with sensory–discriminative characteristics, arousal, feelings of unpleasantness, and motoric responses. It would be inappropriate to make comparisons about the extent to which each pain component is activated by the different types of primary afferents, since different types of pain are so dependent on the parameters of stimulation. For example, if one brief heat stimulus is given, the initial pricking pain is more unpleasant than the second pain. If several heat simuli are given, second pain may summate to a point where it is definitely more unpleasant than first pain.

Classes of Spinothalamic Nociceptive Neurons

It has become increasingly apparent that radical transformations take place between input from primary nociceptive afferents and outputs of second-order sensory neurons (Price & Dubner, 1977; Price et al., 1978). These transformations account for the lack of simple relationships between impulse frequencies in primary nociceptive afferents and pain perception (e.g., the evident lack of a simple one-to-one relationship between C-fiber polymodal nociceptive responses and second pain). The objective of this section is to account for some aspects of pain experience that cannot be explained by the responses of primary afferent neurons. This explanation focuses on the functional characteristics of spinothalamic and trigeminothalamic tract neurons that could be involved in pain. There are two major types of such neurons found in primates that could convey information about tissue injury (Price & Dubner, 1977).

Wide dynamic range (WDR) neurons respond with progressively higher impulse frequencies as stimulus intensities progress from very weak (i.e., <100 mg force) to definitely noxious. Thus, maximum frequencies are evoked in these neurons by either penetration of the skin or noxious skin temperatures above $44°C$. They receive excitatory synaptic effects from large myelinated $(A\beta)$ low-threshold mechanoreceptive (LTM) afferents, $A\delta$ high-threshold mechanoreceptive (HTM) afferents, and C-fiber polymodal nociceptive afferents. As a result of this extensive convergence, these cells respond with increasingly higher frequencies of impulse discharge to touch, firm pressure, and noxious pinching. The responses of many of these cells are monotonic functions of increases in skin temperature within the noxious range $(44–52°C)$, like the perceived magnitude of pain intensity over this same temperature range.

WDR neurons have receptive fields that often have extensive gradients of sensitivity. Although such gradients were first described in anesthetized preparations, they have been confirmed in awake monkeys. These receptive fields usually contain a central zone wherein the neuron responds differentially to gentle touch, firmer pressure, and noxious stimulation. Surrounding this relatively small zone is an area in which the neuron responds differentially to firm pressure ($\geqslant$1 g von

Frey force) and pinch. This area in turn is surrounded by another region in which only definitely noxious stimuli, such as pinch or 49–51°C skin temperatures, will cause impulse discharge. The total receptive field area of these neurons is sometimes quite large, extending across more than one trigeminal division in the case of nucleus caudalis trigeminothalamic neurons and across several spinal dermatomes in the case of spinothalamic tract neurons.

A second type of dorsal horn spinothalamic neuron, termed *nociceptive specific* (NS), is relatively specific for responses to intense mechanical and/or thermal stimuli and is located in both superficial (I–II) and deeper layers (IV–V) of the dorsal horn. This type of neuron is distinguished by receiving excitatory synaptic effects exclusively from one or more types of primary nociceptive afferents. One subcategory of nociceptive-specific neurons is one that receives excitatory input from $A\delta$ HTM, $A\delta$ heat-nociceptive afferents, and C-fiber polymodal nociceptive afferents. As a result of these inputs, this type of neuron responds to firm pressure and pinch with an increasingly higher frequency of impulse discharge. These neurons also respond to noxious skin temperatures. The receptive fields of these neurons are generally smaller than those of wide dynamic range neurons but show a similar gradient of sensitivity. Thus, their receptive fields can sometimes be divided into a central zone, in which firm pressure and pinch result in progressively higher impulse frequencies, and other zones, in which only pinch will cause impulse discharge. Another subcategory of nociceptive-specific spinothalamic tract neuron is unequivocally specific for responses to noxious skin stimuli. It appears to receive input from only $A\delta$ HTM, since it responds only to noxious mechanical stimulation of the skin or to electrical stimulation of $A\delta$ afferents. Its responses do not outlast the stimulus, nor do they summate with repeated application. Therefore, like the $A\delta$ HTM, this type of neuron is likely related to mechanically induced pain such as that evoked by needle prick. Its receptive field does not appear to have a gradient of sensitivity.

The Function of Second-Order Nociceptive Neurons in Awake Primates

The nociceptive stimulus–response functions and other physiological characteristics of WDR and NS neurons make it appear that these neurons are important for pain. However, since nearly all studies of these neurons were performed in anesthetized or spinalized animals, one might wonder whether the physiological properties of these neurons would be different in conscious animals. Furthermore, one might also wonder whether activation of either WDR or NS neurons is sufficient to evoke the experience of pain in awake primates, particularly humans. Two types of experiments have been carried out to answer these questions.

In the first, nucleus caudalis WDR and NS neurons were recorded in awake monkeys trained to make panel releases in order to escape unrewarded noxious heat trials ($\geqslant 45°$C) or to secure reinforcement by detecting the end of an innocuous ($<43°$C) temperature (Hoffman et al., 1981). As is consistent with data recorded from anesthetized animals, WDR and NS neurons recorded from awake behaving monkeys are usually found in layer I or layers IV-V of nucleus caudalis. Receptive fields of the WDR cells vary in area and contain gradients of sensitivity extending from a central zone differentially responsive to touch, pressure, and pinch to an outer zone responsive only to noxious pinch. As data from anesthetized animals show, such neurons are maximally sensitive to heat stimuli in the nociceptive range (above $44°$C) with thresholds of $43-45°$C.

Simultaneous recording of escape behavior and neural responses provides evidence that both WDR and NS are capable of providing information with which to discriminate intensities of stimulation within the noxious range. Escape latencies to $49°$C heat stimuli were all less than 4 sec, whereas latencies on $47°$C trials were all greater than 4.0 sec. The greater increase in discharge of WDR and NS neurons to $49°$C as compared to $47°$C occurred early enough to provide signals related to the shorter escape latencies at $49°$C. Such data indicate that these neurons are capable of discriminating different intensities of noxious stimulation. The extent to which this discrimination can be directly linked to sensory or affective–motivational dimensions requires further experiments.

In the second type of experiment, spinothalamic tract axons within the cervical spinal cord were electrically stimulated in awake humans and the parameters of stimulation were adjusted so as to stimulate *only* the axons of WDR neurons (Mayer, Price, & Becker, 1975). This stimulus condition was inferred by comparing electrical threshold and refractory period of monkey spinothalamic tract axons with similar parameters required to evoke pain in awake patients (Price & Mayer, 1975). The refractory periods and electrical thresholds of WDR neurons (but not of NS neurons) matched the refractory period and electrical thresholds of anterolateral quadrant (ALQ) evoked pain. Since the electrical thresholds of NS axons were higher than current levels required to evoke pain in humans, it appears that activation of WDR neurons is a sufficient condition to evoke pain.

In the context of determining which types of spinal cord ALQ neurons are sufficient to evoke pain, several observations were made that have direct bearing on pain mechanisms in man. First, it is of considerable significance that pain evoked by ALQ stimulation was similar to that evoked by naturally occurring stimuli. Most of the reports were of burning pain, but descriptions of dull aching pain, cramping, and sharp pain were also given. These types of pain were evoked by 50-Hz trains of regularly spaced pulses, a pattern that is not likely to be generated

by natural stimuli. Therefore, it is unlikely that pain is subserved by
some special temporal pattern that depends on the exact intervals of
impulses in spinal cord nociceptive neurons. However, the intensity
of pain was found to be dependent on the overall frequency in ALQ
neurons over a range of 5-100 Hz. A linear relationship was found between stimulation frequency and percentage of subjects reporting pain.
At 25 Hz, 100% of subjects reported pain, whereas none reported pain
at 5 Hz. Similarly, monkey WDR neurons responded to graded noxious
heat with a frequency of 5-25 Hz over a skin temperature range of
44-46.5°C (Price et al., 1978), the range over which most human heat
pain threshold values are distrubuted (Hardy et al., 1952). In contrast,
the frequency of nociceptive-specific responses extends from 5 to
25 Hz over a skin temperature range of 46-48°C. These temperature
values evoke suprathreshold pain in most human subjects. Thus, pain
appears critically dependent on overall frequency in WDR neurons.

These studies also support the concept that central spatial summation is especially critical for pain. When the frequency was held constant (50 Hz), it was found that the perception of ALQ-evoked pain
invariably required larger stimulus intensities and presumably activation
of a larger number of ALQ axons than that required for perceptions of
tingle, warmth, or cooling. The amount of spatial summation was critical since stimulus intensities just sufficient to evoke tingle would do so
even when stimulus frequencies extended up to 500 Hz. In contrast,
when stimulus intensities were increased to activate a critical number
of axons, much lower frequencies (5-25 Hz) evoked pain. These results
fit well with other lines of evidence indicating that pain requires central
spatial summation.

Another finding of this same study was that ALQ-evoked pain was
clearly aversive, although certainly tolerable. Behavioral responses and
reports indicating that the pain was unpleasant (i.e., "bad," "hurts")
were given without provocation or suggestion. Since the currents and
frequencies were adjusted so as to activate mainly the axons of WDR
neurons, these indications of aversion are significant. They lead to the
inference that WDR neurons activate central mechanisms related to
the affective–motivational dimension of pain as well as the central
mechanisms related to sensory discrimination.

Given these sensory and affective effects of stimulation of the spinothalamic pathway, one may begin to question whether all dimensions
of pain are uniformly represented in this pathway or whether there is
some functional separation within the spinothalamic tract. The idea of
functional separation is strongly indicated by the popular assertion
that the paleospinothalamic pathway is more important for affective–
motivational aspects of pain and the neurospinothalamic pathway
carries mainly sensory–discriminative information (Melzack & Casey,
1968; Melzack, 1973). This idea is based mainly on anatomical grounds

(Melzack, 1973); it suggests that the spinothalamic pathway has two components ascending in the brain stem. The medial component of this pathway (paleospinothalamic tract) gives off numerous collaterals to brain-stem structures thought to be involved in arousal (e.g., reticular formation structures) or affect (central grey, tectal area). The lateral component (neospinothalamic tract) is thought to have fewer collaterals to medial brain-stem structures and to project to areas that are mostly involved in sensory–discriminative functions.

There are several lines of evidence that would support a more uniform representation of function within the spinothalamic pathway. First, as we saw earlier, stimulation of spinothalamic tract axons within the cervical spinal cord gives rise to pain with both sensory–discriminative and affective components. Second, numerous lesions have been made within the human cervical spinal cord that only partially interrupt the spinothalamic tract (Nathan & Smith, 1979). Such lesions produce a restricted zone of analgesia in which all of the components of pain are interrupted at once (Nathan & Smith, 1979). Thus, there is no selective loss of aversive components of pain as compared to sensory components. Third, spinothalamic tract axons, whose terminals end within the sensory thalamic nucleus, ventroposteriolateralis (VPL), are now known to have collaterals to medial brain-stem structures such as the central grey (Price et al., 1978). Individual spinothalamic neurons then appear to participate in multiple functions. These neurons, which include WDR and NS types, have physiological characteristics similar to those which *do not* appear to have collaterals to the medial brain stem and to those which *only* project as far as the mesencephalon. Spinal cord afferent neurons with similar physiological characteristics project to varying levels of the brain stem. All of these observations indicate that classic functional subdivisions of the spinothalamic pathway are oversimplified and misleading (Noordenbos, 1959; Melzack, 1973). The spinothalamic pathway appears to contain many neurons that participate in different components of pain and some neurons with more restricted outputs. There does not appear to be a sharp functional subdivision of the different components of pain within the spinothalamic pathway.

Brain Processing of Nociceptive Information

Beyond the level of the efferents emanating from the spinal cord dorsal horn and the homologous components of the trigeminal system, detailed information concerning the processing of nociceptive information has been scant and controversial. Several factors have been responsible for this situation in the studies to be discussed. The most convincing data about pain, particularly concerning brain mechanisms, generally come from studies in man where verbal abilities greatly facilitate the evaluation of the various components involved in the pain experience. However, the conduct of studies in humans presents a number of difficulties:

1. The types of studies that can be done are obviously limited by ethical and practical considerations. For example, although the information yield might be great from single-unit recording studies, these have been few because of the time involved, the need to apply repeated peripheral noxious stimuli, and the necessity of recording from control structures not involved in the normal invasive procedures.
2. Probably the most common disease process leading to stereotaxic invasion of the human brain for pain relief is carcinoma, yet the typically short survival time of these patients renders interpretation of results difficult. On the other hand, patients with long survival times are often afflicted with pain syndromes of idiopathic, psychogenic, or central origin, and observations made on them may not accurately reflect normal processing of nociceptive information.
3. The evaluation of results of lesioning procedures has not utilized consistent criteria for designated success and failure, making comparison of results between studies difficult.
4. Postlesion sensory testing has not been consistently utilized, and when it has been done is typically cursory and qualitative. Thus, a wealth of valuable information about human pain physiology has been lost.
5. Direct histological verification, particularly of stimulation and recording sites, is difficult to achieve.

Medulla and Pons

Information about the neural processing of pain at the medullary level of the neuraxis derives principally from attempts to interrupt spinothalamic fibers for the relief of shoulder and neck pain. A careful review of this work has been given by White and Sweet (1969). Destruction of the spinothalamic tract at the medullary level produces results qualitatively similar to those resulting from anterolateral cordotomy. In a review of nine studies by different investigators, Birkenfeld and Fisher (1963) reported complete relief of pain in 41 of 50 patients and partial relief in 4. Thus, results at the medullary level also appear to be quantitatively similar to those at the spinal level. As with anterolateral cordotomy, medullary tractotomy typically results in at least temporary analgesia to acute pain on the contralateral body surface (White & Sweet, 1969). No evidence emerges from these lesion results that there is any separation in the lateral medulla of the sensory–discriminative from other components of the pain experience.

Simulation of medullary structures in conscious humans has been restricted to attempts to verify electrode placement within the spino-thalamic tract. Both sensory–discriminative and motivational–affective components of pain result from stimulation of the tract (White & Sweet, 1969), thus supporting the conclusion that the nature of pain pathways does not change significantly at this level. No attempt has been made to evaluate the effects of destruction in man of the more medial pontobulbar structures in the vicinity of the nucleus reticularis gigantocellularis (NGC). However, a number of lines of evidence derived from animal experimentation do implicate these more medial structures in the neural processing of pain. Electrical stimulation of the nucleus reticularis gigantocellularis is escaped by animals (Casey, 1971). It should be pointed out that it is very difficult to interpret this type of result, since there are an almost infinite number of reasons for animals to escape brain stimulation, pain or some component thereof being only one. Nevertheless, other experimental approaches do support an involvement of the NGC in pain processing. Lesions in this region result in long-term escape deficits in animals (Anderson & Pearl, 1975). Significantly, the neurons in this region respond either exclusively or differentially to noxious stimuli, and they have wide receptive fields (Pearl & Anderson, 1978). These large receptive fields suggest that the region may be less involved in the sensory–discriminative aspect of pain than in signaling other components.

Mesencephalon

At the mesencephalic level, important information about neural processing of pain in man derives from neurosurgical procedures attempting to alleviate pain by severing either spinothalamic pathways or spinoreticular connections. Studies at this level begin to reveal a divergence of pain pathways with important theoretical and practical significance.

Spinothalamic tractotomy at the mesencephalic level is a procedure that has been for the most part abandoned because of the high incidence of deleterious side effects (White & Sweet, 1969). Those cases that have been reported are highly instructive. Analysis of the review presented by White and Sweet (1969) reveals that this procedure can produce at least temporary relief of clinical pain, although the probability of success, even when the lesion is correctly placed, is lower than at more caudal levels (12 out of 20 cases). Recurrence of pain within a short period after surgery appears likely. Analgesia to acute pain over at least some portion of the body again is less likely than with tractotomy at medullary or spinal levels (13 out of 20 cases), and the analgesia is more likely to recede quickly. Of particular interest are reports (Drake & McKenzie, 1953; White & Sweet, 1969) that the quality of pain sensation to acute noxious stimuli sometimes changes. Pinprick and thermal stimuli can result in reports of deep, diffuse, poorly localized pain after tractotomy.

Examination of the effects of more medial midbrain destruction and stimulation, although not without overlapping effects of spinothalamic tractotomy, is more revealing in the complementary effects observed. Destruction of the midbrain periaqueductal grey matter alone had been done only for the relief of pain of central origin. The procedure seems effective for the relief of this type of pain (Schvarcz, 1977), but its effect on chronic pain of peripheral origin remains unknown. The suffering aspect of central pain has been reported to be affected by this procedure (Schvarcz, 1977). Of particular interest is the observation that lesions restricted to the mesencephalic periaqueductal grey matter do not appear to interfere with localization or detection of acute noxious stimuli, although the sensory sequelae of this lesion have not been analyzed in detail (Schvarcz, 1977).

The most striking effect of electrical stimulation of periaqueductal structures in man is the elicitation of an emotional complex of unpleasantness and fear which often results in the subject's not allowing further stimulation (Nashold, Wilson, & Slaughter, 1969; Schvarcz, 1977). At higher stimulation intensities, reports of frankly painful sensations occur. The pain is typically diffuse, deep, and localized to midline structures, particularly the face (Nashold, Wilson, & Slaughter, 1969; Nashold et al., 1974; Schvarcz, 1977). This is in contrast to midbrain spinothalamic stimulation, which produces sharp, well localized pain referred to the contralateral body surface (Nashold et al., 1974).

In summary, the available evidence from studies in man suggests that a divergence of neural processing of nociceptive information occurs at least as caudally as the mesencephalic level. The lateral mesencephalic structures continue to carry information more concerned with the sensory–discriminative aspects of pain, while the most medial structures appear to be preferentially involved with the emotional and motivational aspects of the sensation. It is important to point out that this separation is certainly not an exclusive one. In fact, it is this overlap of function that probably leads to the unpredictable results of surgical interventions at this level as well as at more rostral levels of the neuraxis. It should also be mentioned that there is clear evidence that medial mesencephalic structures are importantly involved not only in the afferent transmission of nociceptive information but also in the centrifugal control of this system, as will be discussed in detail below. Thus, studies of this area in man are likely to produce complex results and should be interpreted with caution.

Diencephalon

The specialization of neural systems mediating different aspects of the total pain experience is perhaps even more clear from studies of thalamic structures in man. Lesions of the specific sensory nuclei of the thalamus (VPL and VPM) result in at best mediocre relief of chronic pain, and this relief is usually transient (White & Sweet, 1969). The procedure is no longer commonly utilized (Bouchard, Mayanagi, & Martins, 1977). White and Sweet report a case with results similar to the phenomenon discussed above for midbrain lesions in which a specific sensory nucleus lesion resulted in the disappearance of localized pain but was replaced by diffuse aching pain. Some loss of sensibility to pinprick occurs, but this typically is incomplete, and the peripheral field involved is generally smaller than with spinothalamic tractotomies at more caudal levels.

Electrical stimulation of the ventrobasal complex in man typically produces sensations of tingling and numbness but rarely frank reports of pain (Nashold et al., 1974; White & Sweet, 1969). On the other hand, Halliday and Logue (1972) and Hassler (1970) have reported that electrical stimulation of a restricted region in the most ventral aspect of the nucleus ventrocaudalis results in specific localized pains referred to the contralateral body. The reports of pain seem similar to those reported from stimulation of the spinothalamic system at more caudal levels. This report suggests a thalamic specialization for the coding of sensory–discriminative aspects of pain in man. Such a conclusion is supported by electrophysiological studies in animals. A large percentage of neurons in the cat homologue of the ventrocaudal nucleus respond uniquely or differentially to noxious stimuli (Guilbaud, Callie, Besson, & Benelli, 1977), whereas only a very small percentage of neurons in the ventrobasal complex show such responses (Kenshalo, Giesler, Leonard, & Willis, 1980).

It appears that destruction of a variety of medial thalamic structures can have at least a temporary beneficial effect on chronic pain in man. These include the Cm–Pf complex, nucleus limitans, anterior thalamic nuclei, dorsomedial nuclei, and the pulvinar. The results of these interventions are, however, highly variable. Overall, it appears that Cm–Pf, nucleus limitans, and pulvinar lesions are most effective, but the advantage of any one of these over the others is controversial (e.g., cf. White & Sweet, 1969, and Laitinen, 1977). It also may be that the size of the lesion is critical, since enlargement of the lesion can improve the result of an initial smaller lesion (White & Sweet, 1969) and combined medial and lateral lesions appear more effective than either alone (Mundinger & Becker, 1977). These lesions do not appear to alter the response to acute noxious stimuli, although this has not typically been systematically explored.

Stimulation of these thalamic structures does not typically produce pain, but reports of discomfort are common (White & Sweet, 1969). However, stimulation of intralaminar structures (Cm–Pf and nucleus limitans) have been reported to produce pain with a burning (Sano, Yoshioka, Ogashiwa, Ishijima, & Ohye, 1966) or aching (Hassler, 1970) quality and has been referred to large portions of the contralateral and even ipsilateral body surface. Interestingly, one of these groups (Ishijima, Yoshimasu, Fukushima, Hori, Sekino, & Sano, 1975) has recorded from neurons in the human thalamus. They found 20 out of 80 neurons in the Cm–Pf complex that responded to pinprick but not to light touch or joint rotation. No neurons in the dorsal medial nucleus responded in this way.

The Cerebral Cortex

The role of the cerebral cortex in the elaboration of input from several sensory systems has been worked out in considerable detail. Such is not the case with pain. It is clear that the specific somatosensory projection areas are not critical for the relatively normal perception of both chronic and acute pain. SI lesions have consistently had no effect on chronic or acute pain and may even result in hyperpathia (Hassler, 1960; White & Sweet, 1969). Lesions of SII cortex or SI and SII cortex combined do not result in the lack of appreciation of either chronic or acute pain (Hassler, 1960; White & Sweet, 1969), although some hypalgesia has been reported with SII lesions (Hassler, 1970). Electrical stimulation of somatosensory cortex typically does not produce reports of pain (Libet, 1973; White & Sweet, 1969), although Penfield and Boldrey (1937) elicited very real pain sensation from 11 of 426 stimulation sites. Thus, it can be concluded that the cortical projection areas of the specific thalamic nuclei do not code even the sensory–discriminative dimension of pain with the same specificity as at lower levels of the spinothalamic system. This conclusion does not exclude the possibility that other cortical areas participate in the elaboration of noxious inputs, and a few recent electrophysiological studies suggest that this may be so. These experiments have attempted to stimulate selectively nociceptive afferents. Chatrian, Canfield, Knauss, and Lettich (1975) have used tooth pulp stimulation and Carmon, Mor, and Goldberg (1976) have used a laser beam to excite heat nociceptors. These stimuli are synchronous and result in cortical evoked potentials that can be recorded over somatosensory cortex but are maximal at the vertex. Such a result suggests widespread cortical involvement in the processing of this information. The pain-related components have a latency of less than 300 msec, eliminating the involvement of C fibers. In the experiment of Carmon et al. the evoked potential is unlikely to be elicited by prepain sensations, since stimuli that give rise only to a sensation of warmth do not result in an evoked potential. Whether these potentials are related to the perceptual aspects of pain or to a more global variable such as arousal remains to be demonstrated.

Centrifugal Control of Pain Transmission

A major advance in our conception of the neural processing of pain has occurred in the past decade. It has become clear that information about tissue damage is not passively received by the nervous system. Rather, it is filtered, even at the first sensory synapse, by complex modulatory systems (Mayer, 1980). The discovery of these systems has fostered, and in turn been fostered by, the notion that the central nervous system contains endogenous substances, endorphins, that possess analgesic properties virtually identical to opioids of plant and synthetic origin. In this section, we first examine the development of these concepts. We then discuss the existence of opiate and nonopiate central nervous system pain modulatory mechanisms activated by environmental stimuli.

Historical Perspective

It has long been recognized that a simple invariant relationship between stimulus intensity and the magnitude of pain perception is often not present. This was explicitly recognized by earlier models of pain perception despite the lack of direct evidence to support it (Noordenbos, 1959; Melzack & Wall, 1965). The first impetus for the detailed study of pain-modulatory circuitry resulted from the observation that electrical stimulation of the brain could powerfully suppress the perception of pain (Reynolds, 1969; Mayer, Wolfle, Akil, Carder, & Liebeskind, 1971). Further investigation of stimulation-produced analgesia provided considerable detail about the neural circuitry involved (see Mayer, 1979, for a detailed review of this topic). Significantly, several similarities were recognized between these observations and information emerging from a concomitant resurgence of interest in the mechanisms of opiate analgesia. The most important parallel facts revealed by these studies were the following:

1. Effective loci for both opiate analgesia (OA) and stimulation-produced analgesia (SPA) lie within the periaqueductal and periventricular grey matter of the brain stem.
2. OA and SPA are both mediated by the activation of a centrifugal control system that exits from the brain via the dorsolateral funiculus of the spinal cord.

3. The ultimate inhibition of the transmission of nociceptive information occurs at the initial processing stages in the spinal cord dorsal
   horn and homologous trigeminal nucleus caudalis by selective inhibition of nociceptive neurons.

In addition to these correlative observations, studies of SPA produced
direct evidence indicating that there were mechanisms extant in the
central nervous system that depend upon endogenous opiates:

1. Subanalgesic doses of morphine were shown to synergize with subanalgesic levels of brain stimulation to produce behavioral analgesia.
2. Tolerance, a phenomenon invariably associated with repeated administration of opiates, was observed to the analgesic effects of brain
   stimulation.
3. Cross-tolerance between the analgesic effects of brain stimulation
   and opiates was demonstrated.
4. SPA could be antagonized by naloxone, a specific narcotic antagonist.

This last observation, in particular, could be most parsimoniously explained if electrical stimulation resulted in the release of an endogenous
opiate-like factor. Indeed, naloxone antagonism of SPA was a critical
impetus leading to the eventual discovery of such a factor (Hughes,
1975).

Coincidental with work on SPA, another discovery of critical importance for our current concepts of endogenous analgesia systems was
made. Several laboratories, almost simultaneously, reported the existence of stereospecific binding sites for opiates in the central nervous
system. These "receptor" sites were subsequently shown to be localized
to neuronal synaptic regions and to overlap anatomically with loci involved in the neural processing of pain. The existence of an opiate
receptor again suggested the likelihood of an endogenous compound
with opiate properties to occupy it. In 1974, Hughes and Kosterlitz
reported the isolation from neural tissue of a factor (enkephalin) with
such properties. An immense amount of subsequent work has characterized this and other neural and extraneural compounds with opiate
properties. (See Adler, 1980, for a recent review of these studies.) As
with the opiate receptor, the anatomical distribution of endogenous
opiate ligands shows overlap with sites involved in pain processing.

To summarize, the existence of an endogenous opiate analgesia system is suggested by several lines of evidence. Electrical stimulation of
the brain produces analgesia. The anatomical structures and neural
mechanisms involved in SPA parallel those of OA, and strong evidence
exists for the involvement of an endogenous opiate in SPA. The central
nervous system contains opiate binding sites and endogenous ligands
capable of interacting with those sites.

Analgesia Produced by Environmental Stimuli

The demonstration of a well-defined neural system capable of potently blocking pain transmission suggests, but by no means proves, that the function of this system is to dynamically modulate the perceived intensity of noxious stimuli. If, in fact, this system has such a physiological role, then one might expect that the level of activity within the system would be influenced by impinging environmental stimuli. If environmental situations could be identified that produce analgesia, it would give credibility to the idea that invasive procedures inhibit pain by mimicking the natural activity within these pathways. This section reviews the evidence that environmental stimuli activate pain-inhibitory neural circuitry.

A systematic search for environmental stimuli that activate pain-inhibitory systems was begun by Hayes, Bennett, Newlon, and Mayer (1978). They discovered that potent analgesia could be produced by such diverse stimuli as brief foot-shock, centrifugal rotation, and injection of intraperitoneal saline. Two important additional concepts emerged from this work. First was the conclusion that exposure to stress was not sufficient to produce analgesia. Although all environmental stimuli that produce analgesia are stressors, the failure of classical stressors, such as ether vapors and horizontal oscillation, to produce pain inhibition indicated that stress was not the critical variable responsible. Second was the rather unexpected finding that the opiate naloxone did not block environmentally induced analgesias. Therefore, nonopiate systems must exist, in addition to the opiate system described earlier.

Although the stimuli studied by Hayes et al. did not appear to activate an opiate system, investigations that followed found clues that brain endorphins might be involved in at least some types of environmentally induced analgesias. Akil and co-workers (Akil, Madden, Patrick, & Barchas, 1976) studied the analgesic effects of prolonged foot-shock. In contrast to the results of Hayes et al., naloxone did partially antagonize the analgesia. This initial indication of opiate involvement led Akil and co-workers to look for biochemical evidence that foot-shock caused brain opiates to be released. They found that changes in brain opiate levels did indeed parallel the development of foot-shock-induced analgesia. When tolerance developed to the analgesic effects of foot-shock, brain opiate levels returned to control values. In agreement with these results, ^{3}H-leu-enkephalin binding has been reported to decrease as analgesia increases (Chance, White, Kyrnock, & Rosecrans, 1979).

The controversy over the involvement of opiates in foot-shock-induced analgesia was resolved, in part, by Lewis, Cannon, and Liebeskind (1980). They noted that the duration of foot-shock used by Hayes et al. and Akil et al. differed greatly and wondered whether this variable might explain the difference in their results. By comparing the effects of naloxone on analgesia produced by brief versus prolonged foot-shock, Lewis et al. showed that only the latter could be blocked by naloxone. This suggested that different analgesia systems become active as the duration of foot-shock increases.

Concurrently with this work of Lewis et al. (1980), Cobelli, Watkins, and Mayer (1980) made the observation that brief shock restricted to the front paws produced a naloxone-reversible analgesia. In contrast, even high doses of naloxone failed to reduce analgesia produced by shocking the hind paws. Therefore, a nonopiate system seems to be involved in this response.

Conclusions about opiate involvement in neural systems are tenuous when based exclusively on the effects of narcotic antagonists. Narcotic antagonists are known to have effects on nonopiate systems as well (Hayes, Price, & Dubner, 1977). Thus, additional lines of evidence are required to infer opiate involvement. To meet this criterion, Mayer and Watkins (1981) reasoned that if opiates are involved in front-paw foot-shock-induced analgesia (FSIA), then front-paw FSIA should also be reduced in rats that have been made tolerant to opiates. To test whether such cross-tolerance exists between morphine analgesia and front-paw FSIA, rats were infused with either morphine or saline for 6 days. At the end of this time, the rats given morphine were tolerant to this opiate, since 10 mg/kg of morphine no longer produced analgesia. When the rats were tested for front-paw FSIA, analgesia was greatly reduced in morphine-tolerant rats. Since front-paw FSIA shows cross-tolerance with morphine and is antagonized by naloxone, the involvement of an endogenous opiate system in this type of analgesia stands on firm ground.

Using this same procedure, rats were tested to see whether cross-tolerance could be observed between morphine analgesia and hind-paw FSIA. No cross-tolerance occurred. That hind-paw FSIA is not affected by either high doses of naloxone or morphine tolerance demonstrates that this manipulation activates an independent nonopiate analgesia system. Since identical shock parameters were used in the hind-paw FSIA and front-paw FSIA experiments, these results show that the body region shocked, rather than simply exposure to stress, determines whether nonopiate or opiate systems are activated.

That endogenous opiates are involved in front-paw FSIA does not prove that this effect is mediated by the same circuitry as morphine analgesia. Since peripheral, as well as central, opiates are released by foot-shock, a critical question was whether front-paw FSIA could be accounted for by release of opiates from the pituitary or sympathetic-adrenal medullary axis. Mayer and Watkins (1981) did a series of experiments to test whether front-paw FSIA would be abolished by removing the pituitary or adrenal glands or by totally blocking sympathetic response to shock. Hypophysectomy, adrenalectomy, and sympathetic blockade failed to reduce front-paw FSIA. These data strongly suggest that front-paw FSIA, like morphine analgesia, is effected via opiate pathways within the central nervous system.

Based on these results, a search for the neural pathways involved in front-paw FSIA was initiated. Since the spinally mediated tail flick reflex is inhibited by front-paw foot-shock, the circuitry for the observed inhibition either exists entirely within the spinal cord or results from the activation of a centrifugal control system in the brain which then descends to the spinal cord. Thus, the effects of spinal cord lesions on front-paw FSIA were examined. Front-paw FSIA is abolished by lesions of the dorsolateral funiculus (DLF) of the spinal cord (Cobelli, Watkins, & Mayer, 1980). Therefore, front-paw shock, like morphine, activates areas within the brain that inhibit pain via descending pathways within the DLF. Furthermore, it was shown that for front-paw FSIA as well as morphine analgesia, this descending DLF pathway arises from the nucleus raphe alatus (Watkins, Young, Kinscheck, & Mayer, 1981).

At this point, then, front-paw FSIA has been characterized as being a neural, opiate-mediated phenomenon. Analgesia is produced by activating brain sites that inhibit pain by way of descending pathways within the DLF. Yet none of this information pinpoints where the opiate synapse is located. To determine this location, intrathecal catheters were implanted such that the tips ended at the lumbosacral enlargement. In this manner, naloxone could be delivered to the spinal cord level controlling the tail flick reflex, which was the behavioral measure used to assess pain threshold. Immediately prior to front-paw shock, rats were injected either with saline or 1 μg naloxone. Spinal naloxone significantly antagonized front-paw FSIA. This effect is not due to spread of the drug to the brain, since the same dose delivered to the high thoracic cord (further from the level controlling the tail flick reflex yet closer to the brain) failed to reduce front-paw FSIA. These experiments demonstrate than an opiate synapse critical to the production of front-paw FSIA exists within the spinal cord. One intriguing aspect of this naloxone effect is that naloxone can prevent, but cannot reverse, front-paw FSIA. If this opiate antagonist is injected onto the spinal cord immediately after the brief (90-sec) shock, analgesia is not reduced. Naloxone is effective only if it is delivered before the induction of analgesia. This implies that brief activation of this system produces a perserverative activity within the spinal cord that is no longer dependent on continued opiate release. This result suggests that these spinal opiates act as neuromodulators of postsynaptic activity, rather than as classical neurotransmitters.

A parallel series of experiments examined the nonopiate analgesia produced by hind-paw shock (Mayer & Watkins, 1981). This work indicated that this effect is also neurally, rather than hormonally, mediated, since analgesia was not reduced by removal of the pituitary or the adrenal glands. This result led to studies aimed at identifying the neural substrates of hind-paw FSIA. Spinal lesion studies showed that this effect, like front-paw FSIA, is mediated via descending pathways within the DLF. However, since lesions of the nucleus raphe alatus failed to reduce hind-paw FSIA, the neural substrate of this effect is distinct from that of front-paw FSIA. A further difference between the analgesias produced by front-paw and hind-paw shock is that hind-paw FSIA is only reduced, not abolished, by DLF lesions. Therefore, a second pathway must exist to account for the potent analgesia that remains. A comparison of hind-paw FSIA in spinalized and DLF-lesioned animals indicated that an intraspinal, rather than descending, pain-inhibitory system is responsible for the analgesia observed following DLF lesions, since spinalization failed to reduce further the pain-inhibitory effects of hind-paw shock. Thus, segmental circuitry and descending pathways within the DLF account for the entire analgesic response to hind-paw shock.

Plasticity in Analgesia Systems

An intriguing aspect of FSIA is that plasticity exists in the neural circuitry. Using a Pavlovian classical conditioning paradigm, Hayes et al. (1978) found that rats readily associated environmental cues with the delivery of shock, such that they learned to activate their endogenous pain-inhibitory systems when these cues were presented. In that study, the nonelectrified shock chamber served as the conditioned stimulus (CS), grid shock delivered to all four paws served as the unconditioned stimulus (UCS) and tail flick inhibition served as the unconditioned response (UCR). Following CS–UCS pairings, exposure to the nonelectrified grid reliably induced analgesia.

Since it is now known that front-paw FSIA is mediated via a well-defined centrifugal opiate pathway, Mayer and Watkins (1981) used brief front-paw shock as the UCS in a classical conditioning paradigm to determine whether plasticity exists in opiate systems. Exposure to the nonelectrified grid (CS) became capable of producing potent analgesia after this CS was paired with front-paw shock. Classically conditioned analgesia was shown to be antagonized by systemic naloxone, spinal naloxone, and morphine tolerance, demonstrating that animals are learning to activate an endogenous opiate system. Intriguingly, maintenance of the analgesic state again appears to be independent of continued opiate release. Like the situation previously discussed for front-paw FSIA, naloxone can prevent, but cannot reverse, classically conditioned analgesia.

Although, as described above, opiate (front-paw) and nonopiate (hind-paw) FSIA can be differentially elicited, classically conditioned analgesia appears always to involve opiate pathways regardless of the body region shocked during conditioning trials. Classically conditioned analgesia can be antagonized by naloxone regardless of whether front-paw or hind-paw shock is used as the USC. The opiate analgesia produced by these classical conditioning paradigms appears to be neurally, rather than hormonally, mediated, since it is not attenuated by either hypophysectomy or adrenalectomy. Classical conditioning involves supraspinal circuitry, since conditioned analgesia is abolished by bilateral DLF lesions. In addition, Librium markedly attenuates classically conditioned analgesia (Watkins, Young, Kinscheck, & Mayer, 1981). Thus, an affective state, such as fear, may influence the activation of endogenous opiate pain-inhibitory pathways.

Multiple Pain-Inhibitory Systems

These studies of front-paw FSIA, hind-paw FSIA, and classically conditioned analgesia provide strong support for the existence of multiple endogenous pain-modulatory systems within the central nervous system. As reviewed above, at least three systems have been identified. The first two pathways mediate the neural nonopiate analgesia observed following hind-paw shock. These consist of an intraspinal pathway and a descending DLF pathway of supraspinal origin. The third is a neural opiate analgesia that is produced by front-paw shock or by classical conditioning using front-paw or hind-paw shock as the UCS. This opiate analgesia is mediated solely by descending pathways within the DLF and is critically dependent on an opiate synapse within the spinal cord. Thus, front-paw FSIA and classically conditioned analgesia provide the first unequivocal demonstrations of neural opiate pathways activated in response to environmental stimuli.

However, even these three systems do not account for all of the pain-inhibitory responses that have been reported. Presently available evidence indicates that four classes of analgesia exist: neural/opiate, hormonal/opiate, neural/nonopiate, and hormonal/nonopiate.

The neural/opiate class includes the analgesia produced by morphine, electrical brain stimulation, front-paw shock, and classical conditioning. Striking similarities exist between the analgesias induced by these manipulations; none are attenuated by removal of the pituitary or adrenal glands and each is reduced or abolished by naloxone, morphine tolerance, and DLF lesions. Although controversy exists regarding the role of the nucleus raphe alatus in the analgesia produced by electrical brain stimulation and systemic morphine, recent studies (Watkins et al., 1981) have clearly demonstrated that lesions of this area virtually abolish analgesia produced either by morphine microinjection into the PAG or by front-paw shock. Thus this area appears to be involved in at least these neural opiate analgesias.

Analgesia produced by electrical brain stimulation is a special case in that it belongs to two classes: neural/opiate and neural/nonopiate. Although several similarities exist between morphine analgesia and stimulation-produced analgesia (SPA), brain stimulation appears to activate both opiate and nonopiate pain-inhibitory systems. Naloxone has a variable effect on SPA, ranging from no effect to complete reversal. Part of this variability is accounted for by the site of stimulation. Prieto, Giesler, and Cannon (1980) have reported that stimulation sites ventral to the dorsal raphe support a naloxone-reversible analgesia, whereas SPA elicited from more dorsal areas fails to be reversed by this opiate antagonist. That cross-tolerance between morphine analgesia and SPA is incomplete implies that a nonopiate component exists for SPA.

Nonopiate mechanisms are involved in other neural analgesia systems as well. Naloxone and morphine tolerance fail to attenuate the analgesia induced by brief shock of either the hind paws or all four paws. Although the neural substrates of these analgesias have not been as well characterized, it is known that hind-paw FSIA is significantly attenuated by bilateral DLF lesions. Thus, for every analgesic manipulation studied to date, the DLF appears to be a final common pathway for neural pain-inhibitory systems.

In addition, the DLF is involved in the production of at least one hormonal/opiate analgesia. Of the hormonal/opiate class, the effect of DLF lesions has only been examined for acupuncture and was found to partially block the analgesic effect of this manipulation in rabbits (Eh, 1979). Although animal models of acupuncture, as well as the other members of this class, appear to involve endogenous opioids, they are clearly distinguishable from neural analgesias, since removal of the pituitary or adrenal glands attenuates or abolishes the ability of these manipulations to produce pain inhibition (Pomeranz, Cheng, & Law, 1977). However, the underlying bases of these phenomena are far from understood. First, the critical hormone(s) involved in the production of analgesia has yet to be unequivocally identified for any of these manipulations. Second, it is not known whether these humoral agents act directly at the level of the spinal cord to produce pain inhibition or whether they activate supraspinal sites that produce analgesia via descending neural pathways. If the mediation of acupuncture by descending DLF pathways proves to be indicative of this class, then the distinction between hormonal/opiate and neural/opiate analgesia may simply be a difference in the mechanism by which supraspinal pain modulation systems are activated. The endocrine system also appears to be involved in hormonal/nonopiate analgesia, since certain types of nonopiate analgesias are dependent on the integrity of the pituitary gland.

Pain as a Model for Motivational Systems

Our current knowledge of the neural mechanisms involved in pain is extensive. It is of particular interest that the historical development of this field is quite different from that for other motivational systems. The study of pain developed out of classical sensory physiology. However, more recent analysis of the topic has recognized that the sensory component of pain is only one aspect of a complex psychological experience. Pain also has important motivational–evaluative components. In this section, we will review the relevance of such an analysis to the study of other motivational systems.

Two features of pain processing will be discussed: the organization of afferent systems and efferent control over afferent information.

Afferent Processing

Primary afferents that subserve pain activate central neural mechanisms related to all components of pain experience. The magnitudes of aversion, sensation intensity, arousal, and motor responses generally increase as a function of magnitude of stimulation of each class of primary nociceptive afferents. Likewise, many second-order nociceptive neurons (i.e., spinothalamic tract neurons) appear to activate both sensory and affective–motivational components of pain. However, some separation of function may exist at this level, since some second-order nociceptive neurons may project only to medial brain-stem structures concerned with arousal and/or affect. Thus, the spinothalamic system is not an exclusive sensory system but is one that is integrally involved with sensory, affective–motivational, and motoric responses to tissue-threatening stimulation. The separate neurophysiological processing of different components of pain may begin at lower brain-stem levels. In general, it appears that even at the medullary level, medial structures are more involved in the affective–motivational aspects of pain than are more lateral regions. This dichotomy become more apparent at more rostral levels of the neuraxis (mesencephalon and diencephalon). Even at these levels, however, a complete separation of sensory–discriminative, affective–motivational, and arousal components does not occur. An even greater separation may occur at cortical levels. For example, the effect of prefrontal lobotomy has often been interpreted as modulation of only the affective dimensions of the pain experience. These facts about pain may provide new insights into the analysis of other motivational systems. While pain research has generally slighted nonsensory aspects, research on other motivational systems has tended to ignore sensory aspects. Yet it seems clear that at least homeostatic behavior such as feeding, drinking, and temperature regulation have important sensory components. Such components seem likely, as with pain, to be the initiating events in a sequence. The neural processing of this information may diverge into anatomically distinct systems, as it does with pain. The strategies discussed above that have been utilized to separate components of the pain experience should be easily applicable to the analysis of other motivational systems.

Efferent Control

A second aspect of the neural processing of pain that has important implications for the analysis of other motivational systems is the complex and potent centrifugal modulation that exists in pain transmission systems. There exist neural systems, including both opiate-related and nonopiate-related systems, that inhibit transmission of nociceptive information at the level of the first synapse in the somatosensory pathway for pain. Given the neural level at which these systems exert their effects, all components of pain are inhibited at once. Thus, for example, opiate analgesia, stimulation-produced analgesia, and analgesias evoked by somatosensory stimulation all attenuate sensory, affective, arousal, and motoric dimensions of pain together.

On the other hand, there are manipulations and situations in which the affective dimension of pain is selectively attenuated. This type of centrifugal control is more likely to be exerted at suprasinpal levels of processing of nociceptive information. Neural systems involved in this more selective type of control are likely to be influenced by more subtle contextual factors related to an organism's perception of the situation.

Strategies for Identification of Neural Systems Involved in Affect and Motivation

The progress made in elucidating the neural and neurochemical details of centrifugal control systems for pain suggest that such an analysis may be applicable to other motivational systems. It appears clear that, at least in certain circumstances, feeding and drinking are not simple functions of deprivation conditions. Rather, other psychological variables can have potent inhibitory or facilitatory influences on food and water intake. Examination of the neural mechanisms involved in such modulation would provide a more complete description of these psychological experiences. In addition, elucidation of efferent control systems often provides insights into the nature of afferent processing.

Acknowledgment. Portions of this work were supported by USPHS Grant DA-00576 to D.J.M.

References

Adair, E. E., Stevens, J. C., & Marks, L. E. Thermally induced pain: The dol scale and the psychophysical power law. *American Journal of Psychology*, 1968, *81*, 147-164.

Adler, M. W. Minireview: Opioid peptides. *Life Sciences*, 1980, *26*, 497-510.

Akil, H., Madden, J., Patrick, R. L., & Barchas, J. D. Stress-induced increase in endogenous opiate peptides: Concurrent analgesia and its partial reversal by naloxone. In H. W. Kosterlitz (Ed.), *Opiates and endogenous opioid peptides*. Amsterdam: North-Holland, 1976, pp. 63-70.

Anderson, K. V., & Pearl, G. S. Long term increases in nociceptive thresholds following lesions in feline nucleus reticularis gigantocellularis. *Abstract, 1st World Congress on Pain*, 1975, *1*, p. 70.

Bakan, D. *Disease, pain and sacrifice.* Chicago: University of Chicago Press, 1968.

Barrell, J. J., & Price, D. D. The perception of first and second pain as a function of psychological set. *Perception and Psychophysics*, 1975, *17*, 163-166.

Beecher, H. K. *Measurement of subjective responses.* New York: Oxford University Press, 1959, p. 494.

Beitel, R. E., & Dubner, R. Sensitization and depression of C-polymodal nociceptors by noxious heat applied to the monkey's face. In J. J. Bonica and Albe-Fessard (Eds.), *Advances in pain research and therapy* (Vol. 1, *Proceedings of the 1st World Congress on Pain*). New York: Raven Press, 1976, pp. 149-153.

Birkenfeld, R., & Fisher, R. G. Successful treatment of causalgia of upper extremity with medullary spinothalamic tractotomy: Case report and review of the literature. *Journal of Neurosurgery*, 1963, *20*, 303-311.

Bouchard, G., Mayanagi, Y., & Martins, L. F. Advantages and limits of intracerebral stereotactic operations for pain. In W. H. Sweet, S. Obrador, & J. G. Martin-Rodriguez (Eds.), *Neurosurgical treatment in psychiatry, pain, and epilepsy.* Baltimore: University Park Press, 1977, pp. 693-697.

Buytendyck, F. J. J. *Pain.* London: Hutchinson, 1961.

Carmon, A., Mor, J., & Goldberg, J. Evoked cerebral responses to noxious thermal stimuli in humans. *Experimental Brain Research*, 1976, *25*, 103-107.

Casey, K. L. Somatosensory responses of bulboreticular units in awake cat: Relation to escape-producing stimuli. *Science*, 1971, *173*, 77-78.

Chance, W. T., White, A. C., Krynock, G. M., & Rosecrans, J. A. Autoanalgesia acquisition, blockade and relationship to opiate binding. *European Journal of Pharmacology*, 1979, *58*, 461-468.

Chatrian, G. E., Canfield, R. C., Knauss, R. A., & Lettich, E. Cerebral responses to electrical tooth pulp stimulation in man: An objective correlate of acute experimental pain. *Neurology (Minneapolis)*, 1975, *25*, 747-757.

Cobelli, D. A., Watkins, L. R., & Mayer, D. J. Dissociation of opiate and non-opiate footshock produced analgesia. *Society for Neuroscience Abstract*, 1980, *6*, 247.

Collins, W. F., Nulsen, F. E., & Randt, C. T. Relations of peripheral nerve fiber size and sensation in man. *Archives of Neurology*, 1960, *3*, 381-385.

Drake, C. G., & McKenzie, K. G. Mesencephalic tractotomy for pain: Experience with six cases. *Journal of Neurosurgery*, 1953, *10*, 457-462.

Eh, S. Participation of descending inhibition in acupuncture analgesia. *National Symposia of Acupuncture and Moxibustion and Acupuncture Anesthesia*, Beijing, 1979, p. 27.

Graceley, R. H. Psychophysical assessment of human pain. In J. J. Bonica, J. C. Liebeskind, & D. G. Albe-Fessard (Eds.), *Advances in pain research and therapy*. New York: Raven Press, 1979, pp. 805-824.

Gracely, R. H., McGrath, P., & Dubner, R. Validity and sensitivity of ratio scales of sensory and affective verbal pain descriptors: Manipulation of affect by diazepam. *Pain*, 1976, *2*, 19-29. (a)

Gracely, R. H., McGrath, P., & Dubner, R. Ratio scales of sensory and affective verbal descriptors. *Pain*, 1976, *2*, 5-18. (b)

Gracely, R. H., McGrath, P., & Dubner, R. Narcotic analgesia: Fentanyl reduces the intensity but not the unpleasantness of painful tooth pulp sensations. *Science*, 1979, *203*, 1261-1263.

Guilbaud, G., Callie, D., Besson, J. M., & Benelli, G. Single units activities in ventral posterior and posterior group thalamic nuclei during nociceptive and non-nociceptive stimulations in the cat. *Archives of Italian Biology*, 1977, *115*, 38-56.

Halliday, A. M., & Logue, V. Painful sensations evoked by electrical stimulation in the thalamus. In G. G. Somjen (Ed.), *Neurophysiology studied in man*. Amsterdam: Excerpta Medica, 1972, pp. 221-230.

Hardy, J. D. Thresholds of pain and reflex contraction as related to noxious stimuli. *Journal of Applied Physiology*, 1953, *5*, 725-739.

Hardy, J. D., Wolff, H. G., & Goodell, H. *Pain sensations and reactions*. Baltimore: Williams & Wilkins, 1952.

Hassler, R. Die zentralen Systeme des Schmerzes. *Acta Neurochirgica*, 1960, *8*, 354-364.

Hassler, R. Dichotomy of facial pain conduction in the diencephalon. In R. Hassler & A. E. Walker (Eds.), *Trigeminal neuralgia*. Philadelphia: W. B. Saunders, 1970, pp. 123-138.

Hayes, R. L., Bennett, G. J., Newlon, P. G., & Mayer, D. J. Behavioral and physiological studies of non-narcotic analgesia in the rat elicited by certain environmental stimuli. *Brain Research*, 1978, *155*, 69-90.

Hayes, R., Price, D. D., & Dubner, R. Use of naloxone to infer narcotic mechanisms. *Science*, 1977, *196*, 600.

Hoffman, D. S., Dubner, R., Hayes, R. L., & Medlin, T. P. Neuronal activity in medullary dorsal horn neurons of awake monkeys trained in a thermal discrimination task. I. Responses to innocuous and noxious thermal stimuli. *Journal of Neurophysiology*, 1981, *44*, 409-427.

Hughes, J. Search for the endogenous ligand of the opiate receptor. *Neuroscience Research Program Bulletin*, 1975, *13*, 55-58.

Ishijima, B., Yoshimasu, N., Fukushima, T., Hori, T., Sekino, H., & Sano, K. Nociceptive neurons in the human thalamus. *Confinia Neurologica*, 1975, *37*, 99-106.

Johnson, J. E. Effects of accurate expectations about sensations on the sensory and distress of components of pain. *Journal of Personality and Social Psychology*, 1973, *27*, 261-275.

Kenshalo, D. R., Jr., Giesler, G. J., Jr., Leonard, R. B., & Willis, W. D. Responses of neurons in primate ventral posterior lateral nucleus to noxious stimuli. *Journal of Neurophysiology*, 1980, *43*, 1594-1614.

Laitinen, L. V. Anterior pulvinotomy in the treatment of intractable pain. In W. H. Sweet, S. Obrador, & J. G. Martin-Rodriguez (Eds.), *Neurosurgical treatment in psychiatry, pain, and epilepsy.* Baltimore: University Park Press, 1977, pp. 669-672.

Lewis, J. W., Cannon, J. T., & Liebeskind, J. C. Opioid and non-opioid mechanisms of stress analgesia. *Science*, 1980, *208*, 623-625.

Libet, B. Electrical stimulation of cortex in human subjects and conscious sensory aspects. In A. Iggo (Ed.), *Handbook of sensory physiology.* Berlin: Springer-Verlag, 1973, pp. 743-790.

Mayer, D. J. Endogenous analgesia systems: Neural and behavioral mechanisms. In J. J. Bonica, J. C. Liebeskind, & D. Albe-Fessard (Eds.), *Advances in pain research and therapy* (Vol. 3). New York: Raven Press, 1979, pp. 385-410.

Mayer, D. J. The centrifugal control of pain. In L. Ng & J. J. Bonica (Eds.), *Pain, discomfort, and humanitarian care.* Amsterdam: Elsevier, 1980, pp. 83-105.

Mayer, D. J., & Price, D. D. Central nervous system mechanisms of analgesia. *Pain*, 1976, *2*, 379-404.

Mayer, D. J., Price, D. D., & Becker, D. P. Neurophysiological characterization of the anterolateral spinal cord neurons contributing to pain perception in man. *Pain*, 1975, *1*, 51-58.

Mayer, D. J., & Watkins, L. R. The role of endorphins in pain control systems. In H. M. Emrich (Ed.), *Modern problems of pharmacopsychiatry: The role of endorphins in neuropsychiatry.* Basel: Karger, 1981. In press.

Mayer, D. J., Wolfle, T. L., Akil, H., Carder, B., & Liebeskind, J. C. Analgesia from electrical stimulation in the brainstem of the rat. *Science*, 1971, *174*, 1351-1354.

Melzack, R. *The puzzle of pain.* New York: Basic Books, 1973.

Melzack, R., & Casey, K. L. Sensory, motivational and central control determinants of pain: A new conceptual model. In D. Kenshalo (Ed.), *The skin senses.* New York: Charles C. Thomas, 1968, pp. 423-439.

Melzack. R., & Wall, P. D. Pain mechanisms: A new theory. *Science*, 1965, *150*, 971-979.

Müller, J. *Elements of physiology.* Schmerzenburg: Taylor, 1842.

Mundinger, F., & Becker, P. Long-term results of central stereotactic interventions for pain. In W. H. Sweet, S. Obrador, & J. G. Martin-Rodriguez (Eds.), *Neurosurgical treatment in psychiatry, pain, and epilepsy.* Baltimore: University Park Press, 1977, pp. 685-692.

Nashold, B. S., Wilson, W. P., & Slaughter, D. G. Stereotactic midbrain lesions for central dysesthesia and phantom pain: Preliminary report. *Journal of Neurosurgery*, 1969, *30*, 116-126.

Nashold, B. S., Jr., Wilson, W. P., & Slaughter, G. The midbrain and pain. In J. J. Bonica (Ed.), *Advances in neurology* (Vol. 4, *Pain*). New York: Raven Press, 1974, pp. 69-169.

Nathan, P. W., & Smith, M. C. Clinico-anatomical correlation in anterolateral cordotomy. In J. J. Bonica et al. (Eds.), *Advances in pain research and therapy* (Vol. 3). New York: Raven Press, 1979, pp. 921-926.

Noordenbos, W. *Pain.* Amsterdam: Elsevier, 1959.

Pearl, G. S., & Anderson, K. V. Response patterns of cells in the feline caudal nucleus reticularis gigantocellularis after noxious trigeminal and spinal stimulation. *Experimental Neurology*, 1978, *58*, 231-241.

Penfield, W., & Boldrey, E. Somatic motor and sensory representation in the cerebral cortex of man as studied by electrical stimulation. *Brain*, 1937, *60*, 398-418.

Perl, E. R. Myelinated afferent fibers innervating the primate skin and their response to noxious stimuli. *Journal of Physiology*, London, 1968, *197*, 593-615.

Perl, E. R. Afferent basis of nociception and pain: Evidence from the characteristics of sensory receptors and their projections to the spinal dorsal horn. In J. J. Bonica (Ed.), *Pain*. New York: Raven Press, 1980, pp. 19-46.

Pomeranz, B., Cheng, R., & Law, P. Acupuncture reduces electrophysiological and behavioral responses to noxious stimuli: Pituitary is implicated. *Experimental Neurology*, 1977, *54*, 172-178.

Price, D. D. Characteristics of second pain and flexion reflexes indicative of prolonged central summation. *Experimental Neurology*, 1972, *37*, 371-387.

Price, D. D., & Barrell, J. J. An experiential approach with quantitative methods: A research paradigm. *Journal of Humanistic Psychology*, 1980, *20*, 75-95.

Price, D. D., Barrell, J. J., & Gracely, R. H. A psychophysical analysis of experiential factors that selectively influence the affective dimension of pain. *Pain*, 1980, *8*, 137-149.

Price, D. D., & Dubner, R. Neurons that subserve the sensory-discriminative aspects of pain. *Pain*, 1977, *3*, 307-338.

Price, D. D., Dubner, R., & Hu, J. W. Trigeminothalamic neurons in nucleus caudalis responsive to tactile, thermal and nociceptive stimulation of the monkey's face. *Journal of Neurophysiology*, 1976, *39*, 936-953.

Price, D. D., Hayes, R. L., Ruda, M., & Dubner, R. Spatial and temporal transformation of input to spinothalamic tract neurons and their relation to somatic sensation. *Journal of Neurophysiology*, 1978, *41*, 933-947.

Price, D. D., Hu, J. W., Dubner, R., & Gracely, R. Peripheral suppression of first pain and central summation of second pain evoked by noxious heat pulses. *Pain*, 1977, *3*, 57-68.

Price, D. D., & Mayer, D. J. Neurophysiological characterization of the anterolateral quadrant neurons subserving pain in *M. mulatta*. *Pain*, 1975, *1*, 59-72.

Prieto, G. J., Giesler, G. J., & Cannon, J. T. Evidence for site specificity in naloxone's antagonism of stimulation-produced analgesia in the rat. *Society for Neuroscience Abstract*, 1979, *5*, 460.

Reynolds, D. V. Surgery in the rat during electrical analgesia induced by focal brain stimulation. *Science*, 1969, *164*, 444-445.

Sano, K., Yoshioka, M., Ogashiwa, M., Ishijima, B., & Ohye, C. Thalamolaminotomy: A new operation for relief of intractable pain. *Confinia Neurologica*, 1966, *27*, 63-66.

Schacter, S., & Singer, J. Cognitive, social and physiological determinants of the emotional state. *Psychological Review*, 1962, *69*, 379-399.

Schvarcz, J. R. Periaqueductal mesencephalotomy for facial central pain. In H. W. Sweet, S. Obrador, & J. G. Martin-Rodrigues (Eds.), *Neurosurgical treatment in psychiatry, pain, and epilepsy*. Baltimore: University Park Press, 1977, pp. 661-667.

Torebjork, H. E. Afferent C units responding to mechanical, thermal, and chemical stimuli in human non-glabrous skin. *Acta Physiologica Scandinavica*, 1974, *92*, 374-390.

Torebjork, H. E., & Hallin, R. G. Perceptual changes accompanying controlled preferential blocking of A and C fibre responses in intact human nerves. *Experimental Brain Research*, 1973, *16*, 321-332.

Watkins, L. R., Young, E. G., Kinscheck, I. B., & Mayer, D. J. Effect of n. raphe alatus (NRA) and periaqueductal gray (PAG) lesions on footshock induced analgesia (FSIA) and classically conditioned analgesia. *Society for Neuroscience Abstract*, 1981, 7, p. 340.

White, J. C., & Sweet, W. H. *Pain and the neurosurgeon: A forty-year experience.* Springfield, Ill.: Charles C. Thomas, 1969.

Index